Handbook of

Small Animal Dermatology

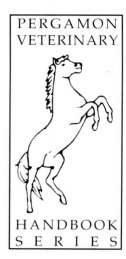

Handbook of
Small Animal Dermatology

by

KAREN A. MORIELLO

Department of Medical Sciences, School of Veterinary Medicine, University of Wisconsin at Madison, USA

and

IAN S. MASON

Veterinary Dermatology Consultants, Sunbury on Thames, Middlesex, UK

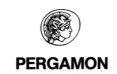

PERGAMON

UK   Elsevier Science Ltd, The Boulevard, Langford Lane,
Kidlington, Oxford, OX5 1GB, UK

USA   Elsevier Science Inc., 660 White Plains Road, Tarrytown,
New York 10591–5153, USA

JAPAN   Elsevier Science Japan, Tsunashima Building Annex, 3-20-12
Yushima, Bunkyo-ku, Tokyo 113, Japan

First edition 1995

Library of Congress Cataloging-in-Publication Data
Moriello, K. A.
   Handbook of small animal dermatology / by K. A. Moriello and I. S. Mason. — 1st ed.
     p.   cm.
   Includes bibliographical references and index.
   1. Dogs — Diseases — Handbooks, manuals, etc.   2. Cats — Diseases —
Handbooks, manuals, etc.   3. Pets — Diseases — Handbooks, manuals,
etc.   4. Veterinary dermatology — Handbooks, manuals, etc.
I. Mason, I. S.   II. Title.
SF992.S55M67   1995

636.089′65–dc20   94-18014

British Library Cataloguing-in-Publication Data
A catalogue record for this book is available from the British Library

ISBN 0-08-042281 0 Hardcover
ISBN 0-08-042280 2 Flexicover

Printed in Great Britain by Redwood Books, Trowbridge

Contents

V **Problem-Oriented Approach to Skin Diseases of Specialised Skin Structures**

VI **Therapeutics**

Preface

As scientific and clinical knowledge advance, veterinary medicine becomes increasingly complex and challenging. This is as true in small animal dermatology as in any other discipline. The expectations and demands of animal owners are also increasing at an almost alarming rate. As a consequence, there exists a need for concise texts and handbooks with readily accessible and clinically relevant information to enable the modern clinician to cope with the almost overwhelming tide of new scientific information and the demands of the pet-owning public.

The *Handbook of Small Animal Dermatology* was written with these factors in mind. The subject is covered using a problem-oriented approach and numerous diagnostic plans, flow-charts and tables are included to enable the busy clinician to extract useful information readily. In addition, this material is supported by detailed text.

The book is divided into sections. The first covers the approach to the animal with skin disease, the structure and function of skin, and a guide to laboratory tests. This section also includes a chapter on the interpretation of histopathology results. The following three sections consider the problem-oriented approach to skin diseases in dogs, cats and non-domestic pets. A section on the diseases of specialised skin structures (ears, anal sacs and nails) is included. The final section covers therapeutics in detail.

We hope that the book will be of interest and value to veterinary practitioners and students and that ultimately it will benefit small animal patients and their owners.

IAN S. MASON and KAREN A. MORIELLO,
SEPTEMBER 1994

List of Contributors

Elizabeth Galbreath DVM Diplomate American College of Veterinary Pathologists, Department of Pathobiological Sciences, School of Veterinary Medicine, University of Wisconsin–Madison, Madison, Wisconsin, USA

Craig Griffin DVM Diplomate American College of Veterinary Dermatology, Animal Dermatology Clinic, 13132 Garden Grove Boulevard, Unit B, Garden Grove, California 92643, USA

Ian Mason BVM, PhD, Cert. SAD, MRCVS, RCVS Specialist in Veterinary Dermatology, Veterinary Dermatology Consultants, 2 Kempton Court, Kempton Avenue, Sunbury, Middlesex, TW16 5PA, UK

Karen Moriello DVM Diplomate American College of Veterinary Dermatology, Clinical Associate Professor of Dermatology, Department of Medical Sciences, School of Veterinary Medicine, University of Wisconsin–Madison, Madison, Wisconsin, USA

Joanne Paul-Murphy DVM Diplomate American College of Zoological Medicine, Clinical Assistant Professor of Special Species Health, Department of Surgical Sciences, School of Veterinary Medicine, University of Wisconsin–Madison, Madison, Wisconsin, USA

Acknowledgements

The authors would like to thank Richard Harvey, Peter Hill, Douglas J. DeBoer, Maron Calderwood-Mays, Robert Dunstan, Cheryl London and Susan Fehrer-Sawyer

Dedications

This book is dedicated to

Ethan, Mark and Doug for holding various aspects of my life together while this book was in preparation

Karen A. Moriello

For my wife Karen with thanks for her infinite patience

Ian S. Mason

How to Use this Book

For each chapter in Sections II and III five basic figures are given to guide diagnosis. The approach should begin with consideration of the animal's history, followed by a full clinical and dermatological examination (*Chapter 2*) to allow the formation of a ranked list of possible disorders and to indicate which diagnostic procedures should be undertaken. The five figures are:

(1) Differential diagnosis, listing possible disorders
(2) Approach: History
(3) Approach: Physical examination

(2) and (3) give examples which may eliminate causes or increase the likelihood that a particular disease is present

(4) Diagnostic plan: A suggested approach to the disease
(5) Problem-oriented diagnostic approach: A flowchart.

I Background Information and Approach to the Animal

1

Clinical Aspects of Cutaneous Structure and Function

IAN MASON

In clinical practice, an understanding of anatomy and physiology is essential to the successful management of disease. This principle is as true for dermatology as any other discipline.

The aim of this chapter is briefly to review skin structure and function, emphasising the clinical significance of the anatomical and physiological features discussed. This chapter reviews the nomenclature of dermatology, thus providing a glossary of dermatological terms.

Functions of Skin (Fig. 1.1)

The skin is essentially a barrier between a mammal and a potentially hostile environment — it keeps the goodies in and the baddies out. 'Goodies' include fluids and electrolytes; 'baddies' are chemical and physical agents and pathogenic and opportunist micro-organisms and parasites. In addition, skin provides sensory perception and temperature regulation, and is involved in the control of blood pressure.

Components of the Skin

The outer part of the skin is the **epidermis,** which is divided into a number of portions. The epidermis rests on and is attached to the **dermis,** which in turn lies on the **subcutis** or hypodermis. Epidermal invaginations form the sweat and sebaceous glands as well as forming the hair follicle (Fig. 1.2). The hair follicle, sweat and sebaceous glands are referred to as the **epidermal appendages.** Hairs and nails are derived from the epidermis and are part of the **adnexa**, which also includes horny structures e.g. nails. Specialised regions of skin in which one or

FUNCTIONS OF THE SKIN	
Barrier	Skin limits loss of water, electrolytes, macromolecules from the animal and excludes chemical, physical and biological agents
Temperature regulation	Insulation (subcutaneous fat, hair), alterations in blood flow and sweating enable regulation of body temperature
Sensory perception	In order to avoid noxious stimuli, receptors for heat, cold, pain, itch and pressure are present
Blood pressure control	Alterations in blood flow to skin allow blood pressure to be modulated
Secretion and excretion	There is limited transepidermal loss of gases, liquids and solutes. Glandular function leads to secretion of sweat and sebum
Flexibility	Elasticity and tensile strength of skin allow movement and provide shape and form
Synthesis	Vitamin D and the adnexa (hair, nails, stratum corneum) are formed by the skin
Storage	The skin forms a reservoir of electrolytes, water, vitamins, fat, carbohydrates and other materials
Immune function	In addition to providing a physical barrier against the ingress of chemicals, and physical and biological agents, the skin has well-developed innate and adaptive immunity. Immuno-surveillance helps prevent persistent infection and neoplasia. The skin surface has antibacterial and antifungal properties
Pigmentation	Skin and hair colour may prevent damage from predators (camouflage) and ultraviolet light (melanin)

FIG. 1.1 Functions of the skin.

Primary hair
Secondary hairs
Epidermis
Sebaceous gland
Dermis
Arrector pili muscle
Apocrine sweat gland
Hypodermis

FIG. 1.2 Structure of the skin.

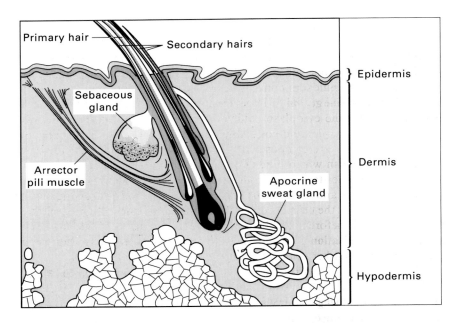

more anatomical components are modified are present. These include the ear, the footpads, the eyelids and other mucocutaneous junctions.

The Interfollicular Epidermis

This section will be concerned with the epidermis between hair follicles. The epidermal appendages and adnexa will be discussed separately. The functions of the epidermis are shown in Fig. 1.3.

The epidermis is a stratified squamous epithelium which is composed predominantly (c. 85%) of **keratinocytes,** although other cell types are present. Keratinocytes are formed by division of the cells of the epidermal basal layer or **stratum basale**. The stratum basale comprises one layer of columnar to cuboidal cells which is tightly adherent to the underlying basement membrane. Following cell division, daughter cells migrate to the outermost part of the epidermis, the **stratum corneum**, via the **stratum spinosum** and **stratum granulosum**, losing their nuclei and becoming packed with keratin (Fig. 1.4). As the cells migrate, they become gradually flattened and hexagonal until they join the proximal layers of the stratum corneum as inert keratinised **squames**.

The cells of the stratum spinosum are characterised by 'spines' which are only visible in tissue processed for histology. This artifactual appearance arises because of the abundance of **desmosomes** between keratinocytes within this layer. Desmosomes hold the cell walls together while the cell walls between desmosomes retract as a result of fixation. Within the stratum spinosum, keratin is formed and is organised into bundles or **tonofibrils**. More mature (i.e. more distal) cells of this layer contain granular membrane bound organelles which are also known as **lamellar bodies**, **Odland bodies** or **membrane coating granules**. These organelles are bound to the cell margin and discharge their contents (mostly **lipid** which is a bi-product

EPIDERMAL FUNCTIONS	
Barrier	Prevents loss of water and electrolytes Limits penetration of bacterial viruses and fungal organisms and their metabolites
Sensory perception	Free nerve endings, Merkel cells
Pigmentation	Camouflage, protects against UV radiation
Immune function	Prevention of parasitic and microbial disease. Surveillance for neoplasia

FIG. 1.3 Epidermal functions.

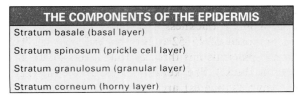

THE COMPONENTS OF THE EPIDERMIS
Stratum basale (basal layer)
Stratum spinosum (prickle cell layer)
Stratum granulosum (granular layer)
Stratum corneum (horny layer)

FIG. 1.4 The components of the epidermis.

of keratinisation) into the intercellular spaces. This process also takes place in the next layer, the stratum granulosum. This intercellular lipid forms a major part of the epidermal permeability barrier.

The stratum granulosum consists of cells which contain **keratohyaline granules**. These are basophilic structures within the cytoplasm which are readily evident in haematoxylin and eosin stained histological sections. They are composed of **profillagrin**, a precursor of fillagrin which binds together keratin bundles. Within the stratum granulosum the cytoplasmic organelles and the nucleus degenerate and become inactive as the cells become more flattened and full of keratin before finally forming the stratum corneum. **Keratinisation** is the term used to describe the maturation of a keratinocyte from the stratum basale to the stratum corneum.

The stratum basale, spinosum and granulosum are known as the **living epidermis**. One of the major functions of the living epidermis is to die usefully as the stratum corneum. This may seem incredible to those who were taught that the stratum corneum is a poorly organised, insubstantial and porous structure. The 'traditional' view of the stratum corneum is borne of the fact that the original descriptions of this structure were made using tissue that had been processed and dehydrated in lipid solvents. The stratum corneum is rich in lipid and depends on it for structural integrity. The destructive effects of conventional histological processing are avoided if frozen sections are examined. The use of this and allied techniques has enabled the true nature of the stratum corneum to be determined. It has been shown that the mammalian stratum corneum is a substantial and highly organised structure comprising tightly packed columns of inert squames embedded in lipid. In the outer layers of the stratum corneum, the cells become loosened and are shed. This process is known as **desquamation**. The rate of desquamation in normal skin matches the rate of cell production so epidermal thickness is maintained.

The stratum corneum is a major barrier to loss of water and electrolytes and is a major part of the cutaneous defences against microbial disease. In the dog, it has a thickness of around 12–15 μm and is composed of 45–52 tightly packed layers. (The living epidermis has three or four layers and is 8–12 μm thick.) The keratinocytes of the stratum corneum (squames) are principally composed of fillagrin and keratin within an insoluble, lipid rich envelope. The intercellular material of the stratum corneum is rich in lipid although some aqueous material is present (see later). The source of the lipid is the lamellar bodies and sebaceous lipid (see later).

Cells other than keratinocytes comprise up to 15% of the epidermis. These cells include dendritic cells such as **Langerhans cells** (5–8% of epidermal cells) and melanocytes (c. 5%). The dendritic processes of the Langerhans cells form a network in the epidermis providing an effective antigen presenting and processing system. Langerhans cell phagocytose antigen and then migrate to the paracortical areas of lymph nodes via the lymphatics. Processed antigen is then presented to antigen specific T-lymphocytes.

Melanocytes are pigment-producing cells which are present in both the epidermis and the hair follicle. Interestingly, the concentration of melanocytes is approximately the same between individuals of the same species, irrespective of the shade or colour of the skin and hair. These cells are of neural crest origin and are principally found in the basal layer of the epidermis and the hair matrix. Pigmentation is important in protecting animals from ultraviolet radiation, for affording camouflage, in reproductive behaviour (e.g. sexual dimorphism) and in social hierarchy. Normal pigmentation of the skin and hair is due to inclusion of melanin pigments into the keratinocytes of the epidermis and hair matrix. The shade and density of pigment is determined by the amounts and types of melanin present. In domestic animals, two forms of melanin are found: **the eumelanins** (brownish-black) and **the phaeomelanins** (yellow to reddish-brown). In humans, a third type of melanin is present in individuals with blond and red hair.

Melanin granules are formed in intracellular melanocyte organelles called **melanosomes**. The biochemical process of melanin formation is complex, involving the oxidation of tyrosine to dihydroxyphenylalanine (dopa). Once formed, melanin granules are incorporated into hair and epidermal keratinocytes by pinocytosis.

Epidermotropic dendritic lymphocytes are also found in the canine epidermis. They bear the Thy-1 marker and act as antigen presenting cells. It is thought that they also have cytotoxic activity and it is possible that they are involved in the development of tolerance.

Merkel cells, which are slow adapting mechano-receptors, are also found in or just below the basal layer of the epidermis but are confined to the **tylotrich pads** (epidermal papillae).

Epidermal immunity

The epidermis is a primary barrier against microbial invasion. Anatomical features of this region impede the penetration of micro-organisms or their potentially toxic secretions and metabolites into the host. The arrangement of inert squames in a lipid-rich matrix prevents the penetration of aqueous substances. The intercellular material of the stratum corneum contains numerous antimicrobial substances such as immunoglobulins, complement and transferrin. These are largely derived from sweat (see skin glands, below).

Keratinocytes themselves play an important role in the immune function of the epidermis. They can no longer be regarded as simply the 'building blocks' of this tissue. They are phagocytic and thought to process antigen more efficiently than the Langerhans cells. They respond to cytokines such as gamma-interferon and they interact with T-lymphocytes. They produce interleukin-1 constitutively and, following antigenic stimulation, can produce a wide range of cytokines which influence the immune response.

The process of desquamation can be important in epidermal immunity. Desquamation leads to shedding of surface pathogens, especially fungi, along with the surface squames.

The Dermal–Epidermal Junction

The dermal–epidermal junction or basement membrane zone is divided into two major sectors, the **lamina lucida** and the **lamina densa**, on the basis of electron microscopical studies (Fig. 1.5).

This region acts as a means of interaction and exchange of both cellular and humoral elements between the epidermis and the underlying dermis. It is important as a structural anchor, holding the epidermis to the dermis, and as part of the cutaneous defences. It lies beneath the interfollicular epidermis and surrounds the hair follicle units and skin glands.

The main structural component is **Type 4 collagen**, which is unique to basement membranes and is organised in a lattice-like arrangement which confers both strength and elasticity to this zone. The epidermal basement membrane also contains **laminin** (a glycoprotein which is involved in the binding of epidermal cells to the collagen) and **bullous pemphigoid antigen**. The function of the latter is unknown, but it is involved in the pathogenesis of the disease from which it derives its name.

Basement membranes do not impede the diffusion of water, electrolytes and other low molecular weight substances as the overlying epidermis is avascular and must rely on diffusion from the dermal blood supply for nutrients and oxygen.

The Dermis

The dermis forms the major component of the skin; its functions are shown in Fig. 1.6. It is a

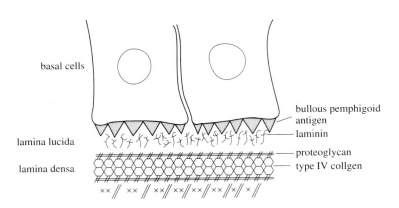

FIG. 1.5 The epidermal basement membrane.

FUNCTIONS OF THE DERMIS
Supports and nourishes the epidermis, hair follicles and skin glands
Confers strength and flexibility to the skin
Immune function — cellular and humoral
Temperature regulation
Sensory perception
Blood pressure control
Synthesis (vitamin D)
Storage

FIG. 1.6 Functions of the dermis.

connective tissue with a fibrous matrix and proteo-glycan ground substance. It contains blood vessels, nerves and lymphatics. Numerous cell types are present including immune cells and the precursors of the fibres.

Dermal connective tissue

The connective tissue matrix comprises mainly **collagen** and **elastic fibres**. The collagen is arranged in bundles which are usually bordered by elastic fibres. In the superficial dermis, the collagen and elastic fibres are fine and irregularly distributed. In the deeper dermis, both types of fibre are thicker and the collagen fibres tend to run parallel to the skin surface. There are fewer elastic fibres in this portion of the epidermis. Collagen forms around 80% of the extracellular connective tissue matrix and provides both strength and elasticity. Collagen fibres are secreted as inactive procollagen and then converted to the active form. Most of the collagen is Types 1 (80–85%) and 3 (15–20%).

Elastic fibres form a network throughout the dermis and are also present in the walls of blood and lymphatic vessels and in the sheaths of the hair follicles.

The proteoglycans and glycoproteins of the ground substance are involved in water and electrolyte balance. They are mostly comprised of hyaluronic acid and dermatin sulphate, with heparin sulphate and chondroitin 4 and chondroitin 6 sulphates. The ground substance surrounds and supports the extracellular matrix and may be involved in promoting growth, differentiation and cellular migration.

Dermal blood and nervous supply and lymphatic drainage

The cutaneous blood supply is well developed and blood flow through the skin exceeds that merely required for the supply of oxygen and nutrients. This excess is to enable the control of blood pressure and temperature regulation. Cutaneous arteries enter the skin from the subcutis and branch to form three plexuses (deep, middle and superficial). Arteriovenous anastomoses are common and enable blood flow and distribution to be closely controlled in the dermis. The distribution of veins parallels the arterial supply.

The lymphatics collect tissue fluid and immune cells and provide a conduit for them to the regional lymph nodes. This is important in maintaining hydrostatic pressure within the tissue and in enabling antigen processing within the lymphatic system.

The nervous supply to the skin is similar to that of the blood vessels. A plexus of nerves lies beneath the epidermis and free nerve endings enter the epidermis itself. Nerve networks are also found in association with the hair follicles and associated glands and the arrector pili muscles. Specialised mechanoreceptors such as **Pacinian corpuscles** are also found in the dermis.

The cells of the dermis

In addition to the cells of the glandular, muscular, nervous and vascular tissues, a variety of cell types are found in the dermis. It is becoming apparent that these cells have complex and interdependent roles in cutaneous metabolism and immunity. They interact with each other and with the other dermal and epidermal tissues both by direct contact and by means of soluble mediators (e.g. cytokines).

Fibroblasts are the cells responsible for the synthesis and degradation of the connective tissue matrix. They secrete collagen but can also produce collagenase and other enzymes which lead to its degradation. They also produce a variety of cytokines which may influence proliferation in the epidermis and have other influences on cutaneous metabolism.

Numerous **mast cells** are present in the epidermis and are usually arranged around blood vessels and the epidermally-derived glands and hair follicles. Mast cell cytoplasm contains large numbers of darkly staining granules. These contain numerous substances, principally histamine and heparin. Other constituents are mediators of inflammation, acid hydrolases and other enzymes.

Mast cells are involved directly in immediate hypersensitivity reactions. Degranulation of these cells occurs following one of several mechanisms, including antigenic challenge, and leads to release of the contents of the cytoplasmic granules and resultant inflammation. Recently it has been shown that mast cells are involved in a more delayed form of hypersensitivity reaction which occurs around 4 hours after exposure to antigen. Mast cells have many characteristics in common with basophils and can be regarded in some ways as tissue basophils. Basophils are ordinarily not found in the skin, although they can be recruited into the dermis as part of an inflammatory response. In some circumstances this may lead to cutaneous basophil hypersensitivity.

Dendritic cells are also found in the dermis. Langerhans cells migrate from the epidermis to the regional lymph nodes via the dermal lymphatics after antigenic stimulation. Melanocytes may also be present in the dermis. Other antigen-presenting cells are also found in the dermis and have been termed **veiled cells**, a term which is also applied to dermal Langerhans cells.

Macrophages are found within the dermis. They are phagocytes and are involved in immune surveillance and antigen processing. They are also capable of secreting cytokines, complement components and antimicrobial substances.

The Hair Follicle and Associated Glands

Bovine, equine and human hair follicles are described as simple: they have only one hair, one sebaceous gland, one sweat gland and arrector pili muscle per follicle. These structures are collectively termed the **hair follicle unit**. In cats and dogs, **compound hair follicles** are present. The compound hair follicle has up to 20 hairs emerging from a common pore, the **hair follicle ostium**. Compound hair follicles are characterised by a large, single, central **primary hair** surrounded by up to five lateral primary hairs. Each of these primary hairs has its own **arrector pili muscle** and **sweat and sebaceous glands**. Each primary hair is also surrounded by smaller **secondary hairs**, secondary hairs which lack arrector pili muscles and sweat glands but may have sebaceous glands.

The arrector pili muscles contract in response to cold environmental temperature, fright or stress. Erection of the hairs increases insulation, so preventing heat loss. 'Raising of the hackles' is important in social interaction between animals.

The hair follicle: Structure and physiology

The structure of the hair follicle is shown in Fig. 1.7. Hair growth commences at the base of the follicle by mitosis of epidermal cells contained in the **matrix** of the **hair bulb**. The **dermal papilla** is a portion of dermis surrounded by the epidermal portion of the hair bulb which it supports and nourishes. Melanocytes are also present in the hair matrix and are responsible for the transfer of pigment into the growing hair.

Hair growth is a complex subject. Its cycle is controlled by many influences, including photoperiod and temperature (i.e. seasonal factors), hormones, nutrition, stress and genetic factors. In cats and dogs, hair growth is mosaic in pattern, occurring throughout the year. There are seasonal effects on hair growth in these species but the distinct shedding of summer and winter coats seen in other species, such as horses, does not occur. However, cats and dogs shed more hair in the spring and autumn. In the spring and early summer, the proportion of hairs in the growing phase is greater than at any other time of the year.

Active hair growth is termed **anagen**. After this phase of growth, a resting phase, **telogen**, occurs. The hairs remain in telogen for some weeks or months before finally being shed. A short transitional stage **catagen** is recognised between these two stages.

Skin glands

A variety of exocrine glands are present within the skin. In non-specialised skin, **sweat** and **sebaceous glands** are present. In specialised regions, such as the ear canal, eyelids and perianal area, modified sweat and sebaceous glands are found. These modified glands have various properties such as the production of pheromones or, in the case of the eyelid glands, contributing to the pre-corneal film.

The sweat glands. Contrary to popular opinion, dogs and cats have sweat glands over the entire body surface. They are not simply confined to the footpads and planum nasale as many people believe.

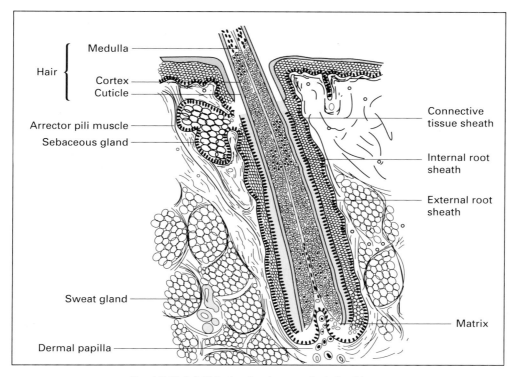

FIG. 1.7 Hair follicle showing the general relationships.

Heat loss via sweating is a significant means of heat loss in humans, horses and pigs. In dogs and cats however sweating is not a major means of thermoregulation. Instead heat loss is via the respiratory tract (panting) and directly from the skin surface without evaporation of fluid. The absence of copious quantities of fluid on the skin surface of overheated dogs and cats when compared with other species may have lead to the erroneous view that dogs and cats do not sweat. In fact, they do sweat continually and this process is of great importance to the animal (Fig. 1.8).

Sweat glands have been erroneously classified as apocrine and eccrine. Apocrine was the term used for glands from which the duct opened directly on to the skin surface, whilst eccrine glands were those with ducts opening into the hair follicle. The constituents of sweat from both types of glands were thought to be different as were the mechanisms of secretion. Recent evidence has shown that the mechanisms of sweat production are common to all sweat glands, irrespective of the anatomical location of the duct. It is for this reason that the terms **epitrichial** and **atrichial** are preferred to describe the two types of sweat gland present in non-specialised skin. Sweat glands with ducts emerging into the hair follicle are termed epitrichial glands; those which emerge directly on to the skin surface are termed atrichial glands. Sweat production is by secretion of preformed sweat and exocytosis of vesicles (**merocrine**) and from necrosis of sweat gland epithelial cells (**holocrine**). Apocrine secretion does not occur.

Sebaceous glands. Sebaceous glands produce a lipid-rich secretion, **sebum**. This, along with the extruded intercellular epidermal lamellar bodies,

FUNCTIONS OF SWEAT
Chemical defence — production or secretion of antimicrobial substances including immunoglobulins, transferrin and sodium chloride
Provision of nutrients (proteins and salts) for the skin microflora
Thermoregulation (pigs, primates and horses)
Provision of moisture to skin to protect against friction, e.g. footpads and eyelids
Maintenance of skin pliability
Excretion of waste products
pH buffering

FIG. 1.8 Functions of sweat.

Contributes to the epidermal water barrier controlling
   water loss and limiting microbial infection
Maintains skin pliability, coat condition and sheen
May form an emulsion with sweat

Fig. 1.9 Functions of sebum.

contributes to the epidermal water barrier. Sebum is
thought to form an emulsion with sweat thus limiting evaporative loss of this aqueous material from
the skin surface. Sweat constituents are vital to the
health and integrity of the skin, particularly with
regard to defence against microbial invasion. The
location of this putative emulsion is the intercellular
spaces of the stratum corneum. The functions of
sebum are shown in Fig. 1.9.

The subcutis. The subcutis hypodermis is a thick
layer comprising lobules of **lipocytes** (fat cells) inter-
spersed with connective tissue. It is the deepest
component of the skin. Its functions are to support
and contour the overlying skin, to act as an energy
reserve and to insulate against heat loss. It also acts
as a protective cushion to absorb trauma — this is
especially important in sites such as the footpad.

Specialised Skin Structures

This review will concentrate on the specialised
structures whose diseases are discussed in *Section V*, namely, the external ear, the anal sacs and
the nails.

The External Ear

The external ear comprises the **pinna** and the **ear
canal**. Its proximal limit is the **tympanic membrane**.

The pinna is a flap of fibrocartilage covered with
skin. The precise shape varies with species and
breed. The skin of the pinna is tightly bound to the
underlying cartilage. The skin is unspecialised
although the skin of the inner surface of the pinna
has fewer hairs. The function of the pinna is to
receive air vibrations and transfer them to the
tympanum via the ear canal.

The ear canal is a tube of cartilage which flares,
funnel-like, distally. It is lined with specialised skin
which has large numbers of modified sweat and
sebaceous (**ceruminous**) glands. These produce wax
and other secretions. The canine ear canal is 5–10

mm in diameter and approximately 2 cm long
though these measurements vary between individuals and breeds. The skin varies in thickness along
the length of the canal, with the skin of the proximal
portion being the thinnest. Numerous glands are
present except in the skin nearest to the tympanum.
The glands are more numerous distally and the
sweat glands are atrichial rather than epitrichial. In
dogs, hairs may be present along the ear canal but
this varies between breeds.

The Anal Sacs

The canine and feline anal sacs are paired diverti-
cula of the rectal wall with an excretory duct which
opens directly into the anus at the mucocutaneous
junction. They are located lateral to the anus and lie
between the external anal sphincter and the smooth
muscle of the rectum.

The anal sacs are lined with a secretory epithelium
which contains numerous modified sweat and sebaceous glands. Anal sac secretions are said to be
involved in social interaction between animals and
for marking territory. Normal anal sacs are emptied
during defaecation when the external anal sphincter
compresses the glands against faeces within the
rectum.

The lumen of the sacs is a reservoir for the secretions of the glands within the epithelium. The anal
sacs are often erroneously referred to as anal glands
but in fact, the glandular tissue is confined to the
lining of the sac. Anal sac secretions are composed of the secretions of modified sweat and sebaceous glands and desquamated epithelial cells. In
normal animals it is serous to slightly viscid, clear
to pale yellow or even brownish. It is somewhat
malodorous!

The Nails

Nails, or claws, are highly complex and specialised structures. Figure 1.10 is a diagrammatic transverse section through a canine digit showing the
relationship between the nail and the underlying
tissues.

The **periosteum** of the **distal phalanx (P3)** of each
toe is continuous with the dermis of the skin immediately proximal to the nail. The epidermis of the
adjacent skin is also continuous with the nail and is
the germinal tissue. The epidermis and dermis are in

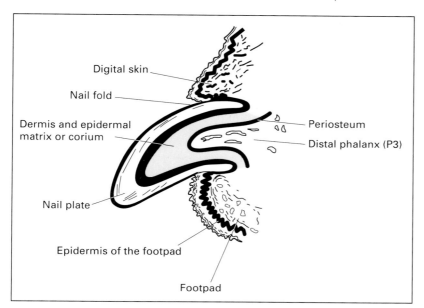

Digital skin

Nail fold

Dermis and epidermal matrix or corium

Nail plate

Epidermis of the footpad

Footpad

Periosteum

Distal phalanx (P3)

FIG. 1.10 Schematic anatomy of the canine claw.

close contact due to interdigitation of fine dermal papillae with epidermal laminae.

Nails are formed continuously following cell division in the nail matrix. The process of nail production is similar to that of keratinisation although the keratinised tissue produced is rather different from the usual product of epidermal growth, the stratum corneum. In contrast with the corneum, nails have little intercellular lipid and the keratin is arranged to impart rigidity and strength to the nail, rather than the flexibility inherent in the non-specialised epidermis.

2

Approach to the Animal with Skin Disease

IAN MASON

In general veterinary practice, dermatological cases form a large proportion of the case load and lead to animal discomfort, pain or even death, as well as being a source of considerable anxiety to owners. Despite this, dermatological cases are seldom afforded the same degree of care and investigation that, say, orthopaedic or neurological cases receive. Few clinicians would hesitate to hospitalise a dog with persistent vomiting with a view to detailed diagnostic testing and yet most clinicians in primary practice are happy to handle complex and serious dermatological cases during routine consulting sessions as out-patients, basing diagnosis on response to empirical, symptomatic therapy.

There is a need for many skin cases to be dealt with in a much more meticulous and detailed fashion in order to attain a specific diagnosis and so advise the client of prognosis and treatment options. Such cases should be identified before the problem becomes chronic and they should be seen again during less busy periods for 30–60 minutes, or referred to a recognised specialist for a dermatological work-up. Practices should consider the establishment of criteria for the identification of these cases. Figures 2.1 and 2.2 illustrate an approach to this problem but it should be recognised that these are guidelines and that the decision about whether to investigate further should be tailored to the specific practice and, just as importantly, the specific case.

Glucocorticoid therapy is a tempting option in the early management of pruritic skin disease. However, it is a temptation that should be resisted until a specific diagnosis has been made. Figure 2.3 summarises reasons for avoiding the inappropriate and premature use of these drugs. The use of glucocorticoids may turn a simple case of flea allergic dermatitis into an idiopathic pruritic recurrent pyoderma with associated iatrogenic hyperadrenocorticism!

GUIDELINES FOR THE MANAGEMENT OF SKIN CASES IN GENERAL PRACTICE

1. Take a brief medical and dermatological history while thoroughly examining the animal. Keep notes of all salient points

2. *If pruritus is present and the lesions primarily affect the dorsum*, implement rigorous flea control (*Chapter 30*)

3. **Glucocorticoid therapy should not be administered at this early stage** (see Fig. 2.3)

4. **Skin scrapings should be taken from all cases**, either during the consultation or in the hospital later, and examined microscopically for evidence of ectoparasites (*Chapter 3*). Other basic tests (microscopy or coat brushings and plucked hairs, cytology etc.) can be considered at this stage

•*If a diagnosis is obtained* in stages 1 to 4, then treat accordingly

•*If no diagnosis is achieved*, then a full history is required (Fig. 2.5). Initially the client can simply fill in a questionnaire but it is likely that direct questioning will be required later for clarification

Further diagnostic tests should be considered at this stage

•*If no diagnosis has been made after two or three consultations, or if the problem recurs* then the **client's** options are:

- Further detailed in-house investigation
- Referral to a specialist
- Long-term symptomatic management

The clinician's guidance of the client's decision should be based on:

- Client's commitment (and finances)
- Severity of the problem
- Clinician's knowledge/enthusiasm

FIG. 2.1 Guidelines for the management of skin cases in general practice.

The Detailed Dermatological Investigation

The most important elements of a meticulous dermatological investigation are:

- a committed and caring owner;
- an enthusiastic and knowledgable clinician;
- *Time*.

Although it is likely that clinicians will differ in their approach to the skin case, the investigation

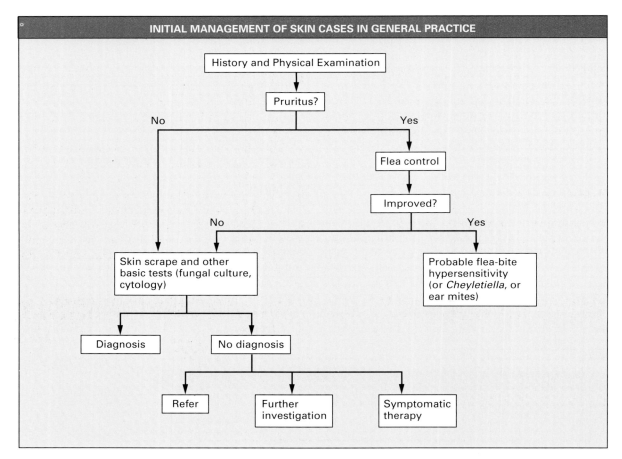

FIG. 2.2 Initial management of skin cases in general practice.

REASONS FOR WITHHOLDING GLUCOCORTICOID THERAPY UNTIL A DIAGNOSIS HAS BEEN MADE

- The client who has seen the unparalleled response to glucocorticoid therapy may be difficult to persuade that these drugs need to be withdrawn later
- Glucocorticoids render diagnosis either difficult or impossible. The use of such drugs changes the clinical picture, the nature of the lesions and results of histopathology and blood analyses
- Dermatological side-effects may be created. Allergic dogs are particularly prone to the development of pyoderma. The immunosuppressive effects of glucocorticoids are likely to make pyoderma an inevitability. They will also mask its presenting signs. Other skin changes include reduction in sebum production and epidermal turnover and long-term effects include calcinosis cutis and demodicosis
- Systemic side-effects may occur (iatrogenic hyperadrenocorticism, diabetes mellitus, subclinical urinary tract infections). These are potentially life-endangering

In almost all cases, therapy will need to be withdrawn at some stage, either because of the development of side-effects, or because the condition becomes refractory to these agents, or because further investigations are required, or a combination of these factors

FIG. 2.3 Reasons for withholding glucocorticoid therapy until a diagnosis has been made.

should always include the following components:

- Dermatological and general medical history.
- Detailed physical and dermatological examination.
- Formulation of a list of differential diagnoses (based on the above).
- Diagnostic tests (*Chapter 3*) and trial therapies (where indicated).
- Definitive diagnosis, prognosis and treatment.

Figure 2.4 summarises this systematic approach.

The problem-oriented sections of this text list differential diagnoses for common clinical presentations and give aspects of the history and examination of these patients which increase or decrease the likelihood of a particular disease being present.

History

The history is probably the most important part of the dermatological investigation: experienced dermatologists spend 20–30 minutes on this part of the investigation alone. Figure 2.5 lists important questions that need to be answered by the client and it is preferable to have these questions on a form so that important aspects are not overlooked. Although it is common practice for clients to fill in these questionnaires themselves, it is better if the clinician does so during the interview: clients are unaware of the significance of certain questions and may inadvertently omit important details.

The animal's breed, sex and age at the onset of the problem may help to increase or decrease the clinician's suspicion that a particular problem is present. Examples of diseases with a strong age, breed and sex predilection are given in Figs 2.6, 2.7 and 2.8.

There are a number of reasons for taking a full medical history in addition to a specific dermatological history. Some serious systemic diseases such as hyperadrenocorticism or other endocrine disorders may present with dermatological signs and a general history may indicate that such diseases should be considered in the differential diagnosis. Drug history (for the dermatological problem and for any

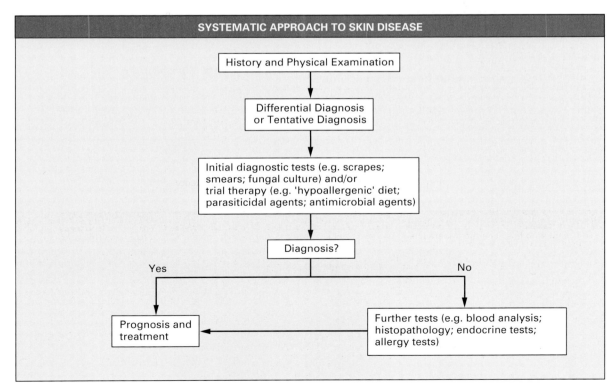

FIG. 2.4 Systematic approach to skin disease.

FIG. 2.5 Dermatology history questions.

DERMATOLOGY HISTORY QUESTIONS	
Patient profile	Species? Breed? Age? Sex? Neutered?
General history	Any evidence of current or previous systemic disease (e.g. diarrhoea, vomiting, lethargy, polyphagia, polydipsia, polyuria, thermophilia, oestrus abnormalities)? Previous and current drug therapy? (This includes vaccines and medicaments administered for non-dermatological disorder) Diet?
Dermatological history	What is /are the skin problem(s) — pruritus, alopecia, scale, odour, other? Age at the onset of the problem? Age at which pet was obtained? Was the animal born in this country or area? Has it been abroad? Was the animal acquired from a breeder, a rescue society, a puppy farm or a pet shop? Are related animals (especially litter-mates) affected? First sign noticed? Sudden/gradual onset? Continuous/intermittent? If intermittent, is this due to therapy or time of year? If seasonal, when? Which body region(s) affected initially? Which region(s) now affected? Pedal or facial dermatitis? Zoonosis/human lesions? Spread to other pets? What other pets are there in the household? Housing? Indoors/outdoors? Flea control (if any)? Recent medication? Response? Relevant exposure to sources of infection — boarding kennels, grooming parlours etc.? Anything else the client wishes to mention?

other disease) is very important as drug-induced problems are becoming recognised with increasing frequency in veterinary medicine (e.g. iatrogenic hyperadrenocorticism, iatrogenic hyperoestrogenism, idiosyncratic drug eruption).

Physical Examination

A full clinical examination should be made along with a detailed dermatological examination. Many internal disorders have dermatological signs and the discovery of a serious systemic disease may affect the client's decisions regarding the investigation and management of the animal's skin disease. Some abnormalities may be detected on physical examination which may assist in the establishment of the differential diagnosis. For example, lymphadenopathy often accompanies demodicosis and chronic pyoderma. Bradycardia can be a feature of hypothyroidism. Conversely, serious systemic disease may affect the diagnostic plan, for example by precluding the use of sedatives or anaesthesia for skin biopsy or other investigations. Internal disease might produce misleading laboratory results.

Dermatological Examination

The entire body surface should be carefully examined by sight, feel and even smell, making sure that no area escapes attention. Good, even lighting is essential and some form of magnification may be of value.

Unless the animal is a giant breed of dog, it should be examined on a table. The animal should be inverted so that lesions on the ventrum can be carefully examined. The examination should also

AGE PREDILECTION FOR SKIN DISEASE	
Age	**Diseases**
Birth to 4 months	Cutaneous asthenia; ectodermal defects; juvenile impetigo; pituitary dwarfism; localised demodicosis
Before 1 year	Demodicosis; food and flea allergy; atopy
1 – 3 years	Hypersensitivity (atopy, food, flea); primary keratinisation disorders; primary idiopathic pyoderma
3 – 9 years	Hypersensitivity; endocrinopathy (hypothyroidism, hyperadrenocorticism)
Over 9 years	Endocrinopathy; neoplasia

FIG. 2.6 Age predilection for skin disease.

include the mucocutaneous areas and the feet (nails, interdigital webs and footpads). Pet owners are often aware of only the most severely affected areas. Note the nature, extent and severity of lesions. Their distribution may be very helpful in narrowing the differential diagnosis: for example,

involvement of the pinnae and elbows might indicate that sarcoptic mange is present, whereas facial and pedal self-trauma are suggestive of atopic dermatitis.

The hair coat and skin surface should be examined for the presence of parasites (fleas, flea faeces,

BREED PREDILECTION FOR SKIN DISEASE	
Breed	**Diseases**
Miniature Dachshund	Acanthosis nigricans
Dobermann Pinscher; Boxer; Persian Cat	Acne
Labrador and Golden Retriever; Boxer; English Setter; Terriers	Atopic dermatitis
Dobermann Pinscher; Whippet; Great Dane; Italian Greyhound	Colour dilute alopecia
Boxer; Bull Terrier; Scottish Terrier; West Highland White Terrier; Shar Pei	Demodicosis
Jack Russell Terrier; Persian Cat	Dermatophytosis
German Shepherd Dog; Rough Collie and Shetland Sheepdog	Discoid lupus erythematosus
Bulldog; Pug; Shar Pei; Persian Cat	Facial intertrigo
Chow Chow; Keeshond; Pomeranian; Miniature Poodle; Siberian Husky; Alaskan Malamute	Growth hormone/castration-responsive dermatosis
Boxer; Dachshund; Great Dane	Histiocytoma
Boxer; Dachshund; Miniature Poodle; Yorkshire Terrier; Boston Terrier	Hyperadrenocorticism
Boxer; Irish Setter; Dobermann Pinscher, Shar Pei	Hypothyroidism
Spaniel; Dobermann Pinscher; West Highland White Terrier; Miniature Schnauzer	Keratinisation disorders
West Highland White Terrier; Basset Hound; Spaniel; Miniature Poodle	*Malassezia* dermatitis
Boxer; Bulldog; Labrador Retriever	Mast cell tumour
Spaniel; German Shepherd Dog	Otitis externa
German Shepherd Dog	Perianal fistula
Abyssinian, Burmese and Siamese Cats	Psychogenic alopecia
Standard Poodle; Samoyed; Hungarian Vizsla	Sebaceous adenitis
Rottweiler; Newfoundland; Dobermann Pinscher	Vitiligo
Siberian Husky; Alaskan Malamute; Dobermann Pinscher	Zinc-responsive dermatosis
This information is based on the author's practice in South-East England. Local gene pools vary and there may be marked disparities between breed incidence of disease in other practices.	

FIG. 2.7 Breed predilection for skin disease.

SEX PREDILECTION FOR SKIN DISEASE	
Sex	**Diseases**
Entire male	Sertoli cell tumour; perianal adenoma; tail gland hyperplasia; castration/growth hormone-responsive dermatosis
Castrated male	Testosterone-responsive dermatosis
Entire female	Sex hormone-related alopecia (or hyperoestrogenism); mammary neoplasia
Spayed female	Oestrogen-responsive alopecia; mammary neoplasia
The terms ovarian imbalance types I and II are simplistic, outdated and inaccurate. Spayed bitches do not have ovaries and therefore they cannot be 'imbalanced'. Moreover, these terms fail to encompass the contribution of adrenal sex steroids and the concepts of hair-follicle cell receptor sensitivity. They are only mentioned here to familiarise the reader with the current terminology.	

FIG. 2.8 Sex predilection for skin disease.

RECORD OF DERMATOLOGICAL EXAMINATION
General: Alopecia Crusts Erythema Excoriations Hyperpigmentation Oedema Odour Papules Pustules Scale Other
Head: Alopecia Crusts Erythema Excoriations Hyperpigmentation Oedema Odour Papules Pustules Scale Other
Dorsum: Alopecia Crusts Erythema Excoriationmentation Oedema Odour Papules Pustules Scale Other
Perineum/perianal: Alopecia Crusts Erythema Excoriations Hyperpigmentation Oedema Odour Papules Pustules Scale Other
Feet/legs: Alopecia Crusts Erythema Excoriations Hyperpigmentation Oedema Odour Papules Pustules Scale Other
Ventrum: Alopecia Crusts Erythema Excoriations Hyperpigmentation Oedema Odour Papules Pustules Scale Other

FIG. 2.9 Record of dermatological examination.

lice and ticks) and a subjective assessment of coat quality (sparse, dry, greasy, alopecic, malodorous) should be made. Alopecia, ease of epilation and the presence of broken hairs should be noted. The skin surface should be systematically examined by parting the hair; any lesions should be recorded. If necessary the coat can be clipped but the client's permission should be obtained first. The texture, thickness and elasticity of the skin should be assessed by palpation. An appropriate record form is illustrated in Fig. 2.9.

There are a number of reasons for such meticulous record keeping. The discipline of filling in the record form forces the clinician to make a full examination. A complete record allows progress to be monitored objectively rather than subjectively and may resolve any dispute between an owner who considers the condition to have worsened and a clinician who knows that the animal's disease has improved. Finally, if the primary clinician wishes to describe the case precisely to a colleague, for example on a pathology request form or in a referral letter, the relevant information can be conveyed accurately.

As with all disciplines, there is a specific vocabulary for the description of dermatological lesions. Two groups of lesions are described: primary and secondary. **Primary lesions** are the most significant diagnostically but may be scant and transient. They arise as a direct consequence of the disease process. **Secondary lesions** result from progression of primary lesions, such as the pustule that develops into an epidermal collarette, or from self-trauma. A glossary of the more commonly encountered terms is given in Fig. 2.10. Knowledge of these terms will facilitate precision in record-keeping but, more importantly, may aid in the formulation of the differential diagnosis; for example, papules, pustules and epidermal collarettes usually indicate that pyoderma is present. Figure 2.10 also briefly indicates the clinical and diagnostic significance of specific skin lesions.

DERMATOLOGICAL LESIONS: A GLOSSARY OF TERMS		
Lesion	**Description**	**Significance**
Primary lesions		
Bulla	Vesicle (q.v.) > 1 cm	Transient so rarely seen. Suggests bullous immune-mediated disease
Cyst	Congenital or developmental. Filled with fluid or keratinaceous debris	May be neoplastic
Macule	Circumscribed area of colour change < 1 cm. Skin thickness normal	Pigmentary disorders, (e.g. vitiligo, lentigo) haemorrhage, vascular engorgement
Nodule	Raised, solid, palpable mass > 1 cm	Neoplastic or inflammatory cell infiltration
Papule	Raised, solid mass < 1 cm	Common. Accumulation of inflammatory cells. Often associated with pyoderma/folliculitis

Continued

DERMATOLOGICAL LESIONS: A GLOSSARY OF TERMS		
Lesion	**Description**	**Significance**
Patch	Macule > 1 cm	Coalescence of papules
Plaque	Elevated area > 1 cm	Pyoderma/folliculitis. Less commonly, bullous immune-mediated disease
Pustule	Elevated, circumscribed. Contains purulent material	Neoplastic (or inflammatory) cell infiltration. Difficult to differentiate from nodule
Tumour	Strictly, a swelling. By popular usage, a neoplastic mass	Immune-mediated, viral, irritant-induced. Urticaria, allergy, oedema
Vesicle	Fluid-filled, circumscribed, elevated, < 1 cm	A large bulla (q.v.)
Wheal	Sharply circumscribed, raised, flat surface	May arise following Type 1 hypersensitivity or exposure to toxins
Secondary lesions		
Comedo	Dilated, keratin-plugged hair follicle (usually hair is lost). Appears dark brown or black	Follicular disease (especially demodicosis); inflammatory or keratinisation defect; hyperadrenocorticism
Crust	Dried exudate (serum, pus, blood)	Pustular disease — pyoderma/folliculitis
Epidermal collarette	Circular, peeling stratum corneum	Sequel to pustule
Erosion	Loss of epidermis (not full thickness). Difficult to distinguish from an ulcer, clinically	Self-trauma (see excoriation). Certain immune-mediated disorders. Heals without scarring
Excoriation	Erosion or ulceration due to self-trauma	Heals without scarring if less than full epidermal thickness
Fissure	Linear cleavage or split	Trauma, swelling, drying
Hyperkaratosis	Increased production or reduced sloughing of stratum corneum	Keratinisation defect. Presents as excess scale, horny projection from footpads
Hyperpigmentation	Increased skin pigmentation	Pigmentary disorders (e.g. lentigo or post-inflammatory)
Hypopigmentation	Reduced skin pigmentation	Sequel to full thickness epidermal damage (traumatic, neoplastic or inflammation)
Lichenification	Thickening. Exaggerated surface 'cobblestone' markings	Non-specific. Any chronic dermatitis
Scale	Accumulation of partially sloughed squames on skin or attached to hairs	Keratinisation defect. Sequel to inflammation
Scar	Fibrous, alopecic, often hypopigmented	Sequel to full thickness epidermal damage (ulcer, severe self-trauma)
Ulcer	Full thickness epidermal defect	Severe and deep vascular, inflammatory or neoplastic disease

FIG. 2.10 Dermatological lesions: A glossary of terms.

3

Diagnostic Testing

KAREN MORIELLO

After completing the history and physical examination of a patient with skin disease, the next step is to choose the appropriate diagnostic tests to confirm or refute the suspected differential diagnoses. *The most important thing to remember when choosing any diagnostic test is to know what question you are trying to answer*. This sounds simple, but it is so often overlooked in clinical practice. Keeping this thought foremost in the mind when choosing tests will be of great help when interpreting test results. This thought pattern is extremely helpful when explaining to the client what tests need to be performed to find the cause of their pet's skin disease.

Another pitfall with diagnostic tests in dermatology, and for that matter in a lot of subspecialties, is that the user often focuses too heavily on the 'face value' of the test results. This can be illustrated by the following example. A dog with a focal area of deep pyoderma on the left hindleg is examined and the following tests are performed: a cytological examination of the exudate; aerobic and anaerobic bacterial cultures; deep fungal cultures; and a skin biopsy. It is strongly suspected that the patient has a staphylococcal infection. The cytological examination of the exudate reveals septic inflammation with degenerative neutrophils, intracellular cocci and macrophages. *Staphylococcus intermedius* is reported as the only organism isolated from the samples submitted for culture. The final diagnosis on the skin biopsy is folliculitis and furunculosis with bacteria. One approach to interpreting these results is to feel as if they do not reveal anything not already known from the clinical examination. On 'face value,' the tests confirmed the existence of a pyoderma but did not add much new information. Another approach, particularly in difficult cases where numerous expensive tests need to be performed, is to look at what the tests did not show. The cytological specimen did *not* reveal rods (possible concurrent Gram-negative infection), neoplastic cells (some neoplastic diseases may mimic infectious processes) or deep fungal organisms (in particular *Blastomyces* spp.). The culture results did *not* identify an unsuspected aerobe or anaerobe or deep fungal organism. Finally, the skin biopsy results did *not* find demodicosis, cutaneous neoplasia, an atypical mycobacterium, deep mycoses, actinobacillosis, a kerion, phaeohyphomycosis or a variety of other conditions. Thus, negative findings help to confirm the suspected diagnosis.

Diagnostic Techniques for Finding Parasites

Skin Scrapings

Indications

All animals with skin diseases should have a superficial and a deep skin scraping performed. Skin scrapings are used primarily to find mites: *Demodex* spp., *Sarcoptes* spp. (Fig. 3.1), *Notoedres cati*, *Cheyletiella* spp. (Fig. 3.2), chiggers, *Dermanyssus gallinae*, *Otodectes cynotis* and others. Additionally, skin scrapings may be useful in diagnosing nematode infestations of the skin, particularly *Pelodera* spp., and larval stages of hookworms. Some mites (e.g. *Sarcoptes* spp.) are very difficult to

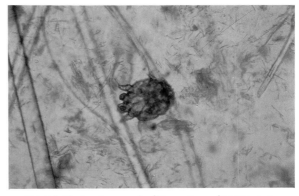

FIG. 3.1 Photomicrograph of *Sarcoptes scabiei* var *canis*.

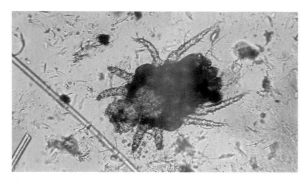

FIG. 3.2 Photomicrograph of *Cheyletiella* spp.

find on skin scrapings and repeat skin scrapings of patients during each follow-up evaluation are recommended.

Pertinent background information

There are two types of skin scrapings: superficial and deep. Superficial scrapings collect material from the superficial layers of the epidermis and do not cause capillary bleeding. *Cheyletiella* spp. are often found in superficial skin scrapings. Deep skin scrapings collect debris from the intrafollicular and superficial dermal areas. Blood must be visible both grossly and microscopically to confirm that a sufficiently deep skin scraping has been taken. *Demodex* mites are best found on deep skin scrapings. The 'right' number of skin scrapings to perform on each patient is somewhere between one and over 100. Realistically, in cases where mite infestations are most strongly suspected, at least 10–15 skin scrapings should be performed; if *Demodex*, *Sarcoptes* or *Notoedres* are suspected, the majority of scrapings should be deep skin scrapings.

Equipment

- Mineral oil
- Glass microscope slides
- Coverslips
- New sterile scalpel blade or skin-scraping spatula

Skin-scraping spatulas are useful because they minimise the chance of accidental laceration. Also, clients are less anxious when a spatula is used for scrapings around the eyes.

Technique

1. Clipping of the hair coat may be necessary. If so, scissors rather than electric clippers should be used. Superficial mites, such as *Cheyletiella* spp., can be lost from the surface if electric clippers are used.
2. The lesion should be moistened with mineral oil to aid the collection of skin debris.
3. The skin-scraping spatula or scalpel blade is held perpendicular to the skin and the skin firmly scraped. If the blade or spatula is held at less than a 90° angle to the skin, skin debris is smeared into the surrounding hair and skin and not collected on the blade. Superficial skin scrapings only collect surface debris and do not cause capillary bleeding.
4. To collect material for a deep skin scraping, the lesion is firmly squeezed between the fingertips and the area scraped until capillary bleeding is seen.
5. The skin scraping material is smeared on to a glass microscope slide; additional mineral oil and a coverslip are added. Coverslips minimise 'microscope oil slicks' and make microscopic examination easier because the entire field is in one visual plane.
6. The specimen is examined first under low magnification with maximum contrast (move the condenser down). Many mites are motile and looking for movement is often useful. Mite movement is often obscured in thick specimens.

Artifacts

Coloured threads are commonly seen in skin scrapings from pruritic animals and may be from carpets and sofas. Fungal spores and pollen grains can be confused with mites. Plant material is often, but not always, coloured. Mites appear transparent and do not have colour to their exoskeleton. *Alternaria* spores are dark brown and are shaped like a macrospore of *Microsporum*; however, superficial macrospores are not visible on skin scrapings. Blood cells mixed in mineral oil will often form round red-brown globular structures. Occasionally, melanin granules from hair shafts will be seen.

Interpretation

Numerous negative deep skin scrapings from appropriate areas should reliably eliminate demodicosis and notoedric mange from the differential list. *Demodex* mites can be part of the normal flora of both dog and cat skin, but it is extremely rare to find *Demodex* mites on skin scrapings. If a *Demodex* mite is found, a case of demodicosis should immediately be suspected. More deep skin scrapings should be taken to confirm the diagnosis of demodicosis. If demodicosis is present, it should be easy to find more mites. *Pelodera* nematodes are also easily found on skin scrapings but hookworm larvae are not. Negative skin scrapings do not eliminate *Sarcoptes* or cheyletiellosis from the differential diagnoses list.

Combing of the Hair Coat, or 'Flea Combing'

Indications

Combing of the hair coat is indicated in any parasitic skin disease or scaling disorder. Combing debris may contain: adult fleas, flea excreta, lice, ticks or *Cheyletiella* mites.

Pertinent background information

Combing is a rapid, inexpensive, atraumatic and often fruitful diagnostic test. The hair coat can be combed while a history is being obtained. It is an especially useful technique for finding parasites on cats, rabbits, ferrets and dogs in which fleas or *Cheyletiella* spp. mites are suspected. Cheyletiellosis is often only manifested by scaling and these mites are more easily found on combings than in skin scrapings.

Equipment

- Hand-held metal or plastic fine-tooth comb

The teeth should be strong enough not to break when pulled through the hair coat and blunt enough not to cause trauma to the skin.

Technique

1. The animal's hair coat is thoroughly combed with special emphasis given to scaly areas of the skin. Hair and scale trapped between the teeth of the comb should be removed periodically and placed in a container.
2. The collected material should be examined with a hand-held magnifying lens. Fleas and flea excreta are usually readily visible. Flea excreta will dissolve when moistened with water into a dark red-brown spot. This is most dramatic if a white paper towel or piece of filter paper is used. Lice are usually found with ease but close examination of the hair shafts for nits should be performed. A small amount of scale should be examined on dark paper because *Cheyletiella* mites are often visible as moving specks. If a parasite is not found easily, the material should be examined more closely with either a dissecting scope or under low power on the microscope.

Artifacts

Soil can be confused with flea excreta and white paper and water can be used to differentiate soil from flea excreta. If the owner has not properly rinsed the animal's coat, a shampoo residue that mimics the excessive scaling observed in *Cheyletiella* infestations may be present. Close examination of these scales is necessary in such cases.

Interpretation

Positive hair combings are diagnostic; negative combings are inconclusive. Cats may remove mites, fleas and lice via grooming. *Cheyletiella* mites can be very difficult to find and may not be visible on either skin scrapings or hair combings.

Acetate Tape Preparations

Indications

Acetate tape preparations are indicated when fleas, lice or *Cheyletiella* spp. infestations are suspected or found.

Pertinent background information

The value of acetate tape preparations in the diagnosis of cheyletiellosis is greatly over-emphasised. In cases where there is a tremendous amount of scale, mites may be found with acetate tape preparations.

If the amount of scale is moderate or scarce, it is not a cost-effective technique. Acetate tape preparations are very useful in flea and louse infestations for 'trapping' parasites to show to clients.

Equipment

- Clear acetate adhesive tape
- Mineral oil
- Glass microscope slides and coverslips

Technique

1. The most common mistake made when performing acetate tape preparations is to collect scale from the hair coat as if one were removing lint from a piece of clothing. The superficial parasites that can be collected with acetate tape are found very close to the skin; it is highly unlikely that *Cheyletiella* mites, fleas or lice will be found on the distal hairs.
2. The skin should be examined until representative scaly lesions are found or until fleas or lice are visible. Scissors should be used to clip hairs, if necessary.
3. The sticky side of a piece of tape is gently and firmly pressed to the base of the hairs and skin.
4. The sticky side of the tape is then pressed on to a glass microscope slide over a drop of mineral oil. Another drop of mineral oil is placed over the acetate tape (non-sticky side) and a coverslip put on to the microscope slide. Sandwiching the acetate tape specimen between two drops of mineral oil greatly improves visual clarity when examining the specimen under the microscope.

Artifacts

The accidental use of frosted acetate tape is the most common cause of inability to see through the tape. If the specimen is not sandwiched between two drops of mineral oil, it will be difficult to see mites clearly. Crinkles are commonly seen if the tape is not carefully placed on the microscope. Coloured threads and pigmented plant and pollen spores are commonly seen.

Interpretation

A positive finding is diagnostic; a negative specimen is inconclusive.

Ear Swabs

Indications

Head pruritus or external ear disease in any animal is a clear indication for performing an ear swab. This technique is used primarily to find *Otodectes cynotis* and other species of ear mites. Occasionally, *Demodex* mites may be found.

Pertinent background information

The pruritus from ear mite infestation is believed to be due to both a mechanical irritation and Type 1 hypersensitivity reaction. Do not discount the finding of even one mite or egg, especially in intensely pruritic adult animals; this is common in animals with hypersensitivity reactions to the mites. Many species of ear mites migrate to the ear margins to deposit eggs, therefore if swabs from the ear canal are negative, skin scrapings from ear margins or the periaural skin are indicated.

Equipment

- Mineral oil
- Glass microscope slide and coverslips
- Cotton-tipped swab

Technique

1. The animal should be firmly restrained and the ear canal gently swabbed with a cotton-tipped swab.
2. The debris should be transferred from the tip of the swab to a microscope slide by gently rolling the swab in a drop of mineral oil.
3. The specimen should be coverslipped before being examined.

Artifacts

The most common artifact is clumps of coagulated dried blood.

Interpretation

A positive finding is diagnostic; a negative finding is inconclusive.

Diagnostic Techniques for Identifying and Culturing Fungi and Bacteria

Wood's Lamp Examination

Indications

A Wood's lamp examination may be useful as a screening tool where *Microsporum canis* infection is suspected. Cats with skin disease and other small mammals presented with hair-loss as the primary problem are the most likely candidates. A positive Wood's lamp examination is only suggestive of an infection; confirmation of infection requires fungal culture and microscopic examination of the fungal colony. The Wood's lamp is most useful in cats with skin lesions; it can be a poor tool to monitor infection status or as a tool to screen cats for subclinical infections.

Pertinent background information

The Wood's lamp is one of the most misused diagnostic tools in veterinary dermatology and it is important to understand the limitations of its use. It is an ultraviolet light with a wavelength of 253.7 nm filtered through a cobalt or nickel filter. When certain strains of dermatophytes infect hairs, fungal metabolites are produced that fluoresce bright green when exposed to this light. Unfortunately, the only species of importance in veterinary medicine which fluoresces under a Wood's lamp is *M. canis*. Not all strains of *M. canis* will fluoresce and, in fact, not all fluorescing strains will fluoresce on all hosts. The lamp must be allowed to warm up for 5–10 minutes before use to ensure that the temperature-dependent wavelength is stable. Infected hairs may need to be exposed to the light for several minutes before they begin to fluoresce.

Equipment

- Wood's lamp

Technique

1. The lamp should be turned on for 5–10 minutes before use.
2. The lamp should be held over the skin lesions for at least 5 minutes before making an interpretation. Positive hairs will glow a bright apple-green

colour. If there is any doubt about the fluorescence, glowing hairs should be plucked in the direction of growth and the proximal end of the hair shaft examined with the Wood's lamp. Dermatophytic fungal growth is often heaviest in the hair follicle and true-positive hairs will fluoresce both intra- and extrafollicularly. These hairs should be used for culture or direct examination.

Artifacts

Only actively infected growing hairs will show positive fluorescence; fluorescence is not seen in scales or fungal culture. False-positive fluorescence may be seen in bacterial infections, which usually show a bluish-white fluorescence. Areas where sebum has accumulated will also give a false-positive reaction, but the colour is a dull blue-green. Fluorescence can be destroyed by soap and topical medications.

Interpretation

A positive Wood's lamp examination is only suggestive of a dermatophyte infection, not diagnostic. Treatment should not be initiated based upon this finding alone and a definitive diagnosis should be obtained via fungal culture. A negative Wood's lamp examination is inconclusive.

Direct Examination of Hair and Scale for Fungal Elements

Indications

Theoretically, direct examination of hair and scale for fungal elements is indicated in any animal in which dermatophytosis is suspected. More practically, this technique is cost- and time-effective only when Wood's lamp-positive hairs are examined. Ectothrix spores may also be visible in animals with generalised *Trichophyton* spp. infections. Because of the infrequency of positive results relative to time invested in performing this technique, it may not be very valuable in a busy practice.

Pertinent background information

As dermatophytes proliferate on anagen hairs, they produce ectothrix spores and fungal hyphae. If one of these hairs is examined microscopically using a clearing agent or mineral oil, these spores are visible and are definitive evidence of a dermatophytosis. Clearing agents are substances which cause background scales, debris and keratin to become swollen and homogenous. Clearing agents are superior to mineral oil because they also make hairs and fungal spores more refractile, so that they are easier to see. The two most commonly used clearing agents are 20% potassium hydroxide (KOH) and chlorphenolac. KOH is readily available and will clear a slide in 15–20 seconds if warmed, or 30 minutes if allowed to stand at room temperature. Chlorphenolac is not commercially available and must be compounded by a chemist or pharmacist. The advantages of this agent are immediate clearing and lack of artifacts.

Equipment

- 20% KOH or chlorphenolac
- Glass microscope slides and coverslips
- Wood's lamp
- Forceps
- Matches

Chlorphenolac can be prepared by mixing the following agents together:

- 25 ml liquid phenol,
- 50 g of chloral hydrate,
- 25 ml of liquid lactic acid.

This should be performed in a fume hood. It will take several days for the crystals to go into solution and the mixture should be stored in a dark-glass bottle. It is stable indefinitely and its superior clearing ability when compared with 20% KOH is definitely worth the difficulty in preparing the mixture.

Technique

1. Suspect hairs are gently plucked in the direction of growth using small forceps. It is important to obtain the intrafollicular portion of the hair and this can be accomplished by gently rolling the hair while plucking. This technique is most fruitful when examining fluorescing hairs.
2. Widely scatter the hairs on a glass microscope slide and place several drops of a clearing agent on them.
3. If chlorphenolac is used, clearing is immediate and the slide can be examined as soon as it is coverslipped. If 20% KOH is used, the slide

should be allowed 30 minutes to clear or it should be gently heated with a match (do not boil!) for 15–20 seconds, coverslipped and then examined. Another technique is to warm the slide on the microscope lamp for 15–20 minutes and place a coverslip on the slide.

4. The slide should be examined first under low magnification. A normal hair should be found and used as a reference. Infected hairs will be visible at low power (4×) and will appear pale, swollen and filamentous (Fig. 3.3). Moving the condenser down will improve contrast and help to find the hairs. If fluorescing hairs were placed on the slide and you cannot find any evidence of infected hairs, dim the lights in the laboratory and re-examine the slide with the Wood's lamp. Often the hairs will continue to glow even after a clearing agent has been used. The microscope stage can be moved until the glowing hair is under the lens. It is important to remember that hairs can be Wood's lamp-positive, but ectothrix spores may not be visible; it is the fungal metabolites that cause the hair to glow, not the ectothrix spores. Once a suspect infected hair is located, it can be examined under higher magnification to make a definitive diagnosis. Fungal spores are very small (usually 2–3 μm in diameter) and may be present in chains in the hair shaft.

Artifacts

Specimens examined with KOH may crystallise and resemble a faecal flotation specimen if left to

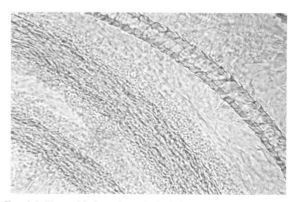

FIG. 3.3 Normal hair and two hairs infected with dermatophytosis as seen with a clearing agent (courtesy of Dr Peter Mac-Williams, University of Wisconsin, School of Veterinary Medicine).

stand. Occasionally, squamous epithelial cells will form 'skeletons' and cholesterol crystals. Oil droplets can resemble budding yeast and threads can look like hairs. These artifacts are minimised with the use of chlorphenolac.

Interpretation

Ectothrix spores or fungal hyphae are definitive evidence of a dermatophyte infection. A negative test is inconclusive.

Dermatophyte Cultures

Indications

A dermatophyte culture is the 'gold standard' for diagnosing a dermatophytosis. It is indicated whenever Wood's lamp examination or direct examination of hair and scale is positive. Although finding ectothrix spores is a clear indication for antifungal therapy, it is important to identify the organism conclusively via culture, for both prognostic and legal reasons. Dermatophyte culture is indicated in cats with any skin disease and in other patients in which hair-loss or hair fragility is a problem.

Pertinent background information

Dermatophytes are commonly cultured on either Dermatophyte Test Medium (DTM) or Sabouraud's dextrose agar. Dermatophyte Test Medium consists of Sabouraud's dextrose agar, antibacterial and antifungal agents to inhibit the growth of contaminants and phenol red (pH indicator). The colour indicator has been added as an aid in identifying dermatophytes; a red colour change is suggestive, though not diagnostic, of a dermatophyte infection.

Dermatophytes initially use the protein in the medium, producing alkaline metabolites which turn the medium red. The red colour disappears when all the protein has been used and the pathogens begin to use the carbohydrate component of the medium. Contaminants use the carbohydrates in the medium first and do not produce a red colour change in the medium until all available carbohydrates have been utilised. This is usually observed at 10–14 days of culture, but may be observed sooner if the plate is heavily overgrown with contaminants. Therefore all plates should be examined daily for the first 14 days.

Pathogenic fungal colonies are pale in colour and never heavily pigmented. The most common pathogens are pale white or buff. Contaminants or saprophytic colonies are commonly pigmented (e.g. brown, black, red, yellow). There are, however, a few common contaminants (*Aspergillus* spp., *Penicillium* spp.) that may mimic pathogens by pale colony growth and a red colour change in DTM. Definitive diagnosis of a dermatophyte on culture is based upon microscopic identification of the organism, not a change in colour in the DTM.

Dermatophyte Test Medium may depress the growth of some dermatophytes and will mask colony pigmentation. Gross colony growth is often slower and less fluffy, when compared with plain Sabouraud's dextrose agar. Microscopically, sporulation may be inhibited, making identification of the organism difficult. Suspect dermatophytes should be subcultured on Sabouraud's agar for identification. In practice, the use of commercial fungal culture plates with dual compartments for both DTM and Sabouraud's dextrose agar are highly recommended to avoid this problem. If these plates are not readily available, they can be produced in-house by using Petri dishes with dual compartments and filling the plates with prepared DTM and Sabouraud's agar.

Commercial DTM is available in either glass jars or flat plates. Glass jars containing DTM slants are not recommended for use. Firstly, the jars are extremely difficult to inoculate with specimens, especially toothbrush cultures. Secondly, it is critical that the lids are not screwed on too tightly or the internal environment becomes anaerobic; dermatophytes are aerobic. Thirdly, if the lids are too tight the internal moisture increases and bacterial and yeast growth are enhanced. Finally, it is extremely difficult to obtain specimens for microscopic examination from these jars.

Equipment

- Dermatophyte test medium and/or Sabouraud's dextrose agar
- Toothbrushes in original packaging or scalp massaging brush
- Alcohol
- Forceps
- Sterile swabs

- Clear acetate tape
- Glass microscope slides and coverslips
- Lactophenol cotton blue stain

Technique

1. If the fungal culture plate has been stored in the refrigerator, allow it to come to room temperature before inoculating. This makes inoculation of the plate much easier.
2. Specimens from cats are best collected using a sterile toothbrush or scalp-massaging brush. The instrument is combed vigorously over the cat's hair coat for several minutes or until hairs are visible in the bristles. Special emphasis should be given to lesional areas, particularly if they are Wood's lamp-positive.
3. The fungal culture plate is inoculated by gently embedding or repeatedly dabbing the toothbrush or scalp brush into the medium. It is important to be gentle or the fungal medium will stick to the bristles and be removed from the plate. Individual Wood's lamp-positive hairs, or hairs from areas where a direct examination for ectothrix spores have been positive, may be cultured instead.
4. Specimens from dogs, rabbits, guinea pigs and other species may be cultured by plucking hairs from the margin of newly developing lesions. Lesions in these species may be cultured using the technique described for cats but increased contamination of the plate may occur. Prior to plucking hairs from the margin of suspect lesions, the area should be gently swabbed with 70% isopropyl alcohol to decrease contaminant growth.
5. Individually plucked hairs should be firmly pressed on to the surface of the medium. Dermatophytes are aerobic organisms so do not embed the hairs.
6. Specimens should be examined microscopically. This is best done by pressing the sticky side of a small piece of clear tape against the edge of the growing colony to collect spores. The tape is then pressed on to a glass microscope slide over a drop of lactophenol cotton blue stain.

Artifacts

Bacteria and yeast can overgrow the plates if incubated over 30°C or 30% relative humidity. Fungal contaminants will commonly overgrow plates if they are held too long or if specimens are improperly collected. A red colour change on DTM is only suggestive, not diagnostic of a fungal pathogen — some colonies of *M. canis* have been identified that did not cause such a colour change. Some common contaminants can mimic pathogens by causing a red colour change and by being pale.

Interpretation

A positive fungal culture is diagnostic for an infection and treatment is warranted. If samples have been properly obtained and cultured, a negative fungal culture is conclusive.

Techniques for Culturing Subcutaneous and Deep Mycoses

Indications

Cultures for subcutaneous or deep mycoses are indicated in patients with draining tracts, nodular lesions and non-healing wounds. In addition, cultures are indicated when cytological examination of exudate is suggestive of a fungal infection.

Pertinent background information

These fungal cultures should not be performed in-house because many of these organisms are potential human health hazards. Additionally, these organisms often require special growth characteristics and so only laboratories familiar with isolating fungal pathogens should be used. Dermatophyte Test Medium cannot be used for these cultures. The laboratory should be provided with a detailed list of the suspect organisms and an adequate sample inoculum. A single swab from a wound is not sufficient. A large piece (at least a 6 mm skin biopsy) of tissue plug for culture and several swabs of the exudate should be submitted. Several unstained glass microscope slides of smears of the exudate should be submitted with the cultures. The reference laboratory can perform Gram stains and special stains on these specimens.

Equipment and facilities

- Diagnostic reference laboratory instructions
- Culture swabs
- Sterile instruments and containers

Technique

1. Disposable latex gloves should always be worn when collecting specimens from animals suspected of being infected with a subcutaneous or deep mycosis.
2. Draining tracts may be cultured using sterile culturettes; however, it is preferable to submit tissue for culture. The skin surrounding a draining tract should scrubbed with an antibacterial scrub (e.g. chlorhexidine) before inserting the tip of the sterile culture swab.
3. Exudative draining lesions are best cultured from skin biopsy specimens to minimise contaminant growth and maximise the opportunity of isolating the pathogen. If it is impossible to biopsy the lesion, then every effort should be made to sample purulent exudate, not blood, from the deepest area of the wound. Aspirates and swabs should be submitted for culture. Do not forget to collect specimens for cytological examination, Gram stain and special stains for the reference laboratory.
4. Nodules and lesions which appear to be granulomatous should be cultured from biopsy specimens. The area immediately over the biopsy site should receive a gentle sterile surgical scrub. Avoid using skin biopsy punches when taking specimens for cultures because it is often impossible to obtain a deep enough specimen. A scalpel blade should be used to remove a deep wedge of tissue from the lesion. The larger the piece of tissue, the better. Nodules can be excised *en masse*. The reference laboratory should be contacted prior to tissue collection for information on how they want the samples submitted.
   Usually laboratories require submission in a sterile container with the specimen kept moist with sterile water. Some laboratories supply transport medium.
5. *Definitive diagnosis of these infections requires proper specimen collection and handling by both the laboratory and clinician. Make sure the laboratory knows exactly what organisms are suspected, not just 'deep fungal culture'.*

Artifacts

Specimens contaminated with normal skin flora are common sequelae to poor specimen collection.

False-negative cultures may occur if the specimen, especially tissue is too small.

Interpretation

Most deep mycoses are diagnosed via cytological or histological examination of tissue specimens. These organisms are rarely, if ever, cultured from uninfected hosts. The isolation of a deep fungal organism via culture should be taken very seriously as this indicates active infection. Laboratory reports of isolates of subcutaneous fungal organisms should be interpreted with caution. A great many of these organisms are saprophytes. Definitive diagnosis of a subcutaneous fungal infection (e.g. agents of phaeohyphomycosis) should be based upon culture and histological or cytological evidence of tissue invasion.

Techniques for Culturing Superficial Bacterial Infections (Pyoderma) (see Fig. 3.4)

Indications

There is a wide range of opinion on when to culture superficial bacterial skin infections. In general, recommendations on when to culture include:

- deep skin infections;
- recurrent bacterial skin infections;
- when several antibiotics have been used previously;
- where corticosteroids have been used recently;
- where there is inadequate clinical response to appropriate therapy; and
- always!

Most bacterial skin infections are not cultured at first presentation to the clinician; antibiotic therapy is selected based upon clinical judgement. In general, it is neither necessary nor cost effective to culture every superficial pyoderma. It is more cost effective to spend the client's money on diagnostic tests that may reveal why the bacterial infection occurred in the first place.

Pertinent background information

Most veterinarians do not perform in-house bacterial cultures; they use diagnostic laboratories. It is important that a laboratory with a microbiologist familiar with veterinary specimens be used; human laboratories may or may not be knowledgeable about veterinary microbiology. Antimicrobial sensitivities and organism speciation should always be performed.

Equipment

- Sterile aerobic culturette swab with transport medium tip
- Sterile 22–27 gauge needle

Technique

1. Find an intact pustule. It is important to remember to avoid touching the pustule with your fingers or else you may contaminate the culture site.
2. It is important to remember not to scrub or wipe the pustule with an antibacterial solution or alcohol or else the culture may be negative for growth.
3. Gently lance open the pustule with the tip of a sterile needle; swab the pustule with the tip of the culturette, and return it to its transport sleeve. It is common to observe only blood when the pustule is ruptured; these cultures almost always reveal pure cultures of *Staphylococcus* spp.

Artifacts

False-negative cultures may result if lesions are cleansed before sampling, not promptly sent to the laboratory, or are heavily contaminated by resident or transient skin flora.

Interpretation

The clinician must be aware of the common transient and resident flora of the species in question. In dogs, the primary pathogen of canine superficial pyoderma is *S. intermedius*. The isolation of *Proteus* spp., *Bacillus* spp., *Escherichia coli*, *Pseudomonas* spp. and *Micrococcus* spp. is not usually significant in the presence of a *S. intermedius* isolate. However, the isolation of one or more of these organisms may be significant if they are present in dogs with deep pyoderma with or without signs of sepsis or in pure culture in animals with overt clinical signs. The interpretation of any bacterial

culture and sensitivity result must be done in light of the patient's clinical signs and history.

Techniques for Culturing Deep Bacterial Infections

Indication

Bacterial cultures are indicated in patients with nodular lesions, draining tracts, non-healing wounds, recurrent cat-bite abscesses, deep pyoderma and cellulitis.

Pertinent background information

A skin biopsy is strongly recommended in patients with deep bacterial infections, especially those with nodules or recurrent/non-healing wounds. Additionally, numerous impression smears should be made of the exudate and lesion and sent along with the cultures and biopsy to the reference laboratory. Some organisms (e.g. *Mycobacterium* spp.)

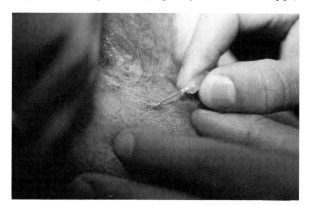

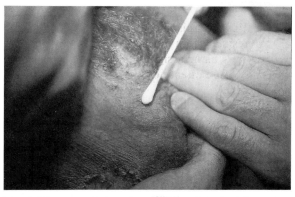

FIG. 3.4 Proper technique for obtaining a superficial bacterial culture.

may be more easily found on cytological examination of tissue impression than on culture. The clinical signs of deep bacterial infections are almost identical to those of the intermediate and deep mycoses. Therefore make sure that an adequate number of specimens is sent to the laboratory for culture.

The most common cause for failure to isolate a pathogen is submission of inadequate specimens. Many pathogens are isolated in the skin beneath or inside of granulation tissue or collagen. There may only be a few organisms per square centimetre of tissue; therefore send large amounts of infected tissue (the host won't miss it). The reference laboratory will macerate the tissue and inoculate appropriate growth plates.

Equipment and facilities

- Veterinary diagnostic laboratory
- Sterile containers
- Sterile surgical equipment
- Sterile culture swabs

Technique

The techniques for culturing deep bacterial infections are similar to those described for culturing subcutaneous and deep mycoses.

Artifacts

See comments for subcutaneous and deep mycoses.

Interpretation

Growth of organisms commonly considered transient or resident flora must be interpreted in light of the patient's clinical signs. Transient and resident flora may cause disease or contribute to it in debilitated hosts.

Techniques for Anaerobic Cultures

Indications

Anaerobic culture is indicated in patients with rapidly progressing tissue destruction, wounds that are extremely malodorous, recurrent abscesses or non-healing ulcerative infections near mucocutaneous junction, or skin diseases that are not responsive to aminoglycosides.

Pertinent background information

Anaerobic cultures are rarely performed in-house and the use of a diagnostic laboratory familiar with handling these specimens is strongly recommended. Most anaerobic infections are due to several organisms that are part of the host's natural flora.

Equipment and facilities

- Veterinary reference laboratory
- Sterile needles and syringes with rubber stoppers
- Anaerobic transport medium
- Sterile surgical instruments

Technique

1. The best technique for isolating anaerobes from abscesses is to aspirate fluid/exudate into a syringe and immediately cap the needle with a rubber stopper. Alternatively, the sample can be collected in an anaerobic transport medium. Each commercial transport medium is slightly different and the laboratory's directions for its use should be followed exactly.
2. The laboratory should be told which organisms are suspected or the sample may be handled incorrectly.

Artifacts

Anaerobic organisms are scant in tissue and often require longer incubation periods than most aerobic organisms. Failure to isolate an organism may be due to inadequate sampling technique or lack of adequate time for growth. Some organisms are extremely fastidious and even short exposure to oxygen can result in a failure to grow.

Interpretation

It is important to be familiar with the normal flora of the patient. Many of the anaerobes that are isolated from cutaneous abscesses/deep pyoderma are from the gastrointestinal tract. If specimen selection is poor, it may be impossible to determine whether the organism is a true pathogen or not. Isolation of the same organism from at least two different cultures strongly suggests that it is pathogenic, whereas growth in only one culture raises suspicion that it may be a contaminant. Most anaerobic infections are due to several organisms.

Collecting Specimens for Cytology

Impression Smears and Fine Needle Aspirates

Indications

Erosive to ulcerative, exudative, pustular, masses/nodules and draining lesions should be sampled.

Pertinent background information

Microscopic examination of exudate or superficial cells from the surface of a lesion can often be diagnostic. Impression smears of exudate should accompany all biopsy specimens and bacterial or deep fungal cultures. Gram stain and special stains may provide valuable information prior to the final culture or biopsy report. Nodular lesions may be inflammatory or neoplastic and should be examined cytologically prior to making any decision regarding further investigations or possible therapy.

Equipment

- Glass microscope slides and coverslips
- 5–10 ml syringe
- 22–23 gauge needles
- Fast Giemsa and Gram stains

Technique

1. Impression smears may be made either from the freshly cut surface of an excised mass or directly from surface of the lesion.
2. When making impression smears from the surface of an excised mass, excess moisture (blood) should be blotted from the surface of a mass before gently touching the surface of the glass microscope slide to the mass. This should be done several times without any twisting or rubbing motion. At least three slides should be prepared. The slide should be held up to the light to ensure that cells have exfoliated on to the slide before placing the tissue specimen into formalin for processing.
3. Impression smears from patients may be collected by directly pressing the glass microscope slide against the lesion. If the lesion is extremely exudative, it may be necessary to spread the material on the slide by making a 'squash' preparation. These are made by sandwiching the exudate between two slides (the collection slide and a second, new slide) and gently pulling the slides apart in a horizontal motion. This technique produces two slides with material for examination. Slides should be air dried before being fixed and stained.
4. Fine needle aspirates of masses or nodules may be made with or without a syringe. It is not necessary to clip the hair from a mass or to scrub the sample site. The mass is gently stabilised in one hand and, using only a needle, stabbed several times. The sample will be collected in the lumen of the needle. To remove the specimen, the syringe is filled with air and the needle reattached. The needle and syringe are held just above a clean glass microscope slide and the contents are quickly 'blown' on to the slide. If the material is very thick, a squash preparation should be made.
5. Alternatively, masses may be aspirated with the needle attached to the syringe. Again, the mass is stabilized in one hand and a needle attached to a syringe is gently inserted into the mass. The mass is stabbed and the syringe barrel is aspirated several times before the needle is redirected. Before redirecting the needle, the negative pressure on the syringe should be released. The needle is redirected at least three to four times in the mass. This technique often results in more artifacts and secondary haemorrhage. The needle must be removed from the syringe before filling the syringe to blow the specimen on to a slide.
6. Slides should be fixed and stained with a modified Wright's stain, fast Giemsa, or new methylene blue stain.

Artifacts

Artifacts in cytological specimens are legion and it is impossible to summarise the possible artifacts that may be seen. The reader is referred to the bibliography for additional information.

Interpretation

Again the reader is referred to a standard text for interpretation of cytological results.

Techniques for Collecting Skin Biopsy Specimens

Indications

The indications for performing a skin biopsy are best summarised by Drs Muller, Kirk and Scott: 'A skin biopsy is indicated in any obvious neoplastic or suspected neoplastic skin disease, in persistently ulcerative diseases, in non-responsive skin diseases, in unusual or apparently serious appearing skin diseases, and in any disease in which a definitive diagnosis is necessary before initiating expensive or dangerous therapy.'

Pertinent background information

In general, skin biopsies are not performed often enough; when they are, poor technique and sample collection minimise their usefulness. Maximum benefit from skin biopsies is obtained when they are used early in the disease — before the underlying disease is treated empirically without the benefit of a diagnosis and before chronic inflammatory changes have occurred in the skin, masking the underlying disease. If one specimen is good, more are better. Several carefully chosen specimens will increase the likelihood of a diagnosis.

Even more important than the number of biopsy specimens submitted for examination is the selection of the lesion itself. The specimen should be representative of the *primary disease process*. For example, ulcerative skin diseases may be caused by infectious agents, neoplastic diseases and autoimmune skin diseases. If the ulceration is caused by an autoimmune disease, the patient should be examined for vesicular or bullous lesions and those lesions should be submitted for biopsy. Histological examination of a skin biopsy specimen of an ulcer from a patient with an autoimmune skin disease is rarely helpful; however, examination of vesicles or bulla from a patient is of value. If, on the other hand, the ulceration is caused by an infectious agent or neoplastic process, perilesional tissue from the ulcer should be examined because the infectious or neoplastic process is very likely to be invading adjacent tissue.

Submitting tissue that is representative of the primary disease process implies a high degree of suspicion of the nature of the underlying skin disease. Unfortunately, this is often not the case. Therefore, when in doubt, submit numerous tissue specimens that represent the range of clinical signs present. Finally, submit a detailed description of the patient including:

- patient profile;
- clinical signs;
- duration, distribution or location of lesion;
- medication history;
- differential diagnoses;
- supporting laboratory data.

Photographs of the patient and the lesions sampled should be submitted with the biopsy, if possible.

Skin biopsy specimens should be evaluated by a *veterinary dermatopathologist*. Specimens should not be submitted to non-veterinary medical laboratories because their pathologists are not trained in comparative skin diseases and few can reliably evaluate tissues from animals.

Equipment

- Local anaesthetic (lidocaine hydrochloride)
- Needles and syringes
- Scalpel blade
- Suture material or skin staples
- Small-toothed forceps
- Sterile surgical instruments
- Wooden tongue depressors
- 4–6 mm skin biopsy punches (optional)
- Michel's fixative for direct immunofluorescence (optional)
- 10% neutral buffered formalin

Technique (see Fig. 3.5)

1. Specimens to be biopsied should be encircled with a felt-tip marker to indicate the location of the local anaesthetic.
2. The surface of the biopsy site should not be scrubbed, wiped or rubbed with water, alcohol or antiseptic. Surface pathology is often critical in making a diagnosis.

3. If it is necessary to clip the hair coat, be very gentle. It is often useful to leave a few long hairs in the area of the biopsy so that the pathologist can orientate the tissue.

4. The biospy site should be anaesthetised by using 2% lidocaine. Approximately 1 ml per site is

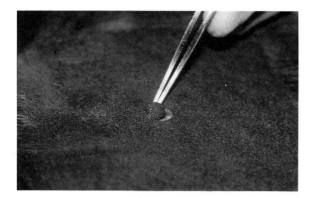

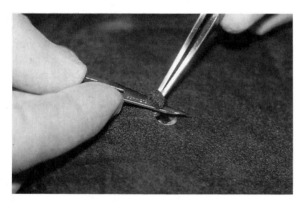

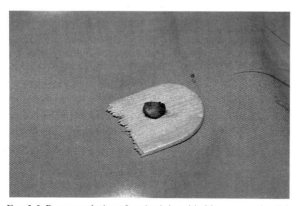

FIG. 3.5 Proper technique for obtaining skin biopsy samples. It is important to grasp the specimen gently by its subcutaneous pedicle and gently sever it from the skin. The biopsy specimen should be placed on a piece of wood or cardboard prior to placing it in formalin.

adequate. Care should be taken to ensure that the lidocaine is injected subcutaneously immediately beneath the specimen. Lidocaine is potentially toxic and a general rule of thumb is not to exceed 1 ml of 2% lidocaine per 5 kg body weight in cats and dogs. In some cats, additional chemical restraint (e.g. ketamine hydrochloride) may be needed. Nasal and footpad specimens are usually obtained using a short-acting general anaesthetic. These areas are very painful to biopsy and it may be difficult or impossible even to inject lidocaine into the subcutaneous tissues.

5. Skin biopsy specimens can be harvested using either a skin biopsy punch or a scalpel blade. The choice of instrument depends upon the type of specimen. Skin biopsy punches are preferred for lesions that are less than 6 mm in diameter, but cannot be used to collect junctional biopsies because it is likely that the pathologist may section the specimen incorrectly. Scalpel blades are preferred when it is desirable to collect both lesional and perilesional tissue via an elliptical incision. The sample can then be correctly sectioned across both lesional and perilesional tissue by requesting that the tissue be sectioned across its length. Elliptical incisions should be used when trying to biopsy intact vesicles, bullae and nodules.

6. The skin biopsy punch is positioned directly over the lesion to be sampled. The punch is gently rotated in *one* direction while gentle downward pressure is exerted. The punch should not be rotated 'back and forth' as this would cause artifacts. The gentle downward pressure and rotation are continued until the punch 'drops' into the subcutaneous tissue. The tissue plug is attached to the body by a small pedicle of subcutaneous tissue and fat and can be freed by cutting this tissue with a scalpel blade.

7. In order to prevent crush artifacts, the tissue plug must be handled very carefully. Small-toothed forceps should be used to grasp the subcutaneous fat pedicle while it is cut with a scalpel blade. The forceps should *never* grasp the biopsy itself. Any blood on the specimen should be gently blotted from the tissue surface. This is very important because excess haemorrhage can obscure the pathologist's view of the tissue.

8. The subcutaneous side of the biopsy specimen is placed on a small piece of tongue depressor and allowed to stand for 30–60 seconds so that it adheres. Mounting of specimens will prevent tissue from curling during fixation. This is a critical step for biopsies from thin-skinned areas of cats, birds or small mammals. If the pathologist is required to section the tissue in a particular direction (e.g. through a pustule), mark the tongue depressor. Tissue that has been fixed in formalin is homogeneous in colour and what appeared clinically as a clear demarcation of normal and abnormal skin may not be visible at all once the tissue has been fixed. After the biopsy has adhered to the wood splint, place it upside down in 10% neutral buffered formalin. The volume of fixative should be at least 10 times the volume of the sample. Allow the specimen to fix for 24 hours before having it processed.

9. Skin biopsy punch sites can be sutured with either a single interrupted suture or a mattress suture.

10. If you choose to use a scalpel blade to perform a skin biopsy, use an elliptical incision that is generous enough to allow you to grasp one edge with forceps when freeing the section from the subcutaneous tissues. Gently blot any blood from both the surface and subcutaneous side of the specimen and mount the tissue specimen on a wooden tongue depressor or piece of stiff cardboard. It is very important to instruct the pathologist as to how the specimen should be sectioned — horizontally or longitudinally. Again, be sure that the specimen is placed in a container with at least 10 times the volume of fixative to specimen.

Artifacts

The most commonly observed artifacts in biopsy specimens over which the clinician has control are shear, haemorrhage and crush.

Interpretation

Interpretation of biopsy specimen reports is discussed in *Chapter 4*.

Diagnostic Procedures for Allergic Patients

Intradermal Skin Testing

Indications

Intradermal skin testing is indicated in patients in which an inhaled allergy (atopy) is suspected. These patients are pruritic or suspected of being pruritic; over-grooming in cats is commonly a clinical sign of pruritus. Intradermal skin testing is generally indicated after other diagnostic tests and therapies have failed to identify the cause of the pruritus.

Pertinent background information

A tentative diagnosis of atopy can be based upon compatible history, clinical signs, and laboratory tests that do not support other differential diagnoses. Intradermal skin testing is used to confirm the diagnosis, to identify potentially important allergens and to initiate immunotherapy (Plate 1). This procedure should be performed on patients whose owners are prepared to be committed to at least 1 year of hyposensitisation for the animal if the test is conclusive.

There is no standard procedure for intradermal skin testing in animals. The allergens in the test kit are supplied by commercial companies and selection of the specific allergens is based upon the region of the country in which one practises. The allergen supplier, veterinary colleagues and human allergists are potential sources for information regarding which allergens are most important in an area. In general, house-dust, house-dust mite, flea and mould allergens are ubiquitous and should be part of any kit. Mixed antigens are best avoided because of potential problems with false-positives and false-negatives. Due to practical and financial considerations, most veterinary dermatologists use between 50 and 70 different allergens. Allergen concentrates are available in either Protein Nitrogen Unit (PNU) or as weight/volume extracts. Most intradermal injections are performed at a concentration of 1000 PNU/ml; however, allergens that may be irritant (e.g. house-dust) are often used at 250 PNU/ml.

Intradermal skin tests are scored either subjectively or objectively using the positive (histamine phosphate) and negative (phosphate buffered saline) controls as references. The subjective scoring scale ranges from 0 (negative) to +4 and allows for interpretation of the degree of induration, erythema and wheal size in the final score. Wheals with a score of 2 or greater are considered significant reactions. Obviously, this method is very subjective. To score individual wheals objectively requires that the mean horizontal and vertical wheal diameters should be measured in millimetres. A 'positive' wheal reaction is defined as any wheal equal to or greater than the mean diameters of the positive and negative controls. This method is more objective but does not allow for such variables as wheal flare, induration and erythema.

A number of factors can cause false-positive and false-negative reactions. The most common cause of false-negative reactions is drug interference. Antihistamines, acepromazine, glucocorticoids (orally, parenterally and topically), griseofulvin and progesterones can all inhibit intradermal skin test reactions. Treatment with acepromazine and antihistamines should be withdrawn for a minimum of 7 days prior to performing an intradermal skin test. Oral and topical glucocorticoids should be withdrawn for a minimum of 4–6 weeks before performing the test. Injectable glucocorticoids can have a prolonged residual effect which may exceed the duration of their therapeutic effect. The most reliable method for determining 'testability' of a patient is to inject intradermal histamine and observe whether or not a wheal reaction occurs; the development of a wheal reaction from histamine injection is not an absolute guarantee that the patient is sufficiently free of the effects of residual glucocorticoids in the skin. The most common causes of false-positive reactions are irritant reactions by the injected antigen or intradermal skin testing in a patient with severely inflamed skin.

There is no agreement among veterinary dermatologists as to the best time of year to test patients. The authors are willing to perform intradermal skin tests on any patient in which it is clinically warranted as long as the patient has symptoms. If the results of the test are negative or equivocal, it is recommended to the owner that the test be repeated at another time of year.

Equipment

- 27 gauge needles and 1 ml syringes
- Tray for syringes
- Black felt-tip marking pen
- Electric clippers with No.40 blade
- Stock allergens
- Sterile diluent
- Empty dilution vials
- Sterile phosphate saline
- Histamine phosphate

Dilute the stock allergens to a skin testing concentration of 1000 PNU/ml. If using house dust allergen, dilute the stock solution to concentrations of 250, 25 and 2.5 PNU/ml. Dilute the positive control, histamine phosphate, to 1:100,000. Allergens should be stored in the refrigerator to minimise bacterial growth and to maintain potency.

Technique

1. Patients may or may not require sedation for intradermal skin testing. Atropine, xylazine hydrochloride, medetomidine, ketamine hydrochloride and diazepam will not interfere with the interpretation of intradermal skin test reactions. Although acepromazine has no effect on erythema and flare, it will decrease wheal size, and therefore it should not be used. Inhalant anaesthetics can be used after induction with barbiturates.

2. The patient is placed in lateral recumbency and the hair from the ventral lateral thorax is gently clipped. The skin over the thorax is the preferred site for testing. Although there are no published reports, anecdotal reports suggest that reactivity varies with testing site. From a practical perspective, it is simply easiest to skin-test flat surfaces on dogs or cats.

3. A black or blue felt-tipped pen is used to mark rows of dots on the skin to indicate each injection site. Red felt-tip pens should be avoided because the colour makes evaluation of erythema or flare difficult in some patients. Rows should be separated from each other by at least 3 cm and each dot in a row should be spaced at least 2 cm apart. This is to prevent positive reaction sites from spreading into each other and complicating scoring.

4. Intradermal injections are performed using a 27 gauge needle and 1 ml syringe. Approximately 0.05 ml of allergen is injected intradermally. By convention, the negative control and positive

control are injected first followed by the test allergens. It is critical to make the injections carefully because any trauma can cause a false-positive reaction. One technique for making an intradermal injection is as follows. Hold the needle and syringe in one hand with your thumb on the syringe plunger and your index and middle fingers resting on the syringe 'wings'. Alternatively, the entire syringe may be held in your palm. It is critical that injections be made in one motion; do not re-grasp the syringe to inject because this often causes haemorrhage in the dermis. Tense the skin near the injection site and, with the bevel of the needle up, inject 0.05 ml approximately 0.5 cm *above* the dot marking the site. The needle should be clearly visible in the superficial dermis. This will allow for the reaction to enlarge, if positive, without spreading beneath the dot. A proper intradermal injection will not dissipate if you gently run your finger across the bleb. Subcutaneous injections are flat and will dissipate quickly when you run your finger across the bleb. Air injected intradermally will give a transient yellow bleb in the dermis.

5. Intradermal skin test sites should be observed throughout the entire test period.

   Although it is conventional to score the sites at 15 minutes post injection, some reactions (especially in cats and ferrets) may fade very quickly. Skin test sites may be scored either objectively or subjectively, as described above. The positive and negative sites are used as reference points. Ideally, intradermal skin test reactions should be examined and scored at 15–30 minutes, 6 hours, 24 hours and 48 hours after injection. In practice, however, most skin tests are scored between 15 and 30 minutes after injection. Immediate reactions are those that occur within 0 to 30 minutes of the injection. Delayed reactions classically occur at 24 or 48 hours post injection and are seen most commonly with intradermal injections of flea antigen. Late phase reactions have been observed at 6 hours after injection. Although their significance is unknown, the author has successfully hyposensitised dogs and cats based on these reactions.

6. Animals with strong intradermal skin test reactions may traumatise the site several hours post injection. These sites apparently are very pruritic and complications of self-trauma include excoriations, areas of pyotraumatic dermatitis and superficial pyoderma. Ice-packs and topical corticosteroids (e.g. triamcinolone acetate cream) may need to be applied to these sites to alleviate the discomfort.

Artifacts

Irritant reactions can occur if the skin testing allergen is contaminated, too concentrated or too cold when injected. Poor intradermal injection technique can cause haemorrhage. The skin of animals with superficial pyoderma or a significant degree of inflammation can be 'over-reactive'. This over-reactivity is usually seen as positive reactions to almost all allergens tested. It can be very difficult in patients with severe skin disease to determine whether the reaction sites are true-positives or just a manifestation of 'over-reactivity' and it is helpful to have at least one irrelevant allergen in your kit for this purpose. This allergen should be something that is not present in your region. For example, orange-tree pollen would be ideal for regions where oranges are not grown, provided that there is no known cross-reactivity with another tree. The commercial allergen company can usually supply this information.

Interpretation

A positive intradermal skin test site simply means that the patient has antibody against the injected allergen. It does not confirm the diagnosis of atopy. The results of an intradermal skin test must be interpreted in light of the patient's history and clinical signs. Intradermal skin tests can be interpreted as negative, positive or equivocal.

Excluding poor injection technique, it is extremely rare to have positive allergen reactions in the absence of a positive histamine control. If this is the case in a patient, re-inject the histamine at another site and question the owner about the recent use of antihistamines and tranquillisers. More commonly, intradermal skin tests are scored as negative because of the lack of reactivity at allergen sites or because the patient has a few weakly positive reactions. A positive intradermal skin test is one in which there are many positive reactions to allergens that are compatible with the patient's history and seasonality of pruritus (see plate 1). It is difficult to recommend a specific minimum number of positive reaction sites because of the importance of interpreting the skin test results in light of patient history. For example, the author has seen several intensely pruritic dogs with year-round pruritus with positive skin test reactions to only house dust or house dust mites. Several of these dogs were successfully hyposensitised using only house dust allergen.

The results of an intradermal skin test are considered equivocal if the patient's clinical signs and history are suggestive of atopy but the results of the test are not diagnostic. Clinically, equivocal intradermal skin tests are those with numerous weakly positive reaction sites. These tests are extremely difficult to interpret because it is hard to distinguish which of the allergen reactions are important to the patient.

If the history and clinical signs of a particular patient are strongly suggestive of atopy, negative or equivocal intradermal skin tests in such patients should be repeated. It is preferable to repeat the intradermal skin test in a different season or time of year. Equivocal intradermal skin tests appear to be most commonly observed in low pollen seasons, i.e. winter and early spring.

In Vitro *Allergy Tests*

Indications

In vitro serum tests for allergies may be indicated if the patient cannot be intradermally skin tested, if there is drug interference, or if a previous intradermal skin test has been negative or equivocal.

Pertinent background information

There are two common methods used to perform *in vitro* tests. The radioallergosorbent test (RAST) uses radioactively labelled antisera. The enzyme-linked immunosorbent assay (ELISA) uses antibodies coupled to enzymes. In both tests, samples of patient serum are placed into different wells, each containing different antigen(s). The patient's serum is allowed to incubate for a specified time and then removed. The wells are rinsed several times to remove any unbound patient serum. Radioactive or enzyme-linked antiserum (antidog IgE) is added to the wells and incubated. In RAST, the radioactivity of the well is measured. In the ELISA test,

the colour change is measured. The more intense the colour or the higher the radioactive count, the more antidog IgE is present in the wells. The amount of radioactivity or colour change supposedly correlates with the amount of allergen-specific antibody from the patient. There is no evidence to suggest that one test method is superior to the other. Many companies perform these tests and there is no standardisation of test results.

Equipment and facilities

- Needle and syringe
- Serum vial
- Submission forms from laboratory

Technique

Each company offers specific instructions on their preferred method of handling the specimen. In general, at least 2–3 ml of patient serum should be sent to the laboratory.

Artifacts

The major problem with both RAST and ELISA serum tests is false-positives. These tests can be positive for allergens to which the animal was never exposed. Additionally, the tests will detect very small concentrations of antibody and it is difficult to determine if these reactions are true-positives or just an indication of previous pollen exposure. Laboratories often use polyclonal antisera that may be measuring IgG, in addition to IgE, further increasing the possibility of false-positive reactions. Mixes of antigens to coat the wells of the test kit are commonly used, but if a mix produces a positive score it is unclear if the patient is positive to one antigen or to all antigens in the mix. This complication is avoided by using a laboratory with single antigen tests.

Interpretations

Most companies will offer an interpretation of the results. It is important to remember, however, that a positive test against a specific allergen or group of allergens is not diagnostic for atopy. Like intradermal skin testing, a positive test merely indicates the presence of antibody against a specific allergen.

Tests for Identifying Food Allergies (Food Trials)

Indications

A food trial is indicated in the evaluation of pruritus and should be performed prior to referring a patient for intradermal skin testing or submitting serum for an *in vitro* diagnostic test.

Pertinent background information

The exact incidence of food allergies in dogs and cats is unknown. The term 'food allergy' is loosely used in veterinary medicine to include food intolerances, food idiosyncrasies and true food hypersensitivities. A **food intolerance** is an abnormal physiological reaction to an ingested food of an idiosyncratic, metabolic, pharmacological or toxic nature. Diarrhoea associated with the ingestion of milk in lactase-deficient individuals is an example. A **food idiosyncrasy** is an abnormal response to an ingested food resembling hypersensitivity but not involving an immune response. Pruritus and urticaria in individuals after ingesting wine, egg whites, shellfish or tomatoes are caused by non-immunological release of histamine and can resemble a true food allergy. A true **food allergy** is an immunological reaction resulting from the ingestion of a food or food additive. The pathogenesis is unproven, although most of the literature cites a Type 1, Type 3 and Type 4 hypersensitivity reaction.

Food allergies in small animals are most reliably diagnosed by the use of an elimination diet, which may be a home-cooked or commercial preparation. The only advantage of a home-cooked diet is strict control over the ingredients. Owner compliance with cooking for their pet is directly related to the detail the owner is given for both preparing the food and administering the diet. Detailed written instructions are an absolute requirement. These should detail ingredients (including trade names and ready sources of micro-nutrients and calcium), cooking methods, storage methods, amount to feed and any instructions that are necessary. There is some clinical evidence to suggest that a home-cooked diet is more reliable than commercial preparations. However, most commercially prepared diets are balanced and complete, minimising the chance of causing a macro-or micro-nutrient deficiency; they are easier for clients to obtain, often less expensive, and usually result in greater client compliance when compared with home-cooked diets.

The choice of diet ingredients depends greatly upon the animal's and the owner's diet history: the initial aim is to avoid ingredients to which the animal has already been exposed. In the United States, lamb has been used for many years with success because most Americans do not eat much lamb and therefore the dog or cat is not likely to have sampled lamb table-scraps. Unfortunately, many commercial companies have recently capitalised on the marketability of lamb-based pet foods by promoting the 'hypoallergenic' nature of such diets. Many of the author's clients report feeding one of these diets to their pet at some time in its life. In general, rabbit, venison, alligator (where available in the USA), goat and lamb are commonly used as the meat source in homemade diets. In commercial pet food diets, whole or by-products of beef, chicken, turkey, pork and fish are common ingredients and are not suitable for a diet trial.

There are many commercial diets marketed for the purpose of food trials or maintenance of a food-allergic pet. It is important to read the label listing the ingredients carefully to determine what is in the diet. In general, meal based dry foods should be avoided during the trial period because meal based diets tend to contain a large amount of animal by-products. Canned diets contain less filler and by-products and may be superior to dry foods during the trial period.

Equipment

- Acceptable food for the trial

An acceptable food is one that is palatable to the pet, that the owner will feed, and that does not contain substances to which the pet has already been exposed.

Technique

1. Food-induced pruritus may result in significant self-trauma and inflammation. If necessary, secondary superficial pyoderma should be treated

prior to initiating the diet or during the first 3 weeks of the diet. If the animal is intolerably pruritic and anti-inflammatory drugs are deemed necessary for humane reasons, antihistamines may be used during the first 2–3 weeks of a food trial. Additionally, soothing baths or cool water soaks are acceptable. Clients are more likely to comply if they do not think that the pet is suffering.

2. While discussing with the client the formulation of an acceptable diet, it is important to discuss what is *not* acceptable. Be specific. During the trial the pet cannot eat any table food (this can be significant problem if there are small children or older people in the house), dog treats, rawhide chew toys, cat food, garbage, flavoured vitamin tablets, chewable heartworm tablets, houseplants (cats mainly) or catnip. Tap water is acceptable.

3. The trial diet (homemade or commercially prepared) should be fed for a minimum of 4–6 weeks. If antibiotics or antihistamines are used during the first 3 weeks, the diet trial should extend for a minimum of 3 weeks after discontinuation of antibiotics or antihistamines. The author instructs the owner to purchase a new food bowl or use a bowl that has not contained the pet's previous diet. This is to prevent contamination of the test diet with food particles from the previous diet.

4. At the end of the diet trial, the patient should be reassessed. Owners will report complete improvement, marked improvement, some improvement or no improvement. Pets that have responded completely should be challenged with their previous diet for a period of 7–10 days. If the improvement was due to the test diet, the pet should relapse when fed the previous diet. If there is no relapse, improvement was coincidental and may have occurred due to antibiotic therapy, change in seasons or location, or some other reason. Owners with pets that show little to no improvement should be encouraged to continue the diet for another few weeks to determine if there will be any further change in the level of pruritus. It may take weeks for the offending allergen to be removed from the skin and weeks for the secondary inflammation to subside. This may delay the obvious benefits of the diet. These clients need continued contact and it is helpful if a technician can call them periodically to obtain progress reports. Somewhere between 3 and 10 weeks is the optimum time for a diet trial, and at some stage during those weeks most clients will have had enough of the trials and tribulations of a food trial. Try to encourage the client to continue with diet trial as long as possible. When they reach the end of their tolerance for the test, ask the client to challenge the pet with its previous diet.

5. It may be useful for clients to 'score' the pet's discomfort as a way of evaluating the effectiveness of the diet. They can use a scale of 1 to 10 to score the level of the pet's pruritus with 1 being a normal pet and 10 being a pet that is so miserable that neither the owner nor the pet can sleep. Clients score the pet's pruritus weekly and keep a record of the number. They should continue to score the pruritus when they challenge the pet with its old diet.

Artifacts

The major danger in any diet trial is the chance that the pet may have access to food other than the test diet during the trial. This danger increases with the length of the diet trial. Another complication is coincidental improvement, which is most likely to occur in atopic patients on long (5–10 week) food trials. The pollen(s) responsible for the pet's atopy may disappear from the environment during the food trial period. Unless the client is willing to wait until winter, it is difficult to avoid the changing pollen season.

Interpretation

Pets that show a complete recovery on an elimination diet and have an exacerbation of the clinical signs when fed the previous diet probably have an allergy or intolerance. If there is no relapse, improvement was coincidental. Pets showing a partial improvement with the diet may have a food allergy concurrent with another allergic disease, most commonly atopy. It is difficult to identify this last group of patients satisfactorily. In the author's experience, a decrease of 50% or more on the owner's pruritus scale is a useful diagnostic criterion. Pets that do not improve on the elimination diet do not have a food allergy.

Patch Testing or Isolation Techniques for Contact Allergies

Indications

Patch testing is indicated for animals in which a contact allergy to a substance is suspected. Patch testing is infrequently performed because allergic contact dermatitis in animals is rare. Isolation of the animal in a controlled environment is an alternative technique for diagnosing irritant or contact allergies but will not distinguish between the two types of reactions.

Pertinent background information

An **irritant contact reaction** is caused by direct chemical damage to the skin. These reactions are believed to be more common than allergic reactions. Irritant reactions are concentration-dependent and tend to occur in all individuals exposed to the chemical. The reactions occur quickly and clinical signs are due to direct chemical damage to the epidermis. **Allergic contact reactions** occur in only a few individuals, take a long time to develop (months to years) and the clinical signs are due to immunological damage to the skin.

Contact dermatitis in animals is uncommon because the hair coat protects the skin. Contact allergies are recognised most frequently in thinly haired areas. The ventral abdomen, perineal area, plantar surface of the paws and periocular areas are commonly affected. If the contact allergen is an aerosol, the conjunctiva may be affected. Contact allergies may be indistinguishable from atopy or food allergy in a pruritic pet.

The diagnosis of a contact allergy can be made by performing a patch test (open or closed) or by isolation techniques. **Patch testing** involves the use of allergens which are applied to the skin. Unless the test material is too concentrated and so causes an irritant reaction, all positive reactions are significant.

Isolation techniques require that the animal be removed from its normal environment for 10–30 days. If the animal's clinical signs resolve while in the new environment and then recur when the animal returns home, one can conclude that an offending substance is present in the old environment. Unfortunately, isolation–provocation testing will not distinguish between atopic or allergic contact dermatitis.

Equipment

Closed patch testing.

- White petroleum jelly
- Sterile non-adhesive gauze squares
- Occlusive adhesive bandage
- Test materials collected from the home or alternatively a commercial human test kit.

(Commercial test kits are not standardised and a control animal should be tested at the same time to ensure that the test materials are not irritant.)

Open patch testing.

- Test materials
- White petroleum jelly
- Elizabethan collar

Isolation–provocation.

- Hypoallergenic shampoo
- Isolation facilities

Technique

Closed patch testing.

1. The hair coat on the lateral or dorsal trunk of the animal is clipped 24 hours prior to the test.
2. The test substance is suspended in petroleum jelly and applied to the skin. If a medication is to be tested, the pure substance and the commercial preparation should be tested. Carpet fibres, plants, cloth etc. can be tested by directly applying them to the skin.
3. The test material is covered with the sterile non-adhesive gauze sponge and the sponge secured with tape at the corners. This step is repeated with all of the test materials, including a control site. This may be a plain, sterile, non-adhesive gauze sponge with or without petroleum jelly. Patch test sites should be well spaced. The test sites are then bandaged with gauze cling and secured in place with an elastic-type bandage. The biggest problem with closed patch testing is slipping of the bandage.
4. The pet should be hospitalised during the test period and the bandage kept in place for 48–72

hours. When the bandage is removed, the test sites may all be uniformly reddened due to the occlusive bandage. The sites should be marked with a felt-tip pen and examined for induration, erythema and vesiculation 30 minutes after removal of the bandage. The pet should be fitted with an Elizabethan collar and the sites re-examined at 24, 48 and 72 hours post bandage removal. If there is any question as to the significance of a positive reaction, it should be biopsied.

5. Closed patch testing can also be performed using a standardised commercial test kit. These contain test materials placed in small wells (Finn Chambers) that adhere to the skin. The hair on the lateral or dorsal trunk is clipped 24 hours prior to the test. Approximately 1 ml of test material is placed into each well. The skin should be wiped with alcohol or ether to remove skin oils and increase adhesion. The wells are placed on the skin and secured with the adhesive strip supplied by the manufacturer for this purpose. An elastic bandage is wrapped around the pet's trunk to further immobilise the bandage and an Elizabethan collar is fitted on the pet. The pet should be hospitalised during this period. The bandage is removed after 48 hours and the sites are marked and examined as described above.

Open patch testing.

1. The hair is clipped over several areas of the pet's body 24 hours prior to performing the test.
2. The test material is rubbed into the skin and examined daily for 5 days. The pet is fitted with an Elizabethan collar and the site is protected from dirt, moisture and trauma. Open patch testing works best with liquid substances and the author has used it frequently to test spray insecticides on pets whose owners are concerned about the substance aggravating or causing skin disease.

Isolation–provocation.

1. The pet should be washed thoroughly in a hypoallergenic shampoo to remove any substances from the hair coat that could be causing the reaction. The pet is then housed in a 'safe' environment in a kennel or veterinary clinic for 10–30 days and examined for resolution of clinical signs.
2. If the pet improves in the new environment, it is returned to the previous environment and carefully monitored for an exacerbation of clinical signs. This usually occurs within 10 days of exposure.

Artifacts

False-positive reactions can occur if the test substance was too concentrated or irritant, if the test was performed on inflamed skin, or if the animal traumatised the site. False-negative reactions can occur if the antigen did not penetrate the skin, if the wrong substances were used in the test, or the site was inadequately occluded (closed patch testing).

Interpretation

All positive reactions are important; however, they may not be clinically relevant. The reaction may, in fact, identify a previous sensitivity or a pending problem. Closed patch test sites can be scored similarly to intradermal skin test reactions. If a commercial patch test kit is used, the charts provided by the company should be examined to determine possible sources of the offending material.

Diagnostic Tests for Endocrine Disorders

Pituitary Adrenocorticotrophin (ACTH) Response Test

Indications

This test is indicated in patients where hypoadrenocorticism (spontaneous or iatrogenic) is suspected or as a screening test for hyperadrenocorticism. It is the preferred screening test for cats with hyperadrenocorticism.

Pertinent background information

The ACTH response test is a crude measure of the responsiveness of the adrenal cortex to exogenous stimulation. Serum samples are collected before and after administration of ACTH and the cortisol concentrations are determined. Oral prednisolone or prednisone should be discontinued for 36–48 hours before performing this test as they will interfere with the assay.

This test is less reliable than the low dose dexamethasone test for screening for hyperadrenocorticism. It is the test of choice for laboratory monitoring of response to mitotane treatment in the management of pituitary dependent hyperadrenocorticism.

Equipment

- Synthetic ACTH (aqueous or gel)
- Needles, syringes
- Serum tubes.

Technique

1. For dogs, a serum sample is collected before, and 1–2 hours after, administration of exogenous ACTH. For cats, a serum sample is collected before, and 30 minutes after, administration of exogenous ACTH.
2. For both dogs and cats, the dose of ACTH gel is 2.2 units/kg IM. If synthetic aqueous ACTH is used, administer 0.25 mg IV for the dog and 0.125 mg IV for the cat regardless of weight.

Artifacts

Oral anticonvulsant medications will elevate cortisol concentrations. Prednisolone and prednisone will cross-react with the assay and erroneously elevate cortisol concentrations. Dexamethasone does not affect the assay. Excited dogs may have elevated basal cortisol concentrations but will have ACTH response tests within normal limits (in the absence of organic disease). Dogs stressed with non-adrenal illness may have abnormal test results.

Interpretation

The reference laboratory should be consulted for normal values. In general, a normal dog will have a post-stimulation cortisol value of at least 2–3 times the baseline value. Dogs with hypoadrenocorticism will show a lack of adrenal responsiveness. This test alone will not differentiate spontaneous and iatrogenic hypoadrenocorticism. In approximately 88% of dogs with pituitary-dependent hyperadrenocorticism, there is hyper-responsiveness to exogenous ACTH. In those with adrenal tumours,

approximately 60% of dogs with hyperadrenocorticism will be hyper-responsive to exogenous ACTH. A normal ACTH response test does not rule out hyperadrenocorticism.

Low Dose Dexamethasone Response Test (LDDRT)

Indications

This is used as a screening test for spontaneous hyperadrenocorticism. It is recommended as a first choice for screening spontaneous hyperadrenocorticism or if the ACTH response test is normal. It is not very reliable in screening cats for hyperadrenocorticism.

Pertinent background information

The low dose dexamethasone response test measures the integrity of the pituitary–adrenal axis. In a normal animal, exogenous administration of small amounts of dexamethasone will cause a decrease in the release of ACTH for at least 8 hours. This results in a decreased production and release of adrenal cortisol and, hence, serum cortisol. In animals with spontaneously occurring hyperadrenocorticism, the administration of small amounts of dexamethasone is insufficient to affect negatively the release of ACTH and, subsequently, adrenal production of cortisol. Dexamethasone does not interfere with cortisol on the serum assay. It is important to remember that dogs with hyperadrenocorticism metabolise dexamethasone much more rapidly than normal dogs; this test is not always diagnostic.

Equipment

- Dexamethasone for intravenous injection
- Needles, syringes
- Serum tubes.

Technique

1. There are two doses of dexamethasone that have been advocated for this test: 0.01 mg/kg and 0.015 mg/kg. Either dose can be used.
2. Blood is drawn for assessment of pre-dexamethasone cortisol concentration and the appropriate dose of dexamethasone is administered

intravenously. Blood is then drawn at 4 or 6 hours and 8 hours after dexamethasone administration.

Artifacts

Anticonvulsant therapy may interfere with suppression. Concurrent administration of other glucocorticoids (prednisolone, prednisone) may falsely elevate cortisol levels. Dogs stressed by non-adrenal illnesses may have abnormal test results.

Interpretation

The reference laboratory should be contacted for normal values. In general there are several possible patterns of test results:

- Cortisol concentrations rapidly decrease to below laboratory normals and remain in this range at least until the 8-hour test sample. These dogs are considered normal. This pattern may be seen in a small number of dogs with early hyperadrenocorticism.
- Cortisol concentrations do not suppress to below laboratory normals throughout the 8-hour test period. This is considered an abnormal test and is supportive of the diagnosis that hyperadrenocorticism is present. A differentiating test is indicated.
- Cortisol concentrations suppress at mid-point in the test, but then escape above laboratory normals. This test is considered abnormal and is supportive of the diagnosis that hyperadrenocorticism is present. The cause is most likely to be pituitary-dependent.

High Dose Dexamethasone Suppression Test

Indications

This test is indicated after the presence of hyperadrenocorticism has been confirmed by either an ACTH response test or an LDDRT.

Pertinent background information

This test is used to differentiate between adrenal tumours and pituitary-dependent hyperadrenocorticism. A much higher dose of dexamethasone is used than in an LDDRT and this dose is capable,

theoretically, of inhibiting ACTH release from the pituitary. In dogs with pituitary-dependent hyperadrenocorticism, this higher dose of dexamethasone will 'turn off' production of ACTH, resulting in a decreased production of cortisol by the adrenal glands. The 'megadose' dexamethasone suppression test is recommended for differentiating adrenal and pituitary-dependent hyperadrenocorticism in cats.

Equipment

- Dexamethasone for intravenous injection
- Needles, syringes
- Serum tubes

Technique

1. There are two doses of dexamethasone that have been advocated for this test: 0.1 mg/kg and 1.0 mg/kg. The author recommends the dose of 0.1 mg/kg IV. The megadose (1.0 mg/kg) may be necessary in some cases of pituitary-dependent hyperadrenocorticism.
2. Blood is drawn for assessment of pre-dexamethasone cortisol concentration and the appropriate dose of dexamethasone is administered intravenously. Blood is then drawn at 4 or 6 hours and 8 hours after dexamethasone administration.

Artifacts

Anticonvulsant therapy may interfere with suppression. Concurrent administration of other glucocorticoids (prednisolone, prednisone) may falsely elevate cortisol levels. Dogs stressed by non-adrenal illnesses may have abnormal test results.

Interpretation

The laboratory should be contacted for normal values. There are several patterns of suppression that may be observed:

- There is a lack of suppression of cortisol concentrations at both the 4 or 6 and the 8-hour sample. This is most supportive of the diagnosis of an adrenal tumour; however this pattern may also be seen in a small number of cases of pituitary-dependent hyperadrenocorticism. If this is the case, the megadose dexamethasone suppression test is recommended. A plasma ACTH concentration may be helpful in differentiating these two diseases. In addition, abdominal radiographs and ultrasound to document the presence of an adrenal tumour are strongly recommended.

- There is adequate suppression of cortisol concentrations by 8 hours post-dexamethasone (50% below the baseline). This is supportive of the diagnosis of pituitary-dependent hyperadrenocorticism.
- There is adequate suppression of cortisol concentrations by 4 or 6 hours post-dexamethasone (50% below the baseline) but not at 8 hours. This is supportive of the diagnosis of pituitary-dependent hyperadrenocorticism.

Endogenous ACTH Plasma Concentrations

Indications

This test is indicated after the presence of hyperadrenocorticism has been confirmed by either an ACTH response test or an LDDRT. In addition, it may be helpful to differentiate between adrenal tumours and pituitary-dependent hyperadrenocorticism after a questionable high dose dexamethasone suppression test has been obtained. It can also be used to differentiate primary from secondary hypoadrenocorticism.

Pertinent background information

A single ACTH measurement is not useful because of the episodic release of this hormone and overlapping values. This test may be helpful for differentiating adrenal and pituitary hyperadrenocorticism in cats.

Equipment

- Cold heparinised syringes
- Ice
- Plastic tubes
- Ability to cold-centrifuge tubes
- Dry ice

Technique

1. The dog should be hospitalised overnight to minimise erroneous results from stress and to allow a sample to be collected between 8 and 9 a.m.

2. The blood sample is collected in a *cold* heparinised plastic syringe that is immediately placed on ice.
3. The blood is transferred to a cold plastic tube and is cold-centrifuged. The plasma must be stored at $-40°C$.
4. The sample should be sent to the laboratory on dry ice.
5. At least two samples, collected 48 hours apart, should be analysed.

Artifacts

Values may be falsely lowered if glass syringes or tubes are used during collection and storage. Samples may be falsely lowered during shipping if the sample is inadequately frozen and packaged. Glucocorticoids may falsely lower values and insulin may falsely increase values.

Interpretation

The reference laboratory should be contacted for laboratory normals. Dogs with adrenal tumours, secondary hypoadrenocorticism and iatrogenic hyperadrenocorticism will have normal to decreased values. Normal to increased values will be seen in dogs with pituitary-dependent hyperadrenocorticism and primary hypoadrenocorticism.

Thyroid Function Tests

Indications

Thyroid function should be tested in dogs suspected of having hypothyroidism.

Pertinent background information

Thyroid function may be evaluated by measuring basal hormone concentrations (free or bound) or by performing a thyrotrophin hormone (TSH) response test. In both cases, measurement of total T4 is most accurate; T3 values are not reliable indicators of thyroid function. All thyroid function tests should be interpreted with caution; specific laboratory tests are used to confirm clinical suspicions and should not be used as a sole diagnostic criterion.

Free T4 concentrations in combination with basal T4 concentrations may be helpful when a

TSH response test cannot be performed. Non-thyroidal skin diseases will not lower free T4 concentrations, but other non-thyroidal illnesses and also glucocorticoids will. Concurrent evaluation of a fasting serum cholesterol concentration may be helpful; serum cholesterol is often elevated in dogs with hypothyroidism.

Equipment

- Needles and syringes
- Serum tubes
- Thyroid stimulating hormone

Technique

1. Samples for assessment of basal hormone concentrations may be collected at any time of the day. It may be useful to collect an adequate amount of serum for also assessing cholesterol concentration if values are difficult to interpret.
2. TSH response tests require 4–6 hours to perform. A serum sample is collected before the administration of TSH. The hormone can be administered either intramuscularly or intravenously. There are several protocols for dosing, administration and sampling. The author uses 0.1 IU/kg IM and takes the post-TSH sample 6 hours after administration.

Artifacts

There are many artifacts which may alter thyroid hormone concentrations. Glucocorticoids and trimethoprim sulpha or ormethoprim sulpha may lower concentrations of thyroid hormones, as may non-thyroidal illnesses, surgery, and anaesthesia. Pyodermas and other skin diseases *do not* affect thyroid hormone concentrations.

Interpretation

The reference laboratory should be contacted for normals.

Sex Hormone Assays

Indications

Sex hormone assays and function tests are indicated in patients with a suspected endocrinopathy and normal adrenal and thyroid function tests.

Pertinent background information

The area of sex hormone dysfunction in dogs is not well understood and there is little conclusive research on the subject. Many of the skin diseases that were originally attributed to 'growth hormone responsive dermatoses' may be, in fact, adrenal sex hormone disorders.

Equipment and facilities

- Needles, syringes
- Plasma and serum tubes
- ACTH gel or aqueous solution
- Reference laboratory capable of performing assays

Technique

1. At least 5 ml of blood is collected in an EDTA tube (2 ml) and a serum tube (3 ml).
2. The whole blood is centrifuged and the plasma is frozen immediately. The serum tube is allowed to clot for 15 minutes and then centrifuged and the serum frozen immediately.
3. ACTH gel or aqueous solution is administered (see ACTH response test, above, for dose).
4. Further samples are collected at 1 and 2 hours after administration of ACTH. At least 5 ml of blood must be collected and handled as described in steps 1 and 2.
5. The samples must be sent on dry ice to the reference laboratory for analysis of cortisol, 11-deoxycortisol, DHEAS, androstenedione, 17-hydroxyprogesterone, progesterone, testosterone and oestradiol.

Artifacts

It is difficult to describe potential artifacts because of the limited knowledge of this test. Test results are most likely to be negatively influenced by inappropriate handling of specimens and shipping.

Interpretation

At present, this test is primarily a research tool and normal values for each breed of dog are non-existent. The laboratory should be contacted for normals and for assistance in interpretation.

4

Dermatopathology for the 'Pathophobe'*

KAREN MORIELLO and ELIZABETH GALBREATH

Introduction

Every text book on veterinary dermatology tells the reader 'Biopsy, biopsy, biopsy!' The key to a diagnosis is the biopsy report. Veterinarians do not perform enough skin biopsies.' These books describe in great detail the mechanics of obtaining the biopsy and sending it to a veterinary dermatopathologist. What is missing is information on interpretation of the report. What is so special or difficult about interpreting a skin biopsy report? As veterinarians we are trained to interpret the results of complete blood counts, serum chemistries, urinalyses, radiographs, electrocardiograms, and a wide assortment of other diagnostic tests. If one gets forgetful or rusty at making these interpretations, there are countless handbooks on clinical diagnosis by laboratory methods, reviews of radiographic interpretation, etc. The purpose of this chapter is give the reader some insight about how to read the description in a written biopsy report and get more information from it than from the one-sentence diagnosis at the bottom of the report. Both the veterinarian and the client pay for all of the words on the page, not just the last line, so why not use them all?

Reading a skin biopsy report is very intimidating. First of all, few people are enthralled with pathology as students and like to avoid memories of 'pyknotic nuclei and intracellular swelling'. Most clinicians are much more comfortable with the 'Diagnosis...'. Secondly, the language of pathology can be a barrier. Like most specialists, dermatopathologists have created their own language and terms to describe pathological changes in the skin. Finally, the art and science of dermatopathology is relatively new and overwhelming. However, the reality is that the average clinician need only learn a few terms and some basic facts to benefit from the information hidden in the 'morphological description' that may influence your diagnosis and treatment plan.

How Tissue is Processed

Clinicians need to have a basic understanding of what happens to a piece of tissue once it is taken from the body. Knowing the 'fate' of the tissue will enable clinicians to know why they may not have obtained the results they expected from the pathologist or diagnostic laboratory. Techniques for obtaining skin biopsy specimens are discussed in *Chapter 3*.

Formalin Fixative

Tissue for biopsy should immediately be placed in a fixative to minimise tissue desiccation and autolysis. Before fixation, any excess blood should be gently blotted from the specimen to prevent the lesion from being obscured by haemorrhage. Tissue shrinkage and curling can be prevented by mounting the specimen on a small piece of wood (tongue depressor) or cardboard.

The most commonly used fixative is 10% neutral buffered formalin. This fixative removes water from the tissue and makes it firmer so that it can withstand processing. Formalin also sterilises tissue and makes it unsuitable for bacterial or fungal cultures. It is very important to use neutral buffered formalin to keep the formalin from degrading. Proper fixation of a 6 mm thick tissue specimen in formalin requires a minimum of 24 hours in a volume of 10–20 parts formalin to one of tissue. Formalin will not penetrate tissue to a depth greater than 1 cm in 24 hours. Very thick specimens should be partially transected at 1 cm intervals to allow for proper fixation or else the pathologist will receive a tissue specimen with a fixed exterior and an autolysed interior. Finally, if tissues are mailed to diagnostic

* The term 'pathophobe' was created by Dr Robert Dunstan, Michigan State University.

45

laboratories in winter, they may freeze during transit. Freezing and thawing of tissue creates significant artifacts that distort the architecture of the tissue and render the specimen worthless for interpretation. Freezing of tissues can be prevented by adding 1 part 95% ethyl alcohol to 9 parts formalin. This will lower the freezing point of the fixative without altering tissue fixation.

Trimming Biopsy Specimens

When a biopsy specimen reaches the diagnostic laboratory, it must be trimmed or sectioned prior to being processed. Tissue is trimmed so that it can be placed into a small plastic cassette measuring 2.6 × 3.2 × 0.5 cm. Tissue cassettes look like small suitcases with two pieces of foam in them. The tissue is placed in the cassette between the two pieces of foam.

Many skin biopsy specimens collected with a punch are cut in half in a plane parallel to the hair follicles. This allows the pathologist to examine the specimen from the epidermis to the subcutaneous fat while visualising the entire hair follicle. In some cases of alopecia, the pathologist may elect to section the biopsy specimen perpendicular to the hair shafts so that a 'Swiss cheese' configuration is seen. Skin biopsies blanch in formalin and if hairs are absent or clipped very closely it may be difficult to orient the specimen. Mounting the specimen on wood or cardboard and leaving some short hairs on the biopsy specimen is very helpful. Small pustules or papules that are easily visible on the live patient, may be invisible in the fixed specimen. If the biopsy is to be sectioned through a papular or pustular lesion, it should be mounted on a wooden or cardboard splint and an arrow drawn in the direction the pathologist should orient and cut tissue section. Nodular lesions larger than 2 × 3 cm do not fit in a cassette even when cut in half. In order to process these specimens, the pathologist must cut the nodule into several transverse sections for processing.

Tissue Processing

After the skin biopsy has been secured in the cassette, it is ready for processing. The process is performed under a vacuum and very small biopsy specimens are at risk of being sucked out of their cassettes and lost. The tissue is dehydrated and infiltrated with paraffin wax, which makes the tissue rigid so that it can be sectioned with a microtome. Infiltration, by means of a machine called a tissue processor, involves several steps and is considered to be one of the most critical stages in tissue processing. It should take 12 to 18 hours but laboratories offering quick turn-around often shorten the process, sacrificing diagnostic quality for speed. Inadequate tissue infiltration creates artifacts, makes tissue examination difficult and affects tissue staining quality.

After being infiltrated with paraffin wax, the biopsy specimen is embedded in a small tub of melted paraffin. The melted wax will fuse with the tissue to form a block that is used for sectioning. It is critical for the histopathologist to orientate the tissues correctly or diagnostic specimens may be not be produced. After the block hardens, it is sectioned on a microtome at thickness of 4–6 μm. Each section is placed on a slide, stained with haematoxylin and eosin (H&E) or other stains, covered with mounting media and a coverslip applied. Most H&E staining is done by machine but special stains are done by hand.

How a Pathologist Generates a Report

Components of the Written Biopsy Report

The standard biopsy report usually has between two and three components and possibly up to four. Typically, the first part of the report is a **histological or morphological description** of the tissue. This is the paragraph that describes the microscopic detail the pathologist has seen. One of the major objectives of this chapter is to help the reader gain more information from this part of the report.

The second part of the standard report is the **morphological diagnosis** of the tissue. This is a one- or two-line series of words that summarise the histological description. Some pathologists working in diagnostic laboratories may choose to use simply the term **diagnosis.** If a causative agent was identified in the tissues a report may contain an **aetiological diagnosis.** For example, if a nodular lesion was biopsied and examined and a deep fungal organism (e.g. *Blastomyces* spp.) was found in the tissues, the aetiological diagnosis would be cutaneous blastomycosis. A pathologist can only make an aetiological diagnosis if agents are found or if changes in the specimen are diagnostic for a disease or syndrome.

Finally, there is the **comment** section of the report. A pathologist may make a comment to answer a specific question posed by the clinician or to aid in the evaluation of the patient (e.g: 'cultures are recommended even though causative agents were not seen on special stains'). To clinicians, this is also where pathologists are annoyingly non-committal by using phrases such as 'consistent with', 'compatible with', 'incompatible with'.

When clinicians read biopsy reports they commonly give only superficial attention to the histological description and, instead, focus their attention on the morphological or aetiological diagnosis. In some cases, all the information needed to make a clinical diagnosis or a therapeutic decision is in the morphological or aetiological diagnosis. Unfortunately, in a great many cases in veterinary dermatology the real clues lie in the histological description and not the morphological diagnosis. For example, one of the authors (KAM) submitted a skin biopsy from a dog with marked scaling and crusting. The histological description noted multifocal areas of parakeratosis including the follicular epithelium. The morphological diagnosis was non-diagnostic: 'Dermatitis, perivascular, neutrophilic and eosinophilic with acanthosis, hyperkeratosis and focal

COMPONENTS OF THE WRITTEN PATHOLOGY REPORT		
Gross description	**Description of the tissues submitted for examination**	**One 6 mm haired skin biopsy sample is submitted for examination**
Histological or morphological description	Detailed description of the microscopic findings. Pathologists either systematically describe the skin from epidermis to dermis or describe the most striking feature first and then other associated findings	Multiple sections of skin are examined. One section has perivascular and periadnexal infiltration of large numbers of neutrophils and some eosinophils in the superficial dermis. Neutrophilic infiltrates focally extend into a follicular sheath with a focus of necrosis in one area. Neutrophils occur within an apocrine gland. There is mild to moderate acanthosis, marked focal spongiosis, and exocytosis with focal epidermitis. Multiple superficial vessels are dilated, lined by swollen endothelial cells and filled with intraluminal neutrophils. Another section of skin has partial ulceration of the epidermis and similar superficial dermal infiltrates admingled with moderate numbers of mononuclear cells. The superficial epidermis has a concave depression in the stratum corneum containing a cross-section of a roughly ovoid mite having a thick integument with spines. Examination of the crust reveals multiple similar mites (*Sarcoptes scabiei*) as well as several ova enmeshed in a milieu of degenerating neutrophils, keratin, and intermingled colonies of cocci
Morphological diagnosis	This is a string of terms used to summarise the histological findings	Hyperplastic spongiotic dermatitis and epidermitis, subacute, diffuse, moderate, with mites
Aetiological diagnosis	This is present when a specific disease or agent is found	Sarcoptic mange
Comments	Pathologists will use this section to answer specific questions that the clinician may have posed, to suggest further tests, or list diseases that are compatible with the histological changes present	The skin condition is attributed to sarcoptic mange
Biopsy reports courtesy of Drs James Cooley and Howard Steinberg, School of Veterinary Medicine, University of Wisconsin-Madison.		

FIG.4.1 Components of the written pathology report.

parakeratosis'. Because the histological description mentioned parakeratosis in the follicular epithelium and this is a feature of zinc-responsive dermatosis, a tentative diagnosis of zinc-responsive dermatitis was made. The dog was treated successfully with zinc supplementation. If the histological description had been ignored, the owners of that dog would still be bathing it daily.

Examination of the Slide

The examination of a skin biopsy slide is very similar to looking at a room full of furniture. You first view the room from a distance and then start focusing on details of the room's contents, finally deciding that you are looking at a living-room decorated in earth tones and furnished in a contemporary style. Other rooms may be very difficult to examine and it may take quite a while before you decide that the style is eclectic. The same approach is used by pathologists when viewing slides.

Pathologists first examine the entire glass slide macroscopically **before** putting it on the microscope stage. This gives them an overall impression of the sample. If the sample is very blue, inflammation may be present because of the staining properties of the nuclei of cells. If a tumour is present, it may be possible to determine if it is raised above the skin surface. Benign skin tumours will often be raised and symmetrical. Malignant tumours often have marked asymmetry. The thickness or thinness of the entire skin specimen (epidermis to panniculus) may be noticeable. Skin biopsies from dogs with hyperadrenocorticism are usually thin and the pathologist may get an impression of this from a 'bird's eye view'.

The next step is the most important. The skin specimen is examined under low magnification ($\times 2$ to $\times 4$ objective). This step is critical because it is here that the pathologist answers the question, 'Is the lesion inflammatory, neoplastic, or neither?' The pattern of the lesion as viewed at low magnification ($\times 2$ or $\times 4$) is used to answer this question. Each of these three lesion types (inflammatory, neoplastic, other) requires a slightly different approach by the pathologist when examining the slide, though there are some similarities. For example, for an inflammatory specimen the pathologist tries to classify the pattern into one of several common patterns that are associated with various diseases. This is called

pattern analysis. The degree of severity (mild, moderate or severe) and the duration (acute, subacute or chronic) are noted, and whether or not the changes are focal, multifocal or diffuse. The dominant cell type is identified. In the case of neoplasms, the organisation of the lesion is assessed. Organised, encapsulated masses tend to be benign while disorganised lesions are more likely to be malignant. Other types of lesions might include atrophy of one or more of the skin components.

Speaking the Language

Before we can discuss the system of **pattern diagnosis** in veterinary dermatopathology, it is necessary to know some of the vocabulary of the specialty. This is important for two reasons. First, some pathologists will describe a slide in exquisite detail and never clearly state the pattern. This is very annoying to clinicians who must make diagnostic and therapeutic decisions on the basis of the biopsy report. However, one can often determine the pattern from the written histological description. The second reason is obvious. If you don't understand the language of dermatopathology, it is impossible to extract all of the relevant information, such as the pattern, or to interpret the report properly and apply it to the patient's skin disease.

The following section has two purposes. The first is to give a working vocabulary of dermatopathology so that we can discuss the system of pattern diagnosis. The second is to provide a glossary of terms for reference. The terms are grouped according to their use in describing a specific structure or anatomic area, rather than alphabetically, because this may be more useful clinically. In addition, we have provided two definitions for each term. The first definition refers to what the pathologist is seeing. The second definition is intended to guide the clinician's interpretation of that term. In other words, when the pathologists writes '....', the clinician should think '.....'.

Common Terms Used To Describe Epidermal Changes

Crust

A crust is a consolidated mass of serum and debris on the surface of the skin. It is usually adherent to the stratum corneum or it may be separated from the tissue during processing. It may contain keratin, sebum, cell debris, serum and often aetiological agents. A crust may be described as **haemorrhagic** (blood — did you blot the specimen?), **serous** (mostly serum), **cellular** (mostly inflammatory cells), **serocellular** (a mixture of serum and inflammatory cells) or **pallisading/laminated** (alternating layers of pus, serum and ortho- or parakeratotic hyperkeratoses).

Clinical relevance. A crust merely implies that there has been an exudative event and that the material has adhered to the tissue. **ALL** crusts from biopsy specimens should be examined carefully because important diagnostic clues may be present. Crusts may contain mite fragments, bacteria, fungal hyphae and spores, and acantholytic cells of pemphigus foliaceus. Bacteria in crusts must be interpreted with care because they may be normal inhabitants. However, they may be clinically relevant when present in an inflammatory lesion and a superficial bacterial infection is suspected.

Hyperkeratosis

Hyperkeratosis is an increased thickness of the stratum corneum or cornified epidermis. It is usually classified as either **orthokeratotic** (epidermal cells without their nucleus) or **parakeratotic** (epidermal cells with their nucleus).

Clinical relevance. Hyperkeratosis implies that there is a disturbance in the orderly production of epidermal cells. For some reason, cells are being produced at a faster rate than normal or they are not being shed from the surface as quickly as they should be. **Orthokeratotic hyperkeratosis** is a non-specific finding that is seen in inflammatory, neoplastic, endocrine or degenerative skin diseases. Grossly, these animals usually have increased scale, crusting and lichenification (gross thickening of the skin). If there is marked orthokeratotic hyperkeratosis and the non-cornified epidermis is described to be of normal thickness, a disorder of keratinisation should be considered.

Parakeratotic hyperkeratosis can be focal, multifocal or diffuse. When parakeratosis is present, it suggests that epidermal turnover rate is very fast or there is a defect in keratinisation. In veterinary dermatology, the most important disease characterised by parakeratosis is zinc deficiency. If the

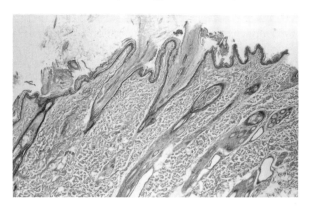

FIG. 4.2 Follicular hyperkeratosis. Note the hair follicles plugged with keratin. This is commonly observed in cases of idiopathic seborrhoea and Vitamin A-responsive dermatoses. Slide courtesy of Dr Maron Calderwood-Mays.

parakeratosis is described as generalised or diffuse and it is present in the epithelium of the hair follicles, the clinician's suspicions of a zinc-responsive dermatosis should be high. It is important to remember that significant inflammation of the skin can be present in the skin of dogs with a zinc-responsive dermatosis and, in contrast, marked parakeratosis can sometimes be seen in inflammatory skin diseases that are not zinc-responsive. Focal and multifocal hyperkeratotic parakeratosis are common in inflammatory lesions and are less likely to characterise a patient with zinc-responsive skin disease.

Follicular hyperkeratosis is a common component of biopsy reports. It describes hair follicles that are plugged or filled with keratin (Fig. 4.2). Hair shafts are usually absent. Follicular hyperkeratosis may be seen in animals with primary seborrhoea, secondary seborrhoea or vitamin A-responsive dermatitis. The follicular hyperkeratosis of vitamin A-responsive seborrhoea is severe, the hair follicle opening (ostium) is usually described as distended, and keratin usually protrudes from the opening. Vitamin A-responsive dermatoses are most common in American Cocker Spaniels and Samoyeds, but can be seen in other breeds. Follicular hyperkeratosis occurs in endocrine diseases as well.

Hypokeratosis

Hypokeratosis is a decreased thickness in the stratum corneum.

Clinical relevance. Hypokeratosis is a rare finding and implies that there is less cohesion between cells than is normally found. It may be a finding in some cases of seborrhoea and exfoliative skin diseases. It is most common in biopsies in which the skin was scrubbed prior to sample acquisition.

Hyperplasia and acanthosis

Epidermal hyperplasia is an increased thickness in the non-cornified epithelium. This increase refers to all layers of the non-cornified epidermis (basal, spinous, granular). Epidermal pegs that project downward into the dermis (**rete ridge formation**) are common in biopsies with epidermal hyperplasia. **Acanthosis** is another term used to describe thickening of the epidermis but it refers specifically to increased thickness of the stratum spinosum (Fig. 4.3).

Clinical relevance. Epidermal hyperplasia and acanthosis are terms that imply chronic skin disease, most often of an inflammatory nature. The increased thickness of the skin is due to the prolonged presence of the disease. This is a common finding in atopic skin disease. It is important to remember, however, that epidermal hyperplasia and acanthosis can be present in some cutaneous neoplasia. Neoplasia may cause secondary inflammation, resulting in a thickening of the epidermis, it may be invading the epidermis and making it appear thickened due to the cellular infiltrate, or it may be producing growth factors which affect the cellularity of the epidermis.

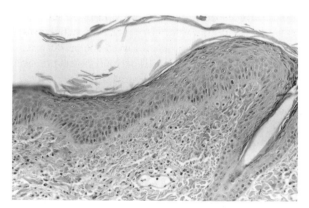

FIG. 4.3 Acanthosis. This is a common finding in many skin biopsy specimens. Note the increased thickness of the non-cornified epidermis; normal dog epithelium is 2–3 cell layers thick. Slide courtesy of Dr Maron Calderwood-Mays.

Hypoplasia and atrophy

Epidermal atrophy refers to a decreased thickness of the non-cornified epithelium due to a decrease in the number of cells. **Atrophy** refers to a decrease in the size of the individual cells and a decreased thickness of the non-cornified epidermis. **Hypoplasia** is usually reserved to describe a congenital defect of the skin.

Clinical relevance. Hypoplasia and atrophy are *very* rare histological findings on skin biopsy specimens. When these changes are found, they may suggest hyperadrenocorticism, sex hormone dermatoses, uncomplicated hypothyroidism, hyperoestrogenism, Sertoli cell tumours, or cutaneous asthenia; they may also be present in some cases of discoid lupus erythematosus.

Hypergranulosis

Hypergranulosis refers to an increase in the thickness of the granular layer. Histologically, this is seen as an increase in the number and size of the keratohyalin granules.

Clinical relevance. Hypergranulosis is a nonspecific finding commonly present in inflammatory skin diseases or diseases of a chronic nature. It is often associated with acanthosis or epidermal hyperplasia.

Necrosis

Necrosis is the death of cells or tissue. It is determined by examination of the nuclear morphology. The term **necrolysis** refers to the separation of dead tissue from the living host.

Clinical relevance. Focal epidermal necrosis may be the result of a drug eruption, microbial infection or lichenoid skin diseases. Diffuse necrosis may be caused by irritant contact dermatitis, burns, loss of blood supply, or an immunological attack on the skin. The two diseases which are infamous for causing epidermal necrosis are toxic epidermal necrolysis and erythema multiforme. Erythema multiforme causes widespread individual cell necrosis while toxic epidermal necrolysis causes widespread necrosis of the epidermis. These diseases are rare.

Intercellular oedema and spongiosis

Intercellular oedema or spongiosis of the epidermis is a widening of the spaces between cells in the stratum spongiosum. The intercellular bridges become very prominent and the epidermis appears spongy or, as the keratinocytes appear, spiny due to widening of the intercellular bridges.

Clinical relevance. Intercellular oedema is commonly present in biopsies from pruritic lesions. It is a prominent feature of several pruritic skin diseases including feline eosinophilic plaque, allergic contact dermatitis, irritant contact dermatitis and atopy. In some cases, intercellular oedema or spongiosis may become severe, resulting in the breakdown of the intercellular bridges and the development of vesicles. Intercellular oedema can also be artifactual.

Intracellular oedema

Intracellular oedema is also known as hydropic degeneration, vacuolar degeneration or ballooning degeneration, depending upon where the affected cells are and what is happening to them. These terms are used inconsistently by pathologists and are confusing. Generically, intracellular oedema refers to an increased cell size, cytoplasmic pallor, and displacement of the nucleus to the periphery of the affected cell. If the intracellular oedema is severe and the cell ruptures, it is called **reticular degeneration**. **Hydropic degeneration** is intracellular oedema of the basal cells. Ballooning degeneration is a type of intracellular oedema in which the cytoplasm of affected cells becomes eosinophilic and swollen without vacuolating, the nuclei condense or enlarge, and there is loss of cohesion between cells resulting in acantholysis.

Clinical relevance. Although this is a non-specific finding, it should alert the clinician that this particular lesion is acute or subacute. The lesion could be an early one in a progressive or chronic skin disease. Hydropic degeneration in basal cells is usually associated with autoimmune or immune-mediated diseases and may be focal or diffuse and involve the hair follicles. The clinician should then consider such diseases as lichenoid dermatoses, drug eruptions, lupus erythematosus, toxic epidermal

necrolysis and erythema multiforme. Reticular degeneration, if severe, may result in intraepidermal vesicles. The clinician should consider irritant and contact dermatitis. Ballooning degeneration is considered a feature of viral skin diseases, but may be a feature of other diseases.

Dyskeratosis

Dyskeratosis is the faulty keratinisation of individual cells. These cells have condensed eosinophilic swollen cytoplasm. Their nuclei stain very dark and they can be difficult to distinguish from dying keratinocytes. If the remaining epidermis is undergoing keratinisation, cells are usually referred to as **dyskeratotic**. If the remaining epidermis is undergoing widespread necrosis, cells are more likely to be called **necrotic keratinocytes**.

Clinical relevance. The presence of these cells in a biopsy report should raise suspicions of diseases where keratinocytes are not being manufactured properly. These would include zinc-responsive dermatoses, vitamin A-responsive dermatosis and 'generic dog food dermatosis'. Dyskeratosis can be a feature in some autoimmune skin diseases such as pemphigus foliaceus, lupus and erythema multiforme. Finally, this is a feature of some neoplastic skin diseases including squamous cell carcinoma, intracutaneous cornifying epithelioma, and papillomas.

Acantholysis

Acantholysis describes a condition in which the keratinocytes lose cohesion between each other, and vesicles, bullae and clefts develop in the epidermis. The cells floating freely in these clefts, vesicles or bullae are acantholytic cells. Acantholysis can occur in the epithelium of the hair follicle and ducts of the glands in the skin.

Clinical relevance. Although acantholysis is a feature of many diseases, the most common and most important disease where it may be seen is pemphigus foliaceus. Acantholysis is only one diagnostic criterion for this autoimmune skin disease, but it is an important one. Acantholysis can be seen in non-autoimmune skin diseases where the disease causes severe spongiosis (intercellular oedema) and the intercellular bridges break. Acantholysis can also be a feature of viral infections and other infectious skin diseases where the agent releases proteolytic enzymes which destroy the intercellular cement. It is also a feature of squamous cell carcinoma and actinic keratosis.

Microvesicles, vesicles and bullae

These terms describe fluid-filled spaces either within the epidermis or just below it. They may or may not be visible grossly. In most cases, the spaces are cell-free.

Clinical relevance. The presence of microvesicles, vesicles and bullae on a biopsy report indicates that severe intercellular and/or intracellular oedema, ballooning degeneration, acantholysis, hydropic degeneration and/or subepidermal oedema are present. Inflammatory, viral, autoimmune, and immune-mediated diseases should be considered. It is unlikely that chronic benign skin diseases are involved in the development of these lesions.

Microabscesses and pustules

Microabscesses and pustules describe intraepidermal and subepidermal spaces filled with inflammatory cells. Histopathology reports usually contain a description of the cell type in the space and the location of the lesion within the epidermis.

Clinical relevance. Microabscesses and pustules are found most commonly in infectious skin diseases, primarily bacterial, and in autoimmune skin diseases such as pemphigus, bullous pemphigoid and systemic lupus erythematosus. It is important that the pathologist describes the cellular infiltrate and states whether it contains eosinophils, neutrophils, acantholytic cells, bacteria etc. This information is needed by the clinician when interpreting the biopsy report.

Exocytosis

Exocytosis describes the migration and infiltration of inflammatory cells into the epidermis. These inflammatory cells migrate through the intercellular spaces and often congregate in masses to form micro- or macro-abscesses (pustules or bullae). Exocytosis may involve neutrophils, eosinophils, mononuclear cells (macrophages or lymphocytes), or even red blood cells.

Clinical relevance. Exocytosis implies inflammation. This may involve infectious agents, parasitic agents, neoplastic diseases or immune-mediated processes. Regardless of the process, chemotactic substances are produced which draw the inflammatory cells to the specific location. This finding is common in pyoderma and ectoparasite infestations. When a pathologist describes red blood cell exocytosis or diapedesis, the clinician should immediately be thinking about haemorrhage. The leaking of red blood cells into the tissue may be microscopic or macroscopic. Vasculitis, coagulation defects and vessel damage from invasive or inflammatory processes should be considered.

Hyperpigmentation, hypopigmentation and pigmentary incontinence

These terms describe changes in the amount and location of melanin in the skin. *Pigmentary incontinence* refers to the presence of melanin granules in macrophages in the superficial dermis.

Clinical relevance. Any comment on the amount of pigment present in the skin must be considered with respect to what is normal. This is one reason why it is important to provide the patient profile on the biopsy submission form.

Hyperpigmentation describes an increase in the visible number of melanocytes and the amount of melanin they are producing. This is a common finding in chronic skin diseases or in local areas of pigmentation, i.e. lentigo in orange cats. It may be present in some neoplastic skin diseases, most notably melanomas. Hyperpigmentation may be present in a number of hormonal skin diseases.

Hypopigmentation refers to less than expected normal pigmentation. It is difficult for a pathologist to assess in the absence of a detailed history.

If melanin granules are seen in macrophages in the superficial dermis, the pathologist will infer that there has been some damage to the basement membrane leading to the death of melanocytes and 'pigment drop-out' into the dermis. Diseases that can cause pigmentary incontinence include discoid lupus erythematosus, toxic chemicals, severe inflammatory diseases and certain endocrine disorders.

Occasionally, the clinician submits a biopsy from an abnormally depigmented area of skin (leucoderma) or hair (leucotrichia) and is annoyed when the pathologist reports that normal skin was examined. It is important to remember that the cause of the depigmentation may precede the development of it by a long period and may no longer be present when the lesion is examined histologically.

Common Terms Used To Describe Dermal Changes

Collagen changes

There are a number of terms used to describe changes in dermal collagen. The majority of them describe degenerative changes or stages of degeneration of collagen fibres. In general, degenerating collagen loses its classic pale eosin-stained colour and becomes more eosinophilic and refractile. It may appear granular or it may completely lose all structural detail. Depending upon the disease process, collagen may even undergo dystrophic mineralisation. Affected collagen fibres have calcium salts deposited within them and are essentially turning to bone. Collagen may appear atrophic or thinner than normal. If dermal collagen atrophy is present, there is usually a comment that the dermis is thinner than expected. Collagen may be described as disorganised or fragmented. These terms describe structural changes in collagen due to altered manufacture by fibroblasts. The orientation of collagen in tissues may be described as vertical, or organised in vertical streaks. This terminology describes collagen that is elongated, thickened and oriented in bundles perpendicular to the epidermis.

Clinical relevance. None of the terms used to describe collagen is diagnostic for any one disease. If the pathologist describes degenerative changes in the collagen, the clinican should recognise that these changes indicate chronicity, possible connective tissue diseases, and inflammation. Collagen degeneration is a feature of feline and canine eosinophilic granuloma. The concurrent presence of atrophic collagen should suggest a possible hormonal skin disease. Although there are many causes for dystrophic mineralisation in tissue, excessive concentrations of plasma glucocorticoids is the most common cause. Hence, dystrophic mineralisation is a clinical hallmark of iatrogenic and spontaneously occurring hyperadrenocorticism. Dystrophic mineralisation may also occur in chronic inflammation, e.g. chronic proliferative otitis externa, neoplasia, foreign body reactions, or in calcinosis circumscripta. Fragmented/disorganised collagen is seen most commonly in developmental collagen diseases such as cutaneous asthenia. Vertical streaking of collagen indicates that this is a chronically rubbed and probably pruritic lesion. It is common in acral lick dermatitis.

Fibroplasia and desmoplasia

Fibroplasia describes the proliferation of apparently normal collagen and blood vessels (granulation tissue). Desmoplasia refers to the dense proliferation of collagen induced by neoplasia.

Clinical relevance. Fibroplasia implies wound healing. Desmoplasia may be used to describe the collagen of a connective tissue tumour or collagen on the periphery of an epithelial tumour. Desmoplasia may also be present in some mesenchymal tumours.

Fibrosis and sclerosis

Fibrosis is a late stage of fibroplasia in which large numbers of densely packed collagen fibres and fibroblasts are present. Blood vessels and inflammatory cells are scarce. Sclerosis is the end point of fibrosis and describes collagen fibres that are thick and eosinophilic in appearance with fewer fibroblasts visible in the tissue.

Clinical relevance. Fibrosis and sclerosis are commonly seen in scar tissue. These terms may be used to describe the collagen fibres in a long-standing lick granuloma.

Pigmentary incontinence

This term has been discussed above under epidermal changes.

Oedema

When oedema is present, lymphatic vessels may be dilated and collagen fibres more widely spaced.

Clinical relevance. Oedema in the dermis suggests that there is inflammation and it may be accompanied by epidermal vesicles and bullae. Severe dermal oedema may make processing of tissue specimens difficult and artifacts may occur because of this oedema. A good dermatopathologist should be able to make a judgement on whether or not a cleft or abnormal separation of the epidermis and dermis is due to a disease process or underlying dermal oedema. Mucinous degeneration must also be ruled out.

Mucinous degeneration

Mucinous degeneration describes an increased amount of 'ground substance' in the dermis. Histologically, this appears as a basophilic amorphous material between the collagen fibres.

Clinical relevance. Localised mucinous degeneration can be found associated with inflammatory skin diseases. Diffuse mucinous degeneration is a feature of acromegaly, lupus erythematosus, idiopathic mucinoses and, according to some authorities, canine hypothyroidism. Diffuse mucinous is normal in the Shar Pei.

Follicular atrophy and follicular dystrophy

Follicular atrophy refers to a small, involuting hair follicle. Follicular dystrophy (or dysplasia) describes hair follicles which appear to be abnormal, incompletely developed hair follicles or abnormal hair development in hair follicles.

Clinical relevance. A large number of diseases of the hair follicles can cause follicular atrophy or dystrophy. Clinically important and common skin diseases where follicular atrophy is often a feature include hypothyroidism, hyperadrenocorticism, post-rabies vaccine alopecia, Sertoli cell tumours, dermatomyositis of Collies and Shetland Sheepdogs, and canine traction alopecia. Follicular dystrophy is a feature of canine colour-dilute alopecia, black-hair follicular dysplasia, idiopathic canine follicular dysplasia and acquired pattern alopecia.

Glandular changes

The glands in the skin may be involved in the skin disease process as 'innocent bystanders' or may be a direct target for the disease's assault, for example sebaceous adenitis. In general there are four common terms used to describe either the apocrine glands or the sebaceous glands: atrophic, cystic, hyperplastic or inflamed. Atrophic glands may be smaller in size or in number. Cystic glands are enlarged and have fluid-filled cavities. Hyperplastic glands are larger in size than expected, are more cellular and may have increased secretory activity. Both sebaceous and apocrine glands can be invaded by inflammatory cells.

Clinical relevance. There are few diseases of importance involving the sweat glands. The most common diseases seen are macroscopic benign cystic structures or malignant sweat gland carcinomas. Microscopically, these glands may become dilated or inflamed as a result of inflammatory skin diseases, especially hormonal and allergic skin diseases. Sebaceous glands may develop hyperplasia/adenomas in allergic skin diseases. Nodular sebaceous hyperplasia or the 'warts' of dogs are common in clinical practice. Glandular inflammation of sebaceous glands is seen at the end of sebaceous adenitis. Atrophy or even total absence of sebaceous glands is a sequela of long-standing sebaceous adenitis.

Blood vessels

The descriptive terms used to describe blood vessels in the dermis include dilatation (ectasia), endothelial swelling, extravasation (diapedesis) of red blood cells, vasculitis and fibrinoid degeneration. In normal tissue, blood vessels are not very prominent and their lumina may only contain one or two red blood cells. When the blood vessels are dilated, they are prominent and filled with red blood cells. The same conditions that cause dilation of blood vessels may also cause the endothelial cells lining the blood vessel to enlarge. Swollen endothelial cells are often seen bulging into the lumen. Extravasation of red blood cells implies that there are free red blood cells in the tissue — cells have escaped into the tissue because of damage to the vessel wall. Vasculitis and fibrinoid degeneration are terms used to describe the blood vessel wall and both refer to inflammation and destruction of the wall.

Clinical relevance. Blood vessel dilatation and endothelial cell swelling are features of many conditions, particularly inflammatory skin diseases. These changes indicate a degree of severity of the pathological changes. Extravasation of blood cells can occur in many inflammatory skin diseases. Changes in the integrity of the blood vessel wall, vasculitis and fibrinoid degeneration, should be taken seriously as these changes may be caused by immune-mediated skin diseases.

Inflammatory Skin Patterns

The type and location of a cellular infiltrate in tissue allows the pathologist to classify skin lesions into patterns. Some patterns are easy to recognise, some patterns are mixed, while others are unrecognisable. Each pattern suggests a range of possible diseases or a specific diagnosis. Pattern analysis is very similar to determining what breed(s) a particular dog may be. When a dog is a purebred, identifying the breed is easy because there are breed standards. Even when a dog is a mixed breed, one can often state with confidence that there is some of this breed or that breed in the dog. However, there are some dogs that defy breed identification.

The most common system of pattern diagnosis used in dermatopathology involves scanning the specimen to determine the predominant changes in the specimen or, more generally, where's the action and what's happening? The system of patterns is subdivided into diseases of the epidermis, dermal–epidermal junction, dermis, adnexa and panniculus. Each of these areas is further subdivided into specific classifications. Because it is not the intent of this chapter to steep clinicians in the details of dermatopathology or bore them, we have taken the liberty of 'lumping' where possible. It is important to remember that several patterns may coexist in the same specimen. Depending upon the pathologist, the final morphological description may either describe the predominant pattern or may report all patterns.

Inflammatory Patterns Of the Epidermis

Pustular/vesicular dermatitis

Pustular/vesicular dermatitis describes an inflammatory pattern in the epidermis that is characterised by pustules and/or vesicles. The pustules/vesicles may be micro- or macroscopic. Pustules or vesicles form in the epidermis when it loses its ability to be cohesive. Spongiosis (intercellular oedema) and acantholysis occur because of inflammation and the influx of inflammatory cells migrating from the superficial dermal blood vessel. The pustules or vesicles may be described as intracorneal or subcorneal (in the cornified epidermis), intraepidermal or intragranular (in the noncornified epidermis) (Fig. 4.4), or suprabasilar. It should be noted whether the pustules or vesicles are focal or diffuse in the skin. Since these lesions form because of inflammatory mediators and the influx of inflammatory cells from the dermis, it is common for there to be a second pattern of inflammation mentioned concomitantly, perivascular dermatitis (see below).

The pustules usually contain neutrophils, but eosinophils may be present depending upon the disease. Since pustules are fragile structures, crusts (scabbed broken pustules) adherent to the epidermis are common. Bacteria may be seen in the pustules or the crusts.

Clinical relevance. Pustular diseases of the epidermis are caused most commonly by infectious agents and include bacterial pyodermas, dermatophytosis

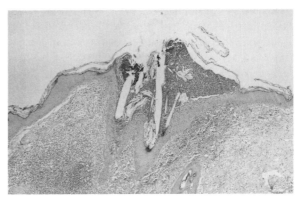

FIG. 4.4 Pustular dermatitis. In this section, note the large intraepidermal pustule. Slide courtesy of Dr Maron Calderwood-Mays.

and mucocutaneous candidiasis (rare). Pustular dermatitis also characterises several autoimmune skin diseases of the pemphigus complex. Pustules may be present in viral skin diseases when vesicles become infiltrated with neutrophils or in neoplastic skin diseases, e.g. microabscesses filled with atypical lymphocytes in epitheliotropic lymphoma.

When a pustular disease of the epidermis is being described, the most important thing for the clinician to determine is whether or not the aetiology of the lesion is infectious or autoimmune. The pathologist is at the mercy of the samples submitted: therefore in pustular diseases a wide variety of lesions should be submitted: intact pustules, samples from the advancing edge of spreading lesions, and crusted lesions with adherent crusts. Microscopically, classic pustules containing neutrophils and bacteria are seen when macroscopic mature intact pustules are biopsied. Acantholytic cells of pemphigus are also most likely to be seen microscopically within intact pustules. Pustules are not always grossly visible in spreading pyodermas or lesions of 'bacterial hypersensitivity'; however, they may be present microscopically if the advancing edge of the lesion is sampled.

Pustular dermatitis is also characteristic of pemphigus foliaceus and pemphigus erythematosus. The pustules of pemphigus foliaceus are quite different in appearance to those of bacterial pyoderma. The pustules occur in waves every 4 to 7 days and are numerous, large, flaccid, and vary in colour from white to yellow to slightly green. An individual pustule may span several hair follicles. Even in a severe bacterial pyoderma it is rare to see large numbers of obvious pustules over the patient's body. The pustules of pemphigus foliaceus typically contain neutrophils, eosinophils and acantholytic cells.

Fungal hyphae or spores within the epidermis may also be seen within the advancing edge of these lesions. Mucocutaneous candidiasis is an ulcerative crusting disease that can mimic systemic lupus erythematosus, drug eruptions, pemphigus vulgaris and bullous pemphigoid. Yeasts and hyphae are most commonly found in crusts and, occasionally, intact pustules.

Necrotising

Necrotising epidermitis describes widespread death of epidermal cells (keratinocytes). The necrosis may be diffuse or focal, depending upon the aetiology. Necrotic keratinocytes appear as brightly eosinophilic cells in the epidermis.

Clinical relevance. A report indicating that there is widespread individual cell necrosis should raise suspicions of erythema multiforme, while widespread necrosis of the epidermis should immediately make the clinician consider toxic epidermal necrolysis (TEN), chemical or thermal burns and superficial necrolytic dermatitis. Toxic epidermal necrolysis and erythema multiforme are usually acute and rapidly progressing. The mucocutaneous junctions are often involved, the animals are systemically ill, and in TEN the skin is painful; clients usually present these animals relatively soon for veterinary medical care. Chemical and thermal burns are common and occur acutely. Veterinary care may be delayed because the hair coat can mask the burns for several days before the client notices the injury. Superficial necrolytic dermatitis is due to poorly characterised internal metabolic disease and patients are presented with various problems. The disease is characterised by widespread slowly progressive mucocutaneous, muzzle, and pedal crusting and the progression is slow.

Exudative and ulcerative epidermitis

These terms describe patterns of inflammation in which large numbers of inflammatory cells accumulate on the surface of the epidermis. This accumulation leads to the formation of crusts.

Clinical relevance. This pattern of inflammation is seen in skin diseases that are characterised by intense self-trauma and secondary exudation. Common skin diseases that have exudation and ulceration as a feature include pyotraumatic dermatitis (hotspots), feline miliary dermatitis and feline indolent ulcer (eosinophilic ulcers).

Spongiotic epidermitis

Spongiotic epidermitis describes skin diseases in which there is marked intercellular oedema in the non-cornified epidermis (spongiosis). Severe spongiosis may lead to the breakdown of intercellular bridges and intraepidermal vesicles.

Clinical relevance. Spongiosis is a characteristic of almost all of the allergic diseases, in addition to many others. There are a few diseases in which spongiosis is the primary abnormal finding and in which the spongiosis is an important diagnostic criterion, including allergic contact dermatitis, irritant contact dermatitis, scabies and feline eosinophilic plaques. The histological changes of allergic contact dermatitis are indistinguishable from those of irritant contact dermatitis. Necrosis of the epidermis may be seen in cases of irritant contact dermatitis, but not in allergic contact dermatitis. Eosinophilic plaques are very common and are a classic example of spongiotic epidermitis. Eosinophils are prominent in the epidermis and in the dermis.

Hyperplastic dermatitis

A hyperplastic pattern of inflammation describes a marked thickening of the non-cornified epidermis (acanthosis). The marked thickening is caused by chronic inflammation and, often, self-trauma. This pattern of inflammation is almost always accompanied by a perivascular infiltrate.

Clinical relevance. Hyperplastic dermatitis could describe almost any chronic skin disease. Clinically, hyperplastic dermatitis is the histological appearance of lichenified skin. One of the most common causes for lichenification is chronic allergy, e.g. flea allergy and atopy. Hyperplastic dermatitis is a feature of acral lick dermatitis, hypothyroidism, canine Sertoli cell tumours (endocrinopathies can also have an atrophied epidermis), actinic keratoses, acanthosis nigricans of Dachshunds, hyperplastic dermatitis of West Highland White Terriers, and psoriasiform-lichenoid dermatitis of Springer Spaniels. It is interesting to note that two endocrinopathies, canine hypothyroidism and Sertoli cell tumours, more commonly have a **thickened epidermis** rather than a **thin epidermis**. This is probably due to secondary conditions, e.g. seborrhoea and bacterial infections that accompany these primary disorders, rather than the disease itself. Diseases of altered keratinisation may or may not have an acanthotic epidermis. In the case of hyperplastic dermatitis of West Highland White Terriers (West Highland White Terrier seborrhoea) and psoriasiform-lichenoid dermatitis of Springer Spaniels, the epidermis is certainly acanthotic. In the Spaniel disease, as the name implies, a second inflammatory pattern is present: a lichenoid infiltrate (see below).

Hyperkeratotic dermatitis

Hyperkeratotic dermatitis describes a dense accumulation of keratin on the surface of the epidermis and the hair follicles. This pattern is seen in diseases in which there is a genetic or metabolic abnormality in the production of the epidermis. The marked hyperkeratosis may or may not be accompanied by marked hyperplasia (acanthosis) of the non-cornified epidermis. When there is marked hyperkeratosis and an epidermis of normal thickness, a primary defect of keratinisation is probably present. It is more difficult, if not impossible, for a pathologist to make a diagnosis of a primary defect of keratinisation when acanthosis and hyperkeratosis are present.

Clinical relevance. Hyperkeratotic dermatitis with or without acanthosis describes the seborrhoeic diseases. Primary seborrhoea, seborrhoeic dermatitis and seborrhoeic dermatitis associated with *Malassezia* spp. will show marked hyperkeratosis, acanthosis and perivascular inflammation. These diseases are usually pruritic, and self-trauma and secondary bacterial infections complicate the histological findings. Vitamin A-responsive dermatoses have similar findings along with severe follicular keratosis. The hair follicles are so stuffed with keratin that it begins to overflow from the hair follicle ostia. Ear margin seborrhoea may look similar histologically to vitamin A-responsive dermatitis. Schnauzer comedone syndrome is characterised by marked to severe follicular hyperkeratosis; however, keratin does not protrude from the hair follicle ostium creating clinical fronds; the ostium appears to be closed. Some cases of sebaceous adenitis may also have marked follicular hyperkeratosis, but the presence of inflammation in the sebaceous gland or complete absence of sebaceous glands differentiates this disease from vitamin A-responsive skin diseases.

Hyperkeratotic dermatitis is also a feature of zinc-responsive dermatoses, except that marked parakeratosis of the epidermis and follicular epithelium is present. 'Generic dog food skin disease', acrodermatitis of Bull Terriers, and superficial necrolytic dermatitis (formerly hepatocutaneous syndrome) may have a similar appearance.

Diseases of the Dermal–Epidermal Junction

Supra- and sub-epidermal vesicular dermatitis

This pattern describes the presence of vesicles above and below the basement membrane of the epidermis. Vesicles may be described as vesicles or clefts in the tissue. The cellular infiltrate may be variable. It is the location of the cleft that aids the pathologist and clinician in making a diagnosis.

Clinical relevance. The most common causes of clefts or vesicles in the deep epidermal or dermal–epidermal region of the skin are autoimmune skin diseases and hereditary or genetic defects in the skin. The age, breed and clinical signs are very important when interpreting a biopsy report describing a vesicular dermatitis. Vesicles at or above the basement membrane zone may or may not be visible grossly. Vesicles below the basement membrane are usually less fragile and tend to be visible grossly because they are less likely to rupture.

Vesicles or clefts at the basement membrane may be seen in discoid or systemic lupus erythematosus and canine dermatomyositis. In lupus, basal cell vacuolation and a lichenoid pattern of inflammation (see below) are also found in 'classic' biopsies. Canine dermatomyositis may be distinguished from lupus because it lacks a lichenoid pattern of inflammation, is associated with follicular atrophy and is most common in young Collies and Shetland Sheepdogs. Pemphigus vulgaris and pemphigus vegetans have vesicles due to acantholysis above the basement membrane (suprabasilar). Vesicles below the basement membrane level (subepidermal) are found in bullous pemphigoid and epidermolysis bullosa.

Lichenoid dermatitis

The histological term 'lichenoid' means band-like and it should not be confused with lichenified (Fig. 4.5). Lichenification is a clinical term which describes a gross thickening of the skin from chronic inflammation. Lichenoid dermatitis describes a pattern of inflammation that is just beneath the epidermis and oriented toward the dermal–epider-

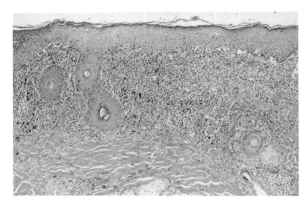

FIG. 4.5 Lichenoid dermatitis. Note the band of inflammatory cells 'hugging' the basement membrane. Slide courtesy of Dr Maron Calderwood-Mays.

mal junction. Some pathologists prefer to use the term interface dermatitis to describe lichenoid patterns that have mild superficial cell infiltrates, and to save the term 'lichenoid' for dense cellular infiltrates. When the pathologist describes a lichenoid pattern of inflammation, it is critical that the basement membrane and basal layer be examined for basal cell vacuolation, pigmentary incontinence and cell type. This will help differentiate the various skin diseases characterised by lichenoid dermatoses.

Clinical relevance. The most common skin diseases characterised by lichenoid (interface) dermatitis are autoimmune skin diseases and cutaneous epitheliotropic lymphomas. The autoimmune skin diseases include discoid and systemic lupus erythematosus, pemphigus erythematosus, oculocutaneous syndrome (previously Vogt–Koyanagi–Harada-like syndrome (VHK)) and erythema multiforme. Discoid and systemic lupus erythematosus are indistinguishable histologically and are characterised by a cellular infiltrate consisting primarily of lymphocytes and plasma cells. Pigmentary incontinence is common. Basal cells are usually vacuolated. The histology of oculocutaneous syndrome is similar to that of lupus except that the cellular infiltrate consists of histiocytes (tissue macrophages). Cutaneous epitheliotropic lymphoma (mycosis fungoides) is characterised by a lymphocytic infiltrate that not only forms a lichenoid band but also invades the epidermis and follicular epithelium. These lymphocytes tend to be large and may accumulate in clusters in the epidermis (Pautrier's microabscesses). Some pathologists have reported that lichenoid bands of plasma cells and neutrophils may be present in lip-fold pyodermas. Finally, a lichenoid band of inflammation may be seen in skin biopsies of actinic (solar) dermatitis and psoriasiform-lichenoid dermatitis of Springer Spaniels.

Inflammatory Patterns of the Dermis

Perivascular dermatitis

A perivascular dermatitis pattern describes the accumulation of cells around the small blood vessels in the superficial dermis (Fig. 4.6). This is the most common inflammatory skin pattern in the skin. Except for panniculitis, all of the other patterns start and end with this pattern; inflammatory cells must use conventional pathways, i.e. blood vessels and lymphatics, to get to the site of inflammation.

Clinical relevance. Allergic and parasitic skin diseases are characterised by a superficial perivascular dermatitis. These diseases include atopy, food allergy, flea allergy, feline miliary dermatitis, scabies, notoedric mange, cheyletiellosis, hookworm dermatitis, pruritic pyoderma, and contact dermatitis. It is nearly impossible to differentiate these diseases based upon a biopsy specimen alone. The cellular infiltrate may help narrow the range of

possibilities but the final diagnosis will be made upon the history and clinical signs. In dogs with atopy, the cellular infiltrate is predominantly comprised of lymphocytes, macrophages and mast cells. Eosinophil infiltrates are variable; some authorities report them as rare and others recognise them more commonly. In food allergy, the findings are similar to atopy except that eosinophils are more prominent. Skin biopsy specimens from flea allergy, scabies, notoedric mange and other cutaneous parasitic infestations are indistinguishable from each other. The presence or absence of eosinophils in the infiltrate can be useful in distinguishing atopy from parasitic skin infestations, since eosinophils are less numerous in atopy. It is important to remember, however, that previous glucocorticoid therapy will alter the histological findings; glucocorticoid use will severely alter the number of perceived eosinophils. Other common histological findings in specimens with perivascular dermatitis are acanthosis due to chronic pruritus, dilatation of sweat glands and sebaceous hyperplasia.

Vasculitis

Vasculitis describes inflammation that is directed at the blood vessels in the superficial or deep dermis. The blood vessel wall may be described as necrotic, the vascular endothelium may be swollen, the blood vessel may be thrombosed, or the wall of the vessel may be invaded by inflammatory cells. The vast majority of attacks on cutaneous blood vessels are due to immune-mediated diseases, especially SLE. There are only a few infectious diseases that primarily affect blood vessels. In many cases, there is little or no pathological change in the epidermis.

Clinical relevance. The most common disease in which cutaneous vasculitis **may** be seen is urticaria or angioedema. Urticaria/angioedema are hypersensitivity reactions and rarely vasculitis is a component of the pathological changes. The most common histological finding in urticaria or angioedema is oedema in the dermis with or without a superficial perivascular infiltrate. In a clinical situation, it is unlikely that skin biopsies would be included in the diagnostic evaluation of patients with urticaria or angioedema as most cases resolve spontaneously. Biopsies are indicated if the episodes are repetitive or extremely severe, or if other clinical

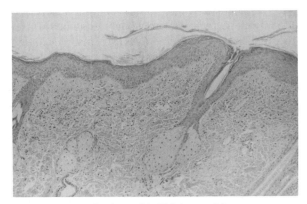

FIG. 4.6 Perivascular dermatitis. This is one of the most common inflammatory patterns. Note the accumulation of cells in the superficial epidermis around blood vessels. Slide courtesy of Dr Maron Calderwood-Mays.

signs are present, i.e. serum exudation from the weals. If vasculitis is found in patients presenting with angioedema or urticaria, an aggressive search for the cause should be pursued. Drug reactions to vaccines, antibiotics, blood transfusions and bacterins can cause vasculitis. Immune-mediated vasculitis is multi-factorial in aetiology and it is reported to be most common on extremities, but not limited to ears, tails and limbs. Leucocytoclastic is a term that is commonly associated with immune-mediated vasculitis. It refers to the invasion of the wall by neutrophils and their subsequent death. Degenerating neutrophils may be described as fragmented around vessels or 'nuclear dust'. Septic vasculitis is rare and may be seen in severe bacterial pyoderma, widespread sepsis and infection with *Rickettsia* spp. The above-mentioned conditions are Type 3 hypersensitivity reactions.

Nodular/diffuse dermatitis

A nodular dermatitis describes an infiltrate of cells that is organised into discrete or easily recognised nodules. Nodular reactions begin as a perivascular, periadnexal or perifollicular dermatitis. The progression may be slow or rapid depending upon the aetiology. The aetiology may also determine where the nodules are located, i.e. dermal or involving adnexa. A diffuse dermatitis describes a widespread infiltrate of cells that is more or less evenly distributed in the dermis. Simply, diffuse dermatitis starts out as perivascular dermatitis that proceeds to nodular dermatitis and eventually becomes confluent in the dermis. Depending upon the severity of the reaction, the infiltrate may even extend into the subcutaneous fat or panniculus. The type of cells in the infiltrate should be determined. A high proportion of neutrophils usually indicates that the inflammatory process is relatively active and new. Pyogranulomatous to granulomatous cell infiltrates indicate that the body has been fighting or walling off the infectious agent or cause for some time. If the nodules are described as being encapsulated, the process is relatively long-standing and the cause difficult to eliminate.

Clinical relevance. Although there are many causes of nodular/diffuse tissue reaction, the presence of this on a biopsy report should scream to the clinician: 'Look for an infectious agent.' The infectious causes are far more numerous and far more likely to lead to serious complications, including death, than the non-infectious causes. Waste no time! Special stains for infectious agents will probably have already been done by the pathologist or should be requested now. Tissue samples should be cultured for aerobic and anaerobic bacteria, deep fungi, and atypical mycobacteria.

Infectious agents or diseases that cause this pattern are: aerobic bacteria (*Staphylococcus* spp., *Nocardia* spp.), *Actinomyces* spp., feline leprosy, atypical mycobacterium, fungal mycetomas, phaeohyphomycetoma, sporotrichosis, blastomycosis, aspergillosis, cryptococcosis, histoplasmosis, coccidioidomycosis and leishmaniasis. Nodular or diffuse reactions can occur secondary to follicular rupture in bacterial folliculitis, demodicosis or dermatophytosis. Feline and canine eosinophilic granulomas can also have this pattern. Eosinophils and collagen destruction are usually prominent in this disease.

Non-infectious causes include foreign body reaction or granulomas. These are usually solitary or well localised. Subcutaneous injections and insect-bites can cause localised granulomatous reactions. Some breeds of dogs, most notably the German Shepherd Dog, frequently have sterile pyogranulomas. The aetiology is unknown and infectious agents are not found. Calcium deposits in the skin can cause nodular and diffuse tissue reactions. Calcinosis circumscripta is an idiopathic nodular disease of giant breeds characterised by calcified nodules. The dystrophic calcification of calcinosis cutis also has a nodular to diffuse tissue reaction pattern.

Finally, there is sebaceous adenitis — an idiopathic, nodular, granulomatous reaction centred around the sebaceous glands of dogs, which eventually destroys the glands. This disease may also be described as a multifocal periadnexal dermatitis.

Nodular/diffuse dermatitis with eosinophils or plasma cells

This inflammatory pattern describes a cellular infiltrate that is organised into discrete nodules or is obscuring the dermis. It is also characterised by a prominent cellular infiltrate consisting of eosinophils and/or plasma cells. Collagen degeneration is common in these lesions.

Clinical relevance. This pattern is seen in skin diseases in which there is an intense hypersensitivity reaction. Such diseases include arthropod-bite granulomas (insect-bite granuloma), feline insect hypersensitivity, feline eosinophilic plaques, feline eosinophilic granulomas, spider-bites, canine eosinophilic granuloma and plasma cell pododermatitis.

Dysplastic and depositional dermatitis

Dysplastic dermatitis describes altered collagen production due to metabolic or inherited diseases. The collagen appears fractured or abnormal and the skin is very fragile. Depositional dermatitis describes the abnormal deposition of minerals or amyloid in the dermis or overproduction of mucin. Definitive diagnosis of depositional diseases usually requires a special stain (Fig. 4.7).

Clinical relevance. The most commonly recognised dysplastic skin disease is cutaneous asthenia (Ehlers–Danlos syndrome). Although the epidermis is normal, the dermal collagen is fragmented and disorganised. In some cases it may appear normal on light microscopy and either electron microscopy or special biochemical analysis of the collagen may be needed to make a definitive diagnosis. Feline skin fragility syndrome is another disease in which the skin is easily torn. It has been seen in cats with naturally occurring and iatrogenic hyperadrenocorticism, feline diabetes mellitus, or following excessive use of megestrol acetate/progestational compounds.

The recognised depositional dermatoses include calcinosis cutis, amyloidosis and cutaneous mucinosis. Calcium can be deposited in the skin via percutaneous or dystrophic mechanisms. The most common cause is associated with either iatrogenic or spontaneous hyperadrenocorticism. Cutaneous mucinosis is caused by an overproduction of mucin in the dermis. This is normal in the Shar Pei. Cutaneous amyloidosis is rare and usually accompanies cutaneous plasmacytomas.

Diseases of the Hair Follicles

Folliculitis, perifolliculitis and furunculosis

Folliculitis describes inflammation in the hair follicle. It is often accompanied by perifolliculitis which is an infiltrate around the hair follicle (Fig. 4.8). Many of the inflammatory cells in perifolliculitis have migrated from the superficial blood vessels

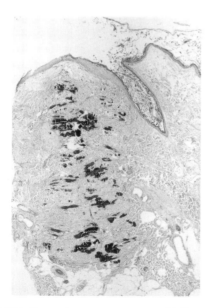

FIG. 4.7 This figure shows two patterns of inflammation — depositional dermatitis and atrophic hair follicles. The darkly stained material in the dermis is calcium (calcinosis cutis). The hair follicles and epidermis are atrophic. This is a biopsy from a dog with endogenous hyperadrenocorticism. Slide courtesy of Dr Maron Calderwood-Mays.

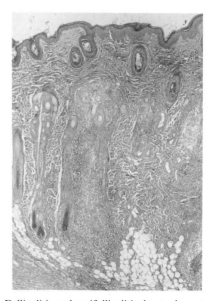

FIG. 4.8 Folliculitis and perifolliculitis due to dermatophytosis. Note the intense inflammatory reaction around the hair follicles. Slide courtesy of Dr Maron Calderwood-Mays.

and into the dermis so they can reach the hair follicle. Furunculosis describes a ruptured hair follicle. Folliculitis and furunculosis may be accompanied by pustular dermatitis and superficial perivascular dermatitis. Many of the diseases that cause folliculitis and furunculosis also affect the epidermis. Inflammatory cells migrate from the cutaneous blood vessels to either the epidermis, dermis and/or hair follicle. Furunculosis may be described as a nodular reaction because ruptured hair follicles surrounded by inflammatory cells appear nodular.

Clinical relevance. The agents most commonly causing folliculitis are bacteria, dermatophytes and demodicosis. Pathologists will not diagnose a fungal folliculitis unless they see spores or hyphae. Anagen hairs are most commonly affected. In contrast, bacterial folliculitis is more common in telogen hairs and bacteria are rare. For the clinician, it is important to recognise that if a pathogen is found it is significant; if it is not found, this does not eliminate a bacterial or fungal infection from the differential diagnosis. Bacterial folliculitis is more common in dogs and fungal folliculitis is most common in cats.

On occasion, pemphigus foliaceus may present with both a pustular and follicular pattern of inflammation. Acantholysis may occur in the follicular epithelium. Although sebaceous adenitis is a nodular reaction, some pathologists prefer to classify it as a perifollicular reaction because of it-s location in the sebaceous gland. The most common causes of furunculosis are bacterial pyoderma, pressure point pyoderma, interdigital pyoderma, dermatophytosis (also called a kerion) demodicosis and ruptured comedones (canine and feline acne).

Atrophic hair follicles

Atrophic hair follicles are those that have been arrested in their development and are smaller in size than expected. Most hair follicles are arrested in either telogen or catagen. The causes may be metabolic, nutritional or even inflammatory.

Clinical relevance. 'Atrophic hair follicles' is what every clinician wants to read on a biopsy report when skin from a dog with a suspected endocrinopathy is submitted. Hypothyroidism, hyperadrenocorticism, canine Sertoli cell tumours, hyperoestrogenism and growth hormone-responsive alopecias may all show atrophic hair follicles. The epidermis may or may not be thinner than expected; the epidermis in hypothyroidism and canine Sertoli cell tumours is often hyperplastic. In post-clipping alopecia and telogen effluvium hair, follicles may be of normal size but in telogen arrest. Other diseases with atrophic hair follicles include post-rabies vaccination alopecia, canine familial dermatomyositis, alopecia areata, scarring or cicatricial alopecia and canine traction alopecia. The hair follicles of feline psychogenic alopecia are normal.

Dystrophic (dysplastic) hair follicles

These are hairs and hair follicles that do not develop normally. The hair follicles may be enlarged or distorted. Abnormally clumped melanin may be present.

Clinical relevance. The clinical signs of dystrophic or dysplastic follicular diseases usually develop very slowly. Hair-loss and seborrhoea are common. The most notable diseases are colour dilute alopecia, black hair follicle dysplasia, canine follicular dysplasia, acquired pattern alopecia and congenital hypotrichosis.

Diseases of the Panniculus

Panniculitis

Panniculitis describes inflammation in either the septal or lobular areas of the subcutaneous fat. Depending upon the agent, inflammation may begin as a septal or lobular pattern and later become diffuse (Fig. 4.9).

Clinical relevance. There is a multitude of causes for inflammation of the subcutaneous fat. Clinically, it is most important to determine whether or not an infectious agent is present. Special stains and tissue for aerobic and anaerobic bacteria, deep fungi and atypical mycobacteria culture are necessary for answering this question. Causes of panniculitis include: trauma, foreign bodies, post-injection reactions, infectious agents, systemic lupus erythematosus, drug reactions, visceral malignancy,

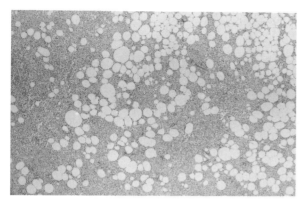

FIG. 4.9 Panniculitis. Note the diffuse infiltrate of cells in the panniculus. Slide courtesy of Dr Maron Calderwood-Mays.

feline pansteatitis, pancreatitis or pancreatic carcinomas, and some are idiopathic. Sterile idiopathic panniculitis is one of the most commonly encountered forms of panniculitis and it is managed with glucocorticoids. However, it is clinically indistinguishable from the other aetiologies and so an aggressive diagnostic evaluation is necessary.

Acknowledgements

The authors would like to thank Dr Maron Calderwood-Mays for her valuable editorial comments. The authors would also like to acknowledge Drs Thelma Gross, Peter Ihrke and Emily Walder for their influence on this chapter; the classification scheme used in this chapter and much of the material presented here are summarised from their book, *Veterinary Dermatopathology: A Macroscopic and Microscopic Evaluation of Canine and Feline Skin Disease*, Masby Year Book.

II Problem-Oriented Approach to Skin Diseases of Dogs

5

Pruritus

IAN MASON

Pruritus is one of the most common reasons for which clients present dogs to the veterinarian. Pruritus, or itch, is defined as an unpleasant sensation of the skin which provokes the desire to scratch. It has a number of causes and treatment can only be instituted once a specific diagnosis has been made. Common causes of canine pruritus are shown in Fig. 5.1.

In order to determine the underlying cause of pruritus, the methodical approach detailed in *Chapter 2* must be applied. Important diagnostic clues may be obtained from the history and physical examination, so narrowing the differential diagnosis and enabling the clinician to rank the likely causes. Figures 5.2 and 5.3 show examples of aspects of the history and physical examination which may eliminate possible causes or increase the index of suspicion that a certain disease is involved. However, the contents of these figures should be regarded as guidelines only, as exceptions will occur. Figures 5.4 and 5.5 illustrate a suggested diagnostic approach for canine pruritus.

Pyoderma is a secondary disorder in the dog and may occur as a complicating factor in any of the disorders listed in Fig. 5.1, thus initiating or exacerbating pruritus. The management of pruritic disorders associated with or complicated by pyoderma is complex. An approach to such situations is presented in Fig. 5.6. Pyoderma is discussed more fully in *Chapter 10*.

Canine Skin Diseases Primarily Associated with Pruritus

Hypersensitivity

Flea allergic dermatitis

Description. Flea allergic dermatitis (**FAD**) is arguably the most common disorder encountered in small animal medicine. The species of flea most frequently associated with skin disease in dogs is *Ctenocephalides felis felis*. Pruritus results from a hypersensitivity reaction following binding of haptens in flea saliva with dermal collagen. The immunology of this disorder is complex and the reader is referred to the bibliography for more information.

FAD can affect virtually any adult dog. It may be seasonal (many cases start in late summer and early autumn) but can occur at any time of year in some geographical regions. Dogs that are intermittently exposed to fleas or that move from a cold (flea-scarce) area to a warmer climate are at most risk. Affected individuals may have a history of infestation with the tapeworm *Dipylidium caninum*, as the flea is the intermediate host of this parasite. Affected animals are often kept with other pets, especially free-ranging cats; in-contact animals may be lesion-free.

Clinical signs. FAD is characterised by moderate to severe pruritus leading to hair-loss, excoriation, hyperpigmentation and scale. Secondary pyoderma

DIFFERENTIAL DIAGNOSIS OF CANINE PRURITUS	
Hypersensitivity (allergy)	Flea-bite hypersensitivity Atopic dermatitis Food intolerance/hypersensitivity Contact hypersensitivity Insect hypersensitivity
Ectoparasitism	*Sarcoptes scabiei* infestation *Cheyletiella* spp. infestation Pediculosis Trombiculidiasis Otoacariasis (*Chapter 27*) Demodicosis (*Chapter 6*)
Infectious causes	Pyoderma (*Chapter 10*) Dermatophytosis (*Chapter 7*) *Malassezia pachydermatis* dermatitis
Miscellaneous causes	Neoplasia (mycosis fungoides / epitheliotropic lymphoma) Contact irritant dermatitis Pyotraumatic dermatitis ('hot spots'; 'wet eczema')

FIG. 5.1 Differential diagnosis of canine pruritus.

often complicates the clinical picture and leads to papule, pustule, scale, crust and epidermal collarette formation. Lesions predominantly affect the dorsal rear quadrant (rump, dorsal lumbar-sacral area and lateral/caudal thighs). Lesions of pyoderma may affect these sites as well as the skin of the ventral abdomen and medial thighs.

Diagnosis. Presence of fleas or flea excrement within material brushed from the coat along with appropriate clinical signs is highly suggestive. Positive reaction to intradermal injection of flea extract

FIG. 5.2 Approach to canine pruritus: History.

APPROACH TO CANINE PRURITUS: HISTORY	
Factor	**Differential diagnosis**
Breed	
Terriers, Labrador and Golden Retrievers, German Shepherd Dog	Atopic dermatitis
Cocker Spaniel, West Highland White Terrier, Miniature Poodle	*Malassezia* dermatitis
West Highland White Terrier, Scottish Terrier	Demodicosis
Age of onset	
Less than 6 months	Ectoparasitism; food intolerance
6 months to 3 years	Atopic dermatitis; demodicosis
More than 5 years	Metabolic/endocrine disease leading to pyoderma
Seasonal pruritus	Atopic dermatitis; flea allergy; trombiculidiasis; biting flies
Pedal/facial pruritus	Atopic dermatitis
Contagion (to people or other animals)	Ectoparasitism; dermatophytosis; fleas
Exposure to wildlife (foxes, hedgehogs, rodents)	*Sarcoptes scabiei* infestation; flea allergy; dermatophytosis
Gastroenteric signs	Food intolerance

FIG. 5.3 Approach to canine pruritus: Physical examination.

APPROACH TO CANINE PRURITUS: PHYSICAL EXAMINATION	
Physical finding	**Differential diagnosis**
Distribution of lesions	
Dorsal rear quadrant	Flea allergic dermatitis
Elbows and pinnae	*Sarcoptes scabiei* infestation
Feet, carpal flexures, face	Atopic dermatitis
Dorsum	*Cheyletiella* infestation
Nature of lesions	
Papules	Pyoderma; *Sarcoptes scabiei* infestation; other ectoparasites; hypersensitivity
Pustules	Pyoderma; demodicosis; pemphigus foliaceus
Follicular plugs/casts	Pyoderma; demodicosis; dermatophytosis; keratinisation disorders ('seborrhoea')
No lesions	Atopy; food intolerance/allergy
Otitis externa	Atopic dermatitis; food allergy; *Malassezia* dermatitis
Conjunctivitis	Atopic dermatitis

FIG. 5.4 Diagnostic plan for canine pruritus.

DIAGNOSTIC PLAN FOR CANINE PRURITUS
1. Rule out ectoparasitism
Focused diagnostic tests: Microscopy of skin scrapings, hair pluckings and coat brushings, flea eradication, trial acaricidal therapy
If no ectoparasites present and no response to flea eradication:
2. Evaluate role of bacterial infection — antibacterial therapy (Fig. 5.6) **3. Investigate allergic skin disease**
Focused diagnostic tests: Flea: Rigorous flea eradication, intradermal test with flea extract; Food: Restriction diet; Atopy: Intradermal skin test
4. If no diagnosis achieved
Further tests: Biopsy; fungal culture; long-term symptomatic therapy

indicates that hypersensitivity is present, although it should be noted that false-negatives are very common. Complete resolution of pruritus following appropriate flea eradication may be impossible to achieve during very warm, humid times of the year.

Treatment. Flea control is discussed in detail in *Chapter 30*.

Prognosis. The prognosis is excellent provided that flea control remains in force. There is some

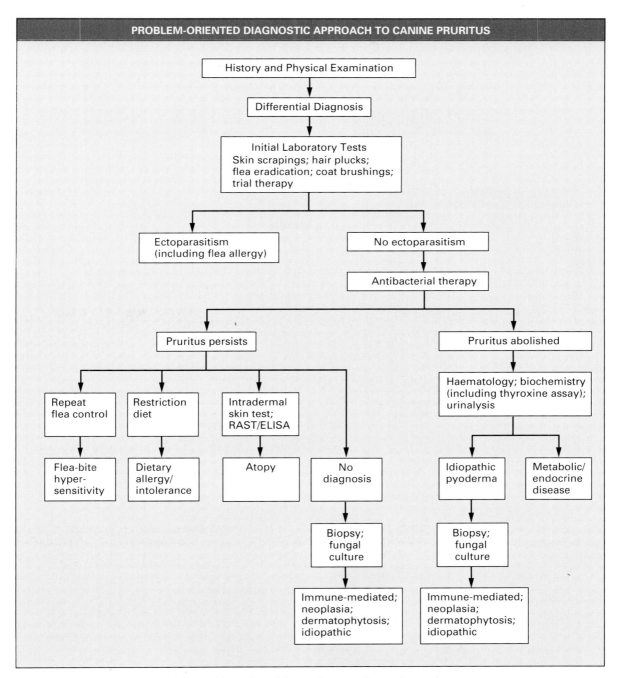

FIG. 5.5 Problem-oriented diagnostic approach to canine pruritus.

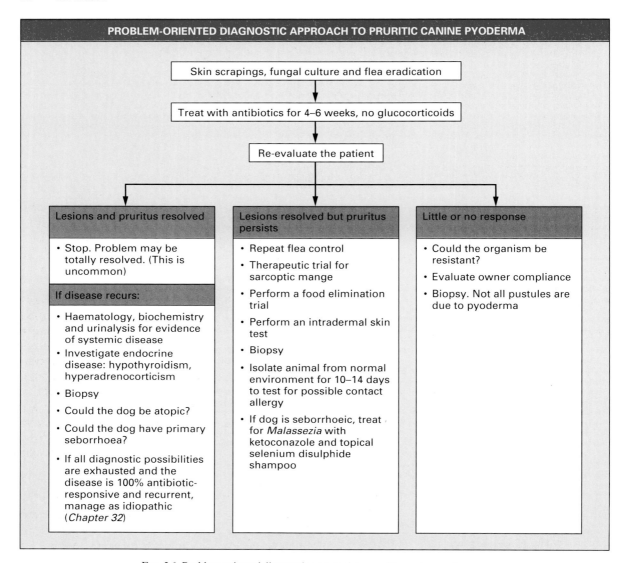

FIG. 5.6 Problem-oriented diagnostic approach to pruritic canine pyoderma.

evidence to suggest that dogs which are continually exposed to fleas may become tolerant. This occurs most commonly in dogs that were exposed to fleas early in life.

Atopic dermatitis

Description. Atopic dermatitis is defined as an inherited predisposition to produce reaginic antibody to inhaled (or possibly percutaneously absorbed) environmental allergens. In sensitised individuals, exposure to these allergens results in disease. The pathogenesis of this complex disease is poorly understood; it involves abnormalities of immunoglobulin production, aberrant T-lymphocyte regulation and possible impaired metabolism of *n*6 series fatty acids. (Readers are referred to the bibliography for further details.) Allergens that are implicated include: house dust; house-dust mites (*Dermatophagoides farinae* and *Dermatophagoides pteronyssinus*); human dander (or shed skin scale); animal dander; pollens from grasses, trees and other plants; fungi; moulds; and feathers. Secondary pyoderma is an almost inevitable complication.

CLINICAL DIAGNOSTIC CRITERIA FOR CANINE ATOPIC DERMATITIS	
Major diagnostic signs	**Minor diagnostic signs**
Pruritus	Onset of symptoms before 3 years of age
Typical morphology and distribution (i) facial and/or digital involvement; or (ii) lichenification of the flexor surface of the tarsal joint and/or the extensor surface of the carpel joint	Facial erythema and cheilitis
	Bilateral conjunctivitis
	Superficial staphylococcal pyoderma
Chronic or chronically relapsing dermatitis	
Family history of atophy and/or the presence of a breed predisposition	
Adapted from: Willemse, T. (1985) Atopic skin disease: A review and a reconsideration of diagnostic criteria. *Journal of Small Animal Practice* **27**, 771–778.	

FIG. 5.7 Clinical diagnostic criteria for canine atopic dermatitis.

Clinical signs. Although most breeds can be affected, some are predisposed to the development of this disorder. Examples include terriers, Labrador and Golden Retrievers, German Shepherd Dogs and English Setters (Fig. 5.8). Most cases occur at between 1 and 3 years of age (range: 6 months to 6 years). The problem may be seasonal at first but most cases either begin as, or become, perennial. This is said to be because affected dogs can expand the range of allergens to which they are hypersensitive.

The pruritus typically affects the feet, face, ventral abdomen and axillae. Occasionally no lesions or mild erythema will be present but in advanced cases lesions due to self-trauma (saliva stains on hairs, excoriation, hair-loss, hyperpigmentation,

lichenification) and pyoderma (papules, pustules, epidermal collarettes, scale) will be observed. Concomitant otitis externa and conjunctivitis may be a feature. In some dogs, recurrent pyoderma is the only sign.

Diagnosis. A clinical diagnosis of atopic dermatitis can be inferred on clinical grounds according to the criteria given in Fig. 5.7, provided that other causes of pruritus (flea-bite hypersensitivity, ectoparasitism, food allergy) have been eliminated from the differential diagnosis. However, it is preferable to perform some form of immunological testing in order both to confirm the diagnosis and to identify the causal allergens. This information may be of value in the clinical management of the case, allowing the formulation of a hyposensitisation vaccine or enabling allergen avoidance.

Treatment. The management of atopic dermatitis involves long-term use of a combination of measures including allergen avoidance, reduction of flare factors (such as staphylococcal pyoderma and flea infestation) and the use of medicaments to manipulate immune function. Hyposensitisation therapy using vaccines is helpful in some instances. The management of allergic skin disease is discussed in detail in *Chapter 31*.

Prognosis. Atopic dermatitis is incurable and requires lifelong management. The prognosis varies between cases. Inexpensive, convenient and safe treatment regimens will often control the problem in dogs with seasonal pruritus. However, in those with non-seasonal signs a combination of glucocorticoids, non-steroidal agents and immunotherapy is needed to control the clinical signs. Such therapy may be costly and time-consuming.

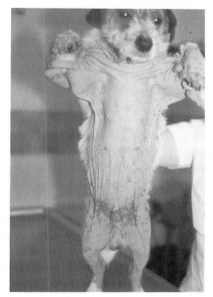

FIG. 5.8 Extensive, erythematous, pruritic alopecia affecting the entire ventrum of a Jack Russell Terrier with atopy. Slide courtesy of Richard Harvey.

Food intolerance/hypersensitivity

Description. Cutaneous reactions to food are uncommon in dogs. The pathogenic mechanisms are unknown and it has been suggested that this disorder may arise from true hypersensitivity to nutrients and food additives, or via non-immunological toxic, idiosyncratic or pharmacological processes. Individual cases may arise due to any one of these mechanisms. It is for this reason that the term 'intolerance' rather than 'allergy' should be applied to reactions to food. *In vitro* measurement of serum-specific antinutrient IgE concentrations is of no value in the diagnosis of this condition as it is extremely unlikely, even in cases due to hypersensitivity, that this disorder is mediated by IgE.

Clinical signs. Any breed can be affected at any age, although most surveys indicate that most dogs develop clinical signs as young adults. The pruritus is non-seasonal. **It is a popular misconception that food allergy occurs soon after a change of diet. Sensitisation may occur rapidly but is just as likely to occur months or years after a new food is introduced.** The clinical signs are usually pruritus and self-trauma leading to excoriation, alopecia, scale and crust. Secondary pyoderma is a complicating factor. Papules, pustules, oedema and erythema may be seen but it is unclear whether these are due to the primary disease or to secondary changes. Pruritus may be generalised or regional. Occasionally pruritus is absent and some cases present simply with otitis externa or recurrent superficial pyoderma.

Diagnosis. The diagnosis of this disorder is discussed in detail in *Chapter 3*. *In vitro* testing is of no value and the only means of diagnosing food intolerance is to feed a restricted diet based on a single, novel protein sources for at least 6 weeks. A clinical improvement is suggestive of this diagnosis; provocative challenge with the original diet is confirmatory.

Treatment. A balanced diet which has been shown not to elicit dermatological signs should be fed indefinitely.

Prognosis. The prognosis is excellent provided that other hypersensitivities do not develop. It is theoretically possible that dogs may develop hypersensitivity to the restricted diet and there have been reports of dogs with this disorder subsequently developing atopy.

Allergic contact dermatitis

Description. Contact allergy is a rare disorder in dogs. This is in contrast to people, in whom contact hypersensitivity is rather more common. The hair coat of animals limits exposure to potential allergens and haptens. In addition, the management of most dogs does not involve direct contact with cosmetics, contact-lens solutions, sun-screens, shaving foams, jewellery and synthetic fabrics.

Pruritus results from delayed hypersensitivity and affects the area or areas in contact with the source of allergen. Allergens include shampoos, soaps, topical medicaments (especially those containing antibiotics), insecticides and disinfectants. A common drug hypersensitivity in humans and other animals is to the antibiotic neomycin. Occasionally the topical treatment of otitis externa with this drug is associated in dogs with worsening of the condition. One possible explanation of this is that contact hypersensitivity has developed.

Materials involved in the manufacture of carpets and other floor coverings (wool, nylon fibre, wooden decking, rubber, plastics, dyes and mordants) may also lead to contact hypersensitivity. However, a recent change of flooring material or carpet is not indicative that contact allergy is involved; usually a prolonged period of exposure to a contactant is needed before sensitisation occurs. Moreover, most carpets are manufactured from similar materials and so it is extremely unlikely that a new carpet would be more immunogenic than any other carpet.

This condition should be distinguished from primary irritant dermatitis (see below). Allergic contact dermatitis affects only sensitised individuals, whereas irritant dermatitis affects all individuals exposed to a substance (provided that they are exposed to it at a sufficiently high concentration). Irritant dermatitis is much more common than allergic contact dermatitis.

Clinical signs. Dogs of any age, breed or sex can be affected. Pruritus, erythema and self-trauma affect contact areas; these are usually the extremities or the relatively hairless ventral abdomen. The disorder may be present throughout the year, but the signs may be seasonal if the dog is managed differently at different times of the year.

The clinical signs include erythema, alopecia, papules, macules, self-trauma and secondary pyoderma.

Diagnosis. Definitive diagnosis is difficult. History and physical examination may yield some clues as to the causal allergen. Elimination of the allergen from the animal's environment for up to 2 weeks should lead to resolution of the clinical signs; re-exposure should lead to recurrence. Contact hypersensitivity is a delayed phenomenon and so recurrence of signs will not occur until 48 hours after re-exposure. If a carpet allergy is suspected, the animal should be confined in an uncarpeted room such as a kitchen; if grass allergy is suspected, the dog should be confined indoors and only walked on a lead on roads or paved walkways. To establish a diagnosis in this way requires considerable dedication on the part of the owner.

Patch-testing, an alternative diagnostic method, is discussed in detail in *Chapter 3*.

Treatment. Prevent access of the affected dog to the substances which have been shown to elicit skin disease.

Prognosis. The prognosis varies. It is not always possible to identify and permanently exclude access to causal allergens.

Primary contact irritant dermatitis

Irritant dermatitis is very similar to allergic contact dermatitis but is much more common. Causal agents include cement dust, freshly laid cement, plaster dust, any acid or caustic substances. Some soaps and detergents may be irritant and there may be variation between individuals regarding the concentration of such substances required to initiate skin disease. History, clinical signs, treatment and prognosis are similar to those for allergic contact dermatitis, although more than one animal in a household may be affected with irritant dermatitis. **Diagnosis** of this condition, with elimination of suspected causal substance and subsequent provocative exposure, is similar to that in contact allergy but recurrence of signs is usually immediate. Patch-

testing is not a suitable technique for the diagnosis of irritant dermatitis.

Insect reactions

Description. Skin reactions to insects are commonly encountered in humans and other animals. Insect reactions result from hypersensitivity or from insect toxins. Flea-allergy dermatitis is an extremely common disorder in small animals and, in the UK, atopy in dogs is most commonly associated with positive intradermal skin test reactions to house-dust mite antigens. Atopy and flea-allergy dermatitis have been considered in detail earlier in this chapter. Other forms of insect-induced skin disease are less well documented but may be more common than is currently suspected. Examples of insect-related skin disease include bee and wasp stings, flea and mosquito bites, and harvest mite infestation (trombiculidiasis).

Clinical features. Insect reactions vary depending on the insect involved, the route of exposure to the allergen or toxin (percutaneous if a bite or sting is involved; via the respiratory tract in atopy) and the immunological status of the host (i.e. whether there has been prior sensitisation).

Bee stings, for example, are usually severe, painful, localised, swollen and sudden in onset. Typically they occur in the summer. Theoretically anaphylaxis is possible in sensitised hosts. Fly- and mosquito-bites may be seasonal and may be local and papular in non-sensitised animals. Pruritus may be present: in sensitised individuals it may be severe and associated with urticaria.

Insect reactions commonly involve areas with sparse or short hairs such as the dorsum of the muzzle, pinnae, ventral abdomen and distal extremities.

Diagnosis. Clearly, history may give important clues that an insect-induced disorder is present. Diagnosis is usually based on elimination of other disorders from the differential diagnosis and on circumstantial evidence. An eosinophilic perivascular dermatitis on histopathology may be supportive evidence that a skin problem is insect-related.

Treatment. Management of insect-induced skin disease varies with the insect involved and the animal's reaction to that insect. Exposure may be prevented by the use of insect repellents and confinement of animals during periods of insect activity (usually dusk and dawn). Topical and systemic antihistamine and glucocorticoid therapy may be required in severe cases.

Prognosis. The prognosis varies with the insects involved, the geographical region and the animal's sensitivity. In some instances anaphylaxis and death may occur.

Ectoparasitism

Sarcoptic mange

Sarcoptic mange, or scabies, is a highly pruritic contagious disorder of dogs and other Canidae. Transient pruritic human lesions may occur. *Sarcoptes scabiei* infestation is by direct contact, though anecdotal evidence indicates that contact with faeces from infested foxes and indirect sources of infestation such as grooming instruments and kennels may be involved in the transmission of this parasite.

History. Severe pruritus and self-trauma, usually affecting the pinnae, elbows and extremities, are typical. Often owners will complain of unexplained pruritus of their own skin or that of a family member. Other dogs in contact with the affected animal may also be pruritic. Anti-inflammatory or even higher doses of glucocorticoids often fail to control pruritus and this is a significant diagnostic pointer towards this disease.

Clinical signs. Papules and crusts especially affect the elbows, pinnae, brisket and limbs. Rubbing the pinnae between forefinger and thumb frequently elicits a scratch reflex if lesions are present at this site. Chronic cases have generalised, hyperpigmented, lichenified lesions with a disagreeable odour (see Plates 2 and 3).

Diagnosis. Diagnosis is based on history, physical examination and microscopy of skin scrapings from papular lesions. In most instances parasites, eggs or mite faeces will be detected provided that a diligent search has been made for them. In some cases a therapeutic trial may be required, provided that the clinical signs and history are compatible with this diagnosis and that skin scrapings have been taken and examined.

Treatment. Detailed information on the treatment of ectoparasitic disorders is given in *Chapter 30*. In the UK only phosmet is licensed for this disease; in the USA, both phosmet and lime sulphur are approved. It is recommended that these products be 'sponged on' and the animal then allowed to dry, without rinsing. Other (unlicensed) products include amitraz and ivermectin.

Long-haired dogs should be clipped prior to therapy and the insecticidal agent should be used strictly as recommended by the manufacturer. There is a case for administration of a short (5–7 day) course of glucocorticoids. Longer courses may give an erroneously optimistic impression regarding progress, which may be particularly misleading if parasites were not detected and trial therapy is being used. The dog's environment should be treated with a suitable insecticide. All dogs in contact with the affected animal should also be treated. In some instances it may be better for the clinician to arrange that the animal is treated in the veterinary clinic by trained staff.

Prognosis. The prognosis for canine scabies is excellent provided that the treatment is administered correctly, that re-infestation does not occur and that the dog does not have another skin disease concomitantly.

Cheyletiellosis

Infestation of dogs with the surface parasites of the genus *Cheyletiella* may lead to pruritus, but these vary in intensity and some dogs may only present with scaling (*Chapter 7*), which is often particularly noticeable. Three parasites may be involved: *C. yasguri*, *C. parasitivorax* and *C. blakei*.

History. Cheyletiellosis is most commonly seen in puppies, especially those from pet shops or breeding establishments. However, dogs are susceptible at any age. Owners may suffer from pruritus and papular eruptions, as this parasite can feed on humans.

Clinical signs. The clinical picture of canine cheyletiellosis is one of variable pruritus and scale; the latter may be particularly evident. Papules are usually present.

Diagnosis. A number of diagnostic techniques have been described, involving microscopy of material from the skin and coat. In some instances, it may be difficult to find the parasites and so it is recommended that the following samples are taken for examination: acetate tape preparations, skin scrapings, hair combings and hair plucks (*Chapter 3*).

Treatment. The treatment of this disease is discussed in detail in *Chapter 30*. In the UK, the only product licensed for the treatment of this disease is selenium sulphide 1%. Three shampoos, each a week apart, are recommended. Other (unlicensed) products include phosmet, amitraz and ivermectin. The dog's environment should be treated with a suitable insecticide. All dogs and cats in contact with the affected animal should be treated. Asymptomatic carrier status may occur.

Prognosis. The prognosis is excellent.

Pediculosis

Lice infestation is known as pediculosis. Lice are host-specific and do not survive for more than a few days in the environment. They can be classified as biting (suborder Mallophaga) or sucking (suborder Anoplura). Species found on the dog include *Trichodectes canis* (biting) and *Linognathus setosus* (sucking). In warm climates, *Heterodoxus spiniger* may be associated with skin disease in dogs.

History. Pediculosis may occur in poorly managed dogs. Overcrowding, dirty kennels and lack of grooming may predispose to this disorder. Old and debilitated animals may be affected.

Clinical signs. The clinical features of pediculosis are variable and infested dogs may be symptomless carriers. Pruritus may be present to a variable degree and scaling may be a feature. Lesions similar to those seen in flea-bite hypersensitivity may be present. Heavy infestations may lead to anaemia.

Diagnosis. Pediculosis may be diagnosed by detection of the parasite in examination of the hairs, preferably with a magnifying lens. Microscopy is needed in order to identify the species involved.

Treatment. Lice are susceptible to most insecticides and antiparasitic shampoos are the treatment of choice. Two or three treatments 10 days apart are recommended. The environment should be treated with a suitable insecticidal agent. Reinfestation may occur unless management is improved.

Prognosis. The prognosis is excellent.

Trombiculidiasis

Infestation with harvest mites, or 'chiggers' is termed trombiculidiasis. In the UK the most common species involved is *Neotrombicula autumnalis*; *Eutrombicula alfreddugesi* may be found in the USA. It is the larvae that are parasitic; the adults live in decaying organic matter.

History. Sudden-onset, moderate to severe pedal pruritus is commonly seen. Harvest-mite larvae only emerge in late summer and autumn and so the disease is only seen at that time of year. It is most prevalent in areas with chalky soil.

Clinical signs. The clinical features are pedal pruritus and saliva staining of feet.

Diagnosis. Trombiculid mites may be seen with the naked eye as bright orange dots between the toes and on the feet, legs and pinnae (especially Henry's pocket). They may be collected by skin scraping. Microscopy confirms the diagnosis.

Treatment. Antiparasitic shampoos are effective but reinfestation may occur. This may be prevented by avoidance of grassland and woods during the appropriate season. If this is not practical, some form of persistent parasiticidal agent is needed (this is one of the few uses for flea collars).

Prognosis. The prognosis is excellent, though the disease may recur the following year.

6

Alopecia

KAREN MORIELLO

Alopecia is defined as the loss of hair from areas of the body in which a normal hair coat is expected. (**Hypotrichosis**, another term that may be used to describe hair-loss or alopecia, is defined as less than the normal amount of hair and is best reserved to describe congenital hair-loss. For the sake of clarity and simplicity, the use of this term will be avoided.)

> The most common cause of hair-loss in the dog is pruritus. If your patient presents with hair-loss and a significant degree of pruritus, the pruritus should be investigated first.

Selected Diseases Associated with Hair-loss in the Dog

Demodicosis

Description. Demodicosis is a parasitic skin disease of dogs. The *Demodex* mite is present normally in the hair follicle and sebaceous glands of dogs and it is believed that the mite is transmitted from the bitch to the puppy in the first few days of life. In the vast majority of dogs, the mite causes no clinical disease. In a small proportion of dogs, the mite proliferates in the hair follicle and sebaceous glands and causes hair-loss, pruritus, scaling, and inflammation, and predisposes the dog to secondary superficial and deep pyodermas. The cause of the proliferation is unknown but it is believed to be due to a local defect in the immune system of the skin.

Clinical signs. There are three clinical syndromes associated with demodicosis in dogs. The first is **localised demodicosis**, which is characterised by focal areas of hair-loss with any combination of erythema, scaling, pruritus, and superficial pyoderma. This disease is called localised demodicosis because mites are found only in the affected area.

This form is most common in puppies. The second clinical presentation is **generalised demodicosis**. Approximately 10% of dogs with localised demodicosis will develop generalised demodicosis. This form of the disease is manifested by any combination of widespread hair-loss, superficial and deep pyoderma, seborrhoea, odour and pruritus. This form is called generalised demodicosis because the lesions are present over the entire body and mites are found in both clinically affected and normal-appearing skin. The third clinical presentation of demodicosis is **adult-onset demodicosis**. In this form, demodicosis develops in adult dogs with no known history of the disease. This form is a cutaneous marker of systemic disease; a thorough search should be made for an underlying disease, e.g. hyperadrenocorticism, iatrogenic hypercortisolism, hypothyroidism or neoplasia.

DIFFERENTIAL DIAGNOSIS OF ALOPECIA IN THE DOG	
Localised lesions	Demodicosis Dermatophytosis Alopecia areata Steroid injection/vaccine vasculitis Post-clipping alopecia Cicatricial alopecia Traction alopecia
Multifocal or diffuse patchy hair-loss	Demodicosis Dermatophytosis Superficial pyoderma Keratinisation defects Sebaceous adenitis Colour dilute alopecia Follicular dysplasia Dermatomyositis
Symmetrical or diffuse alopecia	Demodicosis Dermatophytosis Superficial pyoderma Hypothyroidism Hyperadrenocorticism Sex hormone disorder Pattern baldness, follicular dysplasia Congenital alopecia Telogen effluvium/anagen defluxion Colour dilute alopecia Epitheliotropic lymphoma

FIG. 6.1 Differential diagnosis of alopecia in the dog.

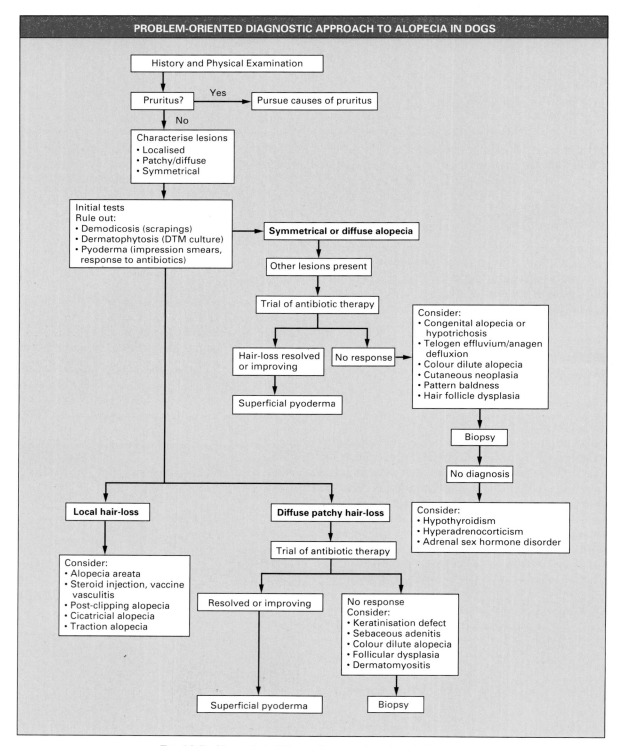

FIG. 6.2 Problem-oriented diagnostic approach to alopecia in dogs.

Diagnosis. Demodicosis is diagnosed by deep skin scrapings. Several skin scrapings should be performed to rule this differential diagnosis in or out.

Treatment. The various treatment strategies for demodicosis are described in *Chapter 30*. If a concurrent pyoderma is present see *Chapter 30*.

Prognosis. The prognosis for localised demodicosis is usually good. The prognosis for generalised and adult-onset demodicosis is less favourable and the owner should be warned that there is a strong likelihood that the dog may not be cured and many dogs will require lifelong therapy to maintain a good quality of life. There is a genetic predisposition for dogs to develop generalised demodicosis. These animals should not be bred. Owners should seriously consider euthanasia if the dog was purchased as a breeding animal, working animal (hunting dog or guide/hearing aid dog) or if the dog's temperament is poor.

APPROACH TO THE PATIENT WITH ALOPECIA: HISTORY	
Factor	**Differential diagnosis**
Presence of pruritus	Pruritic skin diseases (see *Chapter 5*) Superficial pyoderma
Age of onset Less than 1 year	Demodicosis; dermatophytosis; superficial pyoderma; congenital alopecia
Sex Intact females	Sex hormone dysfunction; postpartum alopecia/telogen effluvium
Intact males	Testicular tumours; sex hormone dysfunction
Acute onset	Anagen defluxion; inflammatory skin diseases such as superficial pyoderma
Slow or gradual onset	Endocrine alopecias; follicular dysplasias; bacteria pyodermas; dermatophytosis; demodicosis
Weight gain or distended abdomen	Hypothyroidism; hyperadrenocorticism
Lack of hair regrowth post-clipping	Hypothyroidism; post-clipping alopecia
Polyuria, polydipsia	Hyperadrenocorticism

FIG. 6.3 Approach to the patient with alopecia: History.

APPROACH TO THE PATIENT WITH ALOPECIA: PHYSICAL EXAMINATION	
Physical finding	**Differential diagnosis**
Solitary lesion without inflammation	Alopecia areata; steroid injection; vaccine vasculitis; cicatricial alopecia
Solitary lesion in previous site of ribbon or hairbow	Traction alopecia
Solitary inflammatory lesion	Demodicosis; dermatophytosis; bacterial pyoderma
Multifocal/patchy alopecia with or without scaling	Superficial pyoderma; dermatophytosis; demodicosis; sebaceous adenitis; follicular dysplasia; keratinisation defect
Diffuse alopecia with papules/pustules	Superficial pyoderma; demodicosis; dermatophytosis; colour dilution alopecia
Diffuse alopecia without marked lesions	Endocrine dermatoses; colour dilution alopecia; acquired alopecia; pattern alopecia; congenital alopecia
Diffuse alopecia with marked scaling	Hypothyroidism; Sertoli cell tumour; dermatophytosis; keratinisation defects; colour dilution alopecia
Weight gain or distended abdomen	Hypothyroidism; hyperadrenocorticism
Thin skin and/or comedones	Hyperadrenocorticism

FIG. 6.4 Approach to the patient with alopecia: Physical examination.

Dermatophytosis

Description. Dermatophytosis in dogs is caused most commonly by *Microsporum canis*, *M. gypseum*, and *Trichophyton* spp. It is most common in young dogs, dogs from animal shelters or dogs that are debilitated.

Clinical signs. Dermatophyte infections in dogs are uncommon. Dermatophytosis in dogs may present with a variety of follicularly-oriented signs including variable degrees of hair-loss, scaling and papules and variable pruritus. In contrast to cats, dogs are much more likely to have circular hair-loss areas of 'ringworm lesions'. These lesions may appear identical to lesions of bacterial pyoderma; however, bacterial pyoderma is much more common.

Diagnosis. Definitive diagnosis requires demonstration of the organism via direct examination of hair and scale, fungal culture or skin biopsy. Dermatophytosis cannot be diagnosed on the basis of clinical signs alone. Bacterial pyodermas are commonly misdiagnosed as dermatophytosis.

Treatment. See *Chapter 32*.

Prognosis. The prognosis is excellent. This disease is also a zoonosis.

Alopecia areata

Description. This is a rare skin disease of dogs and is characterised by non-inflammatory hair-loss. It is believed to be caused by an immune attack against hair follicles.

Clinical signs. Alopecia areata is characterised by focal or multifocal areas of well-circumscribed hair-loss. Inflammation is absent. The lesions may enlarge circumferentially and may be confined to one colour of hair. Lesions are most commonly seen on the head and neck of dogs (Fig. 6.5).

Diagnosis. Presumptive diagnosis is made by ruling out dermatophytosis and demodicosis and by compatible histological findings on skin biopsy. Hair follicles are short and deformed and most are in telogen. In early lesions, lymphocytes, macrophages and some neutrophils may be oriented

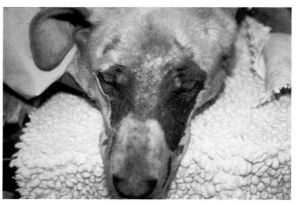

FIG. 6.5 Alopecia areata in a dog.

toward the hair follicle bulb. Older lesions may not show these findings and the diagnosis is more difficult to make.

Treatment. There is no known effective treatment. There are anecdotal reports of dogs responding to topical or intralesional glucocorticoids. The lesions may spontaneously regrow hair. The new hairs may be lighter than normal (leucotrichia).

Prognosis. This disease is not life-threatening and poses no health risk to the dog. The prognosis for hair regrowth is guarded.

Cicatricial alopecia

Description. Cicatricial alopecia is also known as scarring alopecia. It results from permanent hair follicle damage. Potential causes of cicatricial alopecia include physical, chemical or thermal burns; and also severe furunculosis, neoplasia, juvenile cellulitis, lupus or dermatomyositis. In these diseases the hair follicle is permanently destroyed and hair regrowth is not possible.

Clinical signs. Cicatricial alopecia occurs in an area of previous trauma or inflammation. The skin may appear scarred and striae may be visible. The skin may be hyper- or hypopigmented and contracted.

Diagnosis. Definitive diagnosis requires skin biopsy. It is recommended that a skin biopsy is taken from the area of skin with lost hair; it shows total loss of follicles and subepidermal fibrosis.

DIAGNOSTIC PLAN FOR ALOPECIA

At the initial visit, when presented with a dog with the problem of hair-loss, it is important to determine whether the dog is pruritic:
1. *If pruritus is a significant component* of the history or physical examination, the diagnostic plan for pruritus described in *Chapter 5* should be pursued
2. *If pruritus is absent or minimal,* the most representative pattern of the hair-loss is then determined (localised, diffuse/patchy, symmetrical or diffuse)

Localised Alopecia

1. *If the area of hair-loss is focal,* demodicosis and dermatophytosis must be considered. This is especially important in puppies and young dogs

Focused diagnostic tests: Skin scrapings for demodicosis and a dermatophyte culture. Because dermatophytosis is uncommon in dogs, it is most cost-effective to perform a dermatophyte culture in young patients or when the lesion has obvious scaling or broken hairs present. Dermatophytosis should be considered more seriously if the dog has recently been acquired from an animal shelter

2. *If the skin scrapings and fungal culture are negative* (or dermatophytosis is not seriously contemplated), consider hair follicle destruction, damage or telogen arrest. Localised areas of steroid atrophy of hair follicles can occur where subcutaneous glucocorticoids have been administered. In rare cases, a vaccine-induced vasculitis develops at the site of a vaccination injection. Traction alopecia develops in the area where decorative hair ribbons, bows, rubber bands or ornaments have been placed

Focused diagnostic test: A skin biopsy is necessary for a definitive or presumptive diagnosis of the above-mentioned conditions

Multifocal or Patchy Hair-loss

1. A multifocal or patchy distribution of hair-loss is most characteristic of bacterial pyoderma, demodicosis or dermatophytosis

Focused diagnostic tests: Skin scrapings are required to rule out demodicosis. A dermatophyte culture should be performed if the patient is young or debilitated, if hairs in the area of the lesions are broken or frayed, or if the hairs are Wood's-lamp positive

2. *If skin scrapings and the dermatophyte culture are negative,* or if dermatophytosis is not considered, a superficial bacterial pyoderma should strongly be considered

Focused diagnostic tests: A therapeutic trial of oral antibiotics and topical antibacterial shampoos for 21 days is necessary to rule out a bacterial pyoderma (see *Section VI*)

3. The patient should be re-examined at the end of the 21-day treatment to evaluate the response to therapy. *If there is a marked improvement and hair regrowth is obvious,* the problem was a superficial pyoderma. (Some cases of short-coat folliculitis may require more than 21 days of therapy before significant growth of hair is evident; therapy should be individualised for the patient. In these cases, however, the owner invariably reports that new hair-loss has ceased.) Therapy should be continued for at least 1 week post clinical cure; as a rule of thumb the author usually plans to treat superficial pyoderma for at least 21 days with a mean treatment time of 30 days. If there has been no improvement disorders of keratinisation, hair follicle growth or dermatophytosis should be considered

Focused diagnostic tests: A skin biopsy is necessary for a definitive diagnosis. Several representative skin biopsies should be submitted for examination

Symmetrical or Diffuse Alopecia

1. *If the hair-loss is associated clearly with lesions (papules, pustules, seborrhoea) or inflammation,* consider dermatophytosis, demodicosis and bacterial pyoderma

Focused diagnostic tests: Skin scrapings for demodicosis and a dermatophyte culture should be performed. Dermatophytosis is uncommon in dogs; however, a dermatophyte culture is recommended if the dog is young or debilitated, if hairs are broken or frayed, or if the hairs are Wood's-lamp positive

2. *If the skin scrapings and dermatophyte culture are negative,* or if dermatophytosis is not seriously considered, a superficial pyoderma should strongly be suspected

Focused diagnostic tests: A therapeutic trial of systemic antibiotics and topical antimicrobial shampoos for 21 – 30 days is indicated

3. The patient should be re-examined at the end of the treatment period to evaluate the response to therapy. *If there is a marked improvement and hair growth is obvious,* the problem was a superficial pyoderma. Therapy should be continued for at least 1 week post clinical cure. *If there is no improvement,* disorders of keratinisation or hair follicle growth and endocrine alopecias should be considered

Focused diagnostic test: At this point, a skin biopsy should be performed to rule in or rule out disorders of keratinisation, cutaneous neoplasia or hair follicle disorders

Continued

DIAGNOSTIC PLAN FOR ALOPECIA
4. *If the skin biopsy report indicates either normal skin or 'compatible with endocrine alopecia'*, pursue diagnostic testing for endocrine alopecia
Focused diagnostic tests: There are two approaches that may be taken at this stage. The first is to perform a haematological test, serum biochemistry panel and urinalysis to look for abnormalities which may support either hypothyroidism or hyperadrenocorticism. The second is to pursue diagnostic endocrine testing based upon either clinical suspicion or frequency of occurrence in the general population. The frequency of occurrence of the endocrine disorders in the general dog population are as follows: hypothyroidism, hyperadrenocorticism and adrenal sex hormone dysfunctions

FIG. 6.6 Diagnostic plan for alopecia.

Treatment. There is no known treatment.

Prognosis. If cicatricial alopecia is present, the hair-loss will be permanent. The condition causes no major medical problems and is merely cosmetic.

Traction alopecia

Description. Traction alopecia is a rare condition that is seen exclusively in small-breed dogs whose owners elect to have them wearing hair ornaments (bows, rubber bands etc). It is believed that the tension on the hairs caused by these devices cause interferes with the blood supply to the hair root.

Clinical signs. A focal area of hair-loss develops in the area where a hair ornament was placed or attached. Lesions are most common on the head and ears. Small-breed dogs that frequent grooming parlours are predisposed. Scaling may be present along with follicular plugging. The shape of the hair-loss may mimic the device, i.e. round for areas where rubber bands were placed and linear in areas where hairslides were worn.

Diagnosis. A tentative diagnosis can be made based upon the history and the physical findings. A skin biopsy is useful to confirm the diagnosis and as a prognostic aid as to whether or not hair will regrow. Histologically, hair follicles are extremely small and in telogen phase. The hair follicle epithelium may be reduced to a single cord of cells. Follicular keratosis may be present.

Treatment. There is no known treatment. Hair ornaments should be only loosely attached in the hair coat.

Prognosis. Hair regrowth may occur if the hair follicles are not permanently destroyed.

Post-rabies vaccination alopecia

Description. Post-rabies vaccination alopecia is a rare disease of dogs that is due to an idiosyncratic hypersensitivity reaction to the subcutaneous deposition of rabies vaccine. Similar lesions have been reported anecdotally after canine distemper vaccination.

Clinical signs. Clinical signs are not usually visible until 2–3 months after vaccination. A small alopecic macule develops at the site of the vaccination. Lesions vary between 2 and 10 cm in diameter. Early lesions show annular areas of alopecia, mild erythema, scaling and some hyperpigmentation. Unfortunately, these signs are often missed by the owner. Inflammation is absent in older lesions and there may be a few hairs in the lesion. This disease has a predilection for toy or small-breed dogs, and Poodles are especially at risk.

Diagnosis. Definitive diagnosis requires a skin biopsy. The most diagnostic samples are obtained from the margin of the lesion and a long elliptical skin biopsy should be submitted. Histologically, hair follicles are severely atrophic and are in telogen phase. Nodular inflammation may be present in the panniculus.

Treatment. There is no known treatment.

Prognosis. The alopecia may be permanent. Skin biopsy may be prognostic for hair regrowth but clients are best warned that the hair-loss is persistent. Subcutaneous administration of rabies vaccine is best avoided in small and toy breeds, especially Poodles.

Post-glucocorticoid injection alopecia

Description. This is a temporary type of alopecia that occurs at the site of subcutaneous glucocorticoid administration. It is frequent in dogs that have received repositol glucocorticoid injections.

Clinical signs. A circular patch of alopecia occurs at the site of a previous subcutaneous injection of glucocorticoids. The skin may appear thinner and scaling may be present.

Diagnosis. Diagnosis is most frequently based upon history and clinical signs. Skin biopsy will reveal atrophic hair follicles in telogen.

Treatment. None is necessary. The lesion will resolve spontaneously in several months.

Prognosis. Prognosis is good. It is advisable to avoid repeating subcutaneous injections of glucocorticoids in dogs with a history of this reaction.

Post-clipping alopecia

Description. Post-clipping alopecia is a relatively common clinical syndrome. It occurs most often in German Shepherd Dogs, Chow Chows, Siberian Huskies, Alaskan Malamutes, Keeshonds, and Samoyeds. Although this type of alopecia may occur anywhere on the body, the author has seen it most commonly in dogs that have been clipped for surgery, especially in the lumbosacral area. Other authors have seen it most commonly on the foreleg in areas clipped for cephalic venipuncture. The pathophysiology of this syndrome is not known but it is hypothesised to be due to vasoconstriction of the blood vessels in the skin that are no longer insulated by the hair coat. Alternatively, it is has also been suggested that the skin temperature of sledge dogs is higher than in other dogs and that the loss of the coat may itself produce a temperature drop sufficient to cause vasoconstriction.

Clinical signs. In this syndrome, the hair coat does not completely regrow as expected in the area that has been clipped. If an extensive area has been clipped, partial hair regrowth may be seen in the periphery of the clipped area. Some guard (primary)

hairs may regrow in the area and mild scaling is commonly observed. Total hair regrowth may take 6 to 12 months and the hairs may be darker in colour than before. Normal pigmentation of the hairs will return with the next hair cycle.

Diagnosis is made most often on the basis of history and clinical signs. It is important to rule out hypothyroidism and hyperadrenocorticism from the differential diagnosis list. Histologically, the hair follicles are arrested in catagen; however, a few may be in telogen. The hair follicles are of normal size.

Treatment. There is no specific therapy. Anecdotal reports suggest that hair regrows after vigorous brushing of the area, massage and covering of the lesion with a tight-fitting cloth dog sweater. These activities increase the skin temperature and increase blood perfusion to the skin, supporting the suggested pathophysiology of the disease.

Prognosis. Prognosis is good. The haircoat will eventually regrow after 6 to 12 months.

Dermatomyositis

Description. Dermatomyositis is a heritable disease of the skin and muscle. The exact pathogenesis is unknown and it is believed to be an autoimmune disease. It is most commonly diagnosed in Collies and Shetland Sheepdogs, although clinical findings consistent with the diagnosis have been reported in Chow Chows and German Shepherd Dogs.

Clinical signs. Most of the clinical signs are usually evident by 6 months of age. Very early lesions may be seen by 7 to 12 weeks of age. Initial lesions begin as pustules and vesicles that ulcerate and crust. The face, tail and extremities are the most common sites for the lesions, which may also be seen on the ear tips. There is no noted pain or pruritus associated with the lesions. They may wax and wane and may regress completely.

Marked scarring of the skin is noted and hair-loss may be permanent. Hair-loss is patchy and occurs in areas where the skin lesions were seen (face, extremities, tip of the tail). Skin lesions tend to flare at or around the time the muscles are affected: the temporal and masseter muscles atrophy and affected dogs also have difficulty swallowing and eating. Severely affected dogs may be stunted in growth, have a megaesophagus, be lame and have marked widespread muscle atrophy. Infertility has also been noted.

Diagnosis. This is a disease of young dogs. Skin scrapings and dermatophyte cultures should be obtained to rule out parasites and dermatophytosis as a cause for the hair-loss. Definitive diagnosis requires finding compatible histological changes in both skin and muscle and abnormal electromyographic changes. A presumptive diagnosis can be made on clinical signs, history and skin biopsy. The best sites for biopsy are early lesions showing erythema, hair-loss and vesicles. Histologically, the most common findings are scattered degeneration of basal cells in the epidermis and outer root sheath, vacuolation of the basement membrane, vesicles and follicular atrophy. Appropriate sites for muscle biopsy are best found via electromyography rather than by random sampling.

Treatment. There is no effective treatment. Affected dogs should be kept out of the sunlight and should not be used for breeding. Anecdotal reports have indicated that large doses of vitamin E (400 IU per day, orally) may be useful.

Prognosis. Good to guarded. Mildly affected dogs may have only cosmetic defects. More severely affected dogs may have chronic problems, particularly due to the muscle atrophy, and euthanasia may be indicated. The full extent of the muscle involvement may not be evident for a long time — a year or greater. This is a heritable disease and test breeding supports an autosomal dominant mode of inheritance with variable expressivity. Affected dogs and all siblings should be neutered and not allowed to breed.

Canine follicular dysplasia

Description. Canine follicular dysplasia is a poorly understood group of syndromes. It is an uncommon cause of alopecia in the dog and is characterised by the acquisition of an altered hair coat. Anecdotally, there appear to be various breed predispositions and the condition may be hereditary.

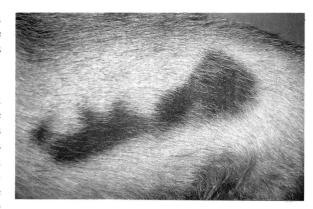

FIG. 6.7 Idiopathic flank alopecia (follicular dysplasia) in a Miniature Schnauzer.

Clinical signs. In general, canine follicular dysplasia begins with deteriorating hair coat quality. The hair may become rough and seborrhoeic and may show changes in colour in areas where hair-loss is beginning. Hair-loss may involve both primary and secondary hairs, or be limited to primary hairs (guard hairs). Hair-loss may be patchy, widespread or bilaterally symmetrical. The disease occurs most commonly on the trunk and tends to spare the face and extremities. The disease may wax and wane for months but it is usually progressive and hair-loss is usually permanent (Fig. 6.7).

Diagnosis. Definitive diagnosis requires a skin biopsy and specimens should be taken from areas of maximal hair-loss or change. **In addition, a skin biopsy from a normally haired site should be submitted for comparison**. Histologically, the most important changes are found in the hair follicle. The follicular infundibulum is almost always markedly hyperkeratotic and pigmentary incontinence may be found around the base of the hair bulb. The structure of the hair follicle itself is structurally abnormal. The specific hair follicle changes are believed to be breed-specific.

Treatment. There is no effective treatment but some dogs may respond to oral isotretinoin or etretinate (1 mg/kg daily).

Prognosis. The owner should be told that the hair-loss is probably permanent. There may be transient hair regrowth, but follicular dysplasia is a progressive disease. If the dog's signs do respond to isotretinoin or etretinate, therapy is expensive and lifelong.

Hypothyroidism

Description. Hypothyroidism is the most common endocrine skin disease of dogs. The vast majority of cases are caused by primary thyroid dysfunction (lymphocytic thyroiditis or idiopathic thyroid atrophy). Thyroid hormone is necessary for normal cell metabolism. In the skin, thyroid hormone is needed for the initiation of anagen in hair follicles.

Clinical signs. The dermatological signs of canine hypothyroidism are extremely variable (Figs 6.8–6.10). In some cases, the dog may have no obvious signs of hypothyroidism except for a history of recurrent pyoderma, persistent seborrhoea and chronic otitis externa. In other cases the signs may be very dramatic. The classic bilaterally symmetrical alopecia so commonly associated with this disease in the literature is a relatively uncommon finding in practice. Most clients present dogs for veterinary consultation long before they become totally alopecic. It is more common for clients to complain of 'rat-tail', thinning of the hair coat (loss of guard hairs), or hair-loss in areas of repeated trauma or wear, such as the neck where collars rub. The coat may have a 'puppy-like' appearance. The quality of the hair coat is usually affected and a dry, brittle coat with easily epilated hairs is a common clinical finding. Some clients simply complain about an increased presence of hair

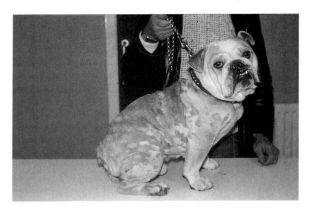

FIG. 6.9 Patchy multifocal alopecia on the trunk of an English Bulldog with hypothyroidism and secondary pyoderma. Although hypothyroidism is not a pruritic disorder, the secondary pyoderma may lead to pruritus Slide courtesy of Richard Harvey.

in the house and the need to sweep or vacuum rugs more often. Lichenification of the skin, comedones and secondary seborrhoea are common findings. Pruritus is not typical of uncomplicated hypothyroidism but it may be present in dogs with secondary superficial pyodermas or *Malassezia* dermatitis. Miscellaneous changes include sagging of the facial skin, poor wound healing and easy bruising. Clinically obvious signs usually develop in middle-aged dogs but the disease may occur in dogs of any age.

Diagnosis. Skin biopsy alone is rarely helpful in making a definitive diagnosis (Fig. 6.11). A skin

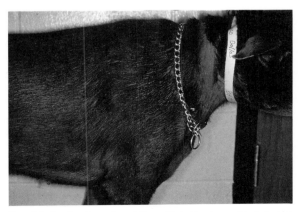

FIG. 6.8 Canine hypothyroidism. Note the loss of hair in the area of the collar.

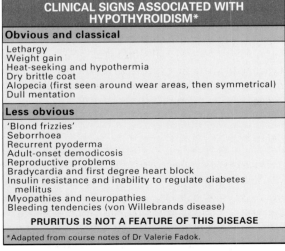

CLINICAL SIGNS ASSOCIATED WITH HYPOTHYROIDISM*
Obvious and classical
Lethargy Weight gain Heat-seeking and hypothermia Dry brittle coat Alopecia (first seen around wear areas, then symmetrical) Dull mentation
Less obvious
'Blond frizzies' Seborrhoea Recurrent pyoderma Adult-onset demodicosis Reproductive problems Bradycardia and first degree heart block Insulin resistance and inability to regulate diabetes mellitus Myopathies and neuropathies Bleeding tendencies (von Willebrands disease)
PRURITUS IS NOT A FEATURE OF THIS DISEASE
*Adapted from course notes of Dr Valerie Fadok.

FIG. 6.10 Clinical signs associated with hypothyroidism.

DIACNOSTIC TESTS FOR CANINE HYPOTHYROIDISM	
Non-specific tests	
Haematology	Non-regenerative anaemia
Biochemistry panel	May see hypercholesterolaemia
Skin biopsy	May see changes associated with endocrinopathy, mucinosis, or it may be normal
Specific tests of thyroid gland or hormone activity	
Basal T4 concentrations	May be affected by non-thyroidal illness, glucocorticoids, sulpha drugs >15µg/l dog is probably euthyroid 10 to 15 µg/l may be hypothyroid or euthyroid <10 µg/l dog is probably hypothyroid **Reference laboratory should be consulted for normals and values should not be interpreted in isolation of the patient's clinical signs and history**
TSH response test	Normal dogs will show at least a doubling of basal concentrations. The post-TSH concentration should be within the normal range. Dogs with basal concentrations in the normal range may not show a doubling; these dogs are considered euthyroid
Free T4	Used in combination with total T4 this may help confirm the diagnosis of hypothyroidism. Non-thyroidal systemic diseases will lower free T4
Thyroid biopsy	This is the ultimate diagnostic test but is not a very practical test
Antithyroglobulin antibodies	This test is useful in the genetics of screening dogs or breeds with suspected heritable hypothyroidism. These antibodies are seen to correlate with the lymphocytic thyroiditis
Less useful diagnostic tests for hypothyroidism	
T3 concentrations	Not reliable as a screening tool
K value test	This is a mathematical equation using T4 and cholesterol. This test is time-consuming and it is questionable as to whether or not it adds much diagnostic assistance
Semi-quant CITE T4	Not as reliable as a quantitative measurement. Treatment is life-long in this disease and is not without possible side-effects. **DO NOT SKIMP ON DIAGNOSTIC TESTING**
Response to therapy	**THIS IS NOT RECOMMENDED AND IS UNRELIABLE.** Almost all dogs will improve clinically when they receive thyroid hormone supplementation, but if they are truly euthyroid, they will relapse

FIG. 6.11 Diagnosis tests for canine hypothyroidism (adapted from course notes of Dr Valerie Fadok).

biopsy from a patient with symmetrical alopecia may be helpful in identifying a histological pattern consistent with an endocrine alopecia but ancillary diagnostic tests are needed for a definitive diagnosis. (See *Chapter 3* for information on endocrine testing.)

Treatment. Treatment is lifelong and not without possible side effects; therefore, a definitive diagnosis is required. The replacement hormone therapy of choice is thyroxine (T4) orally, 0.5 mg/m^2 b.i.d. Tailoring the dosage on the basis of m^2 is preferred because it will minimise underdosing of small dogs and overdosing of large dogs. After a patient has been receiving replacement therapy for 4–8 weeks, a 'post-pill' serum sample should be obtained **6 hours** after administration to determine if adequate concentrations of hormone are present in the blood. The post-pill test results should be in the high normal range or at least slightly above the normal range. Based upon the findings, the dosage can be increased or decreased. Dogs that are clinically overdosed are usually hyperactive, tachycardic and polyphagic.

Clients often ask if the medication can be administered once a day. In many cases this is possible but it is advisable to wait until the dog is clinically normal and adequate serum concentrations of replacement therapy have been documented. It is recommended that clients administer replacement hormone therapy in the morning to mimic naturally occurring hormone cycles.

If the dog maintains clinical normalcy after 3 or 4 months of once-a-day replacement therapy, it may be continued on a once-a-day basis indefinitely. Serum concentrations of thyroid hormones should be measured annually. Deterioration of a patient should raise suspicions that the dog is not receiving the proper dose, that the formulation may have changed or that a new disease is present.

Prognosis. Prognosis for a normal quality of life is excellent. This disease requires lifelong therapy and monitoring but it responds well to therapy. Most dogs will show marked improvement in mental attitude within weeks of initiating therapy. Regrowth of hair may take several months.

Hyperadrenocorticism

Description. Hyperadrenocorticism may be caused by either endogenous production or exogenous administration of excess glucocorticoids. Endogenous production is caused by either an autonomously functioning adrenal tumour or bilateral adrenal hypertrophy resulting from pituitary adenoma (pituitary-dependent). Excess administration of glucocorticoids is referred to as **iatrogenic hypercortisolaemia**. The old terminology 'iatrogenic hyperadrenocorticism,' is best avoided since it implies overproduction of glucocorticoids by the adrenal glands. The clinical signs of this disease syndrome are produced by the effect of glucocorticoids on fat and glucose metabolism and the catabolic nature of the hormone (Plate 4).

CLINICAL SIGNS ASSOCIATED WITH HYPERADRENOCORTICISM*

Obvious and classical

Polyuria, polydypsia, polyphagia
Bilaterally symmetrical alopecia
Thin skin with decreased elasticity
Wrinkled skin, tissue paper appearance
Prominent vasculature
Bruising
Comedones
Pendulous abdomen
Calcinosis cutis

Less obvious

Adult-onset demodicosis
Adult-onset pyoderma, especially with large flaccid pustules or atypical presentation
Chronic or recurrent dermatophytosis
Urinary tract infections
Hypertension
Pulmonary thromboembolism
Sloughing nails
Ear margin necrosis
Glomerulonephritis
Recurrent pancreatitis
Diabetes mellitus refractory to treatment
Neurological signs
Muscle weakness or pseudomyotonia

*Adapted from course notes of Dr Valerie Fadok

FIG. 6.12 Clinical signs associated with hyperadrenocorticism.

Clinical signs. The dermatological signs of hyperadrenocorticism are similar, regardless of aetiology (Fig. 6.12). Bilaterally symmetrical alopecia that spares the head and legs is common. The hair coat is thin and sparse. The skin is markedly thinner and subcutaneous vasculature is often prominent. Alterations in the pigmentation (hyper- or hypopigmentation) of the skin and hair coat may be seen. Delayed wound healing, bleeding disorders, comedones, scaling, phlebectasia and calcinosis cutis may also be seen. Hyperadrenocorticism is seen most frequently in older dogs and there appears to be a predilection for females to develop adrenal tumours. Unless polydipsia and polyuria are present early in the disease, prompting clients to seek veterinary care, many clients will present dogs with much more markedly pronounced hair-loss with this disease in comparison with hypothyroidism. Glucocorticoids may have a much more dramatic effect on the hair follicle than can thyroid hormone concentration.

Diagnosis. Definitive diagnosis of both the existence of the disease and the source is critical for appropriate treatment (Fig. 6.13).

Treatment. Iatrogenic hypercortisolaemia is treated by withdrawal/discontinuation of the exogenous administration of glucocorticoids. Cessation of therapy may be abrupt or slow, depending upon the duration and amount of glucocorticoids the patient has been receiving. The author recommends performing an ACTH-response test as a means of determining how soon the exogenous glucocorticoids can be withdrawn. If the test shows some adrenal responsiveness, the glucocorticoids can be stopped abruptly. The owner can be told to watch for signs of adrenal insufficiency (weakness, vomiting, depression, anorexia) and instructed to administer glucocorticoids (0.5 mg/kg *per os*) if the signs occur. In the author's experience, signs of adrenal insufficiency are rare in dogs when ACTH-response tests show adrenal responsiveness. If, on the other hand, the ACTH-response test shows no adrenal responsiveness, glucocorticoids should be withdrawn more slowly over several weeks. Intermittent ACTH-response tests should be performed to monitor the patient's adrenal status.

Adrenal tumours are best treated via surgical excision of the affected adrenal gland. This surgery can be difficult to perform and these animals can be very fragile to manage post-operatively.

Pituitary-dependent hyperadrenocorticism is best treated by the administration of cytotoxic drugs such as mitotane. The treatment and management of this disease requires a thorough understanding of the pathophysiology of this disease, the adrenal glands and the pharmacology of these drugs.

DIAGNOSTIC TESTS FOR HYPERADRENOCORTICISM	
Screening tests (answers the question: 'Is hyperadrenocorticism present?')	
ACTH stimulation test	Measures pre- and post-cortisol concentrations in response to exogenous administration of ACTH. Affected dogs will hyper-respond. This test is less reliable than the LDDST, but takes only 2 hours to perform
Low doses dexamethasone suppression test (LDDST) (0.01–0.15 mg/kg)	This is the test of choice for screening. This test measures pre-and post-cortisol concentrations in response to exogenous administration of a small dose of dexamethasone. Normal dogs will show appropriate suppression by or at 8 hours post-drug. Dogs with hyperadrenocorticism will not show suppression of cortisol concentrations or will suppress at 4–6 hours and escape by 8 hours. This test takes 8 hours to perform and is not 100% reliable
V test	This is a combination test that uses the high dose dexamethasone suppression test and the ACTH response test. This test is not recommended for use
Urinary cortisol/creatine ratio in nmol/l and mmol/l respectively (To convert mg/dl to mmol/l, multiply by 0.088)	Morning urine samples (n=2) are analysed for urine cortisol and creatine and the ratio is determined. If the ratio is ≤ 35, hyperadrenocorticism is not present. This test is good for discriminating normal and affected dogs, but false positives are seen in dogs with polyuria and polydipsia associated with other diseases. This test may be more useful to monitor therapy
Cortisol-induced alkaline phosphatase	This test is easy and inexpensive. False positives may occur in dogs with non-adrenal diseases. There is no overlap between normal dogs and dogs with hyperadrenocorticism
Non-specific tests	
Haematology	Leucocytosis with left shift, eosinopaenia, lymphopaenia, monocytosis
Biochemistry panel	Elevated alkaline phosphatase, alanine aminotransferase and cholesterol. Hyperglycaemia, elevated BUN/SUN and elevated creatinine
Urinalysis	Low specific gravity, possible bacteraemia, inflammatory cells (variable)
Abdominal radiographs	Calcification of adrenals
Abdominal ultrasonography	Bilaterally enlarged adrenal glands, calcification of adrenal gland, unilateral adrenal masses
CT scans and MRI scans	Pituitary tumours > 1 cm in diameter, best used to evaluate adrenal tumours to look for evidence of metastasis. Expensive and difficult to obtain in private practice
Skin biopsies	Thin skin, calcinosis cutis, suggestive of endocrinopathy
Discriminating tests for hyperadrenocorticism (answers the question: 'What is the cause — adrenal or pituitary?')	
High dose dexamethasone suppression test (0.1 mg/kg)	This test measures pre- and post-cortisol concentrations in dogs that have received dexamethasone. In theory, dogs with pituitary-dependent hyperadrenocorticism (PDH) will show adequate suppression (at least 50% decrease from baseline concentration) by 8 hours. Adrenal tumours do not show any suppression
Mega dose dexamethasone suppression test (1.0 mg/kg)	This test is used in dogs suspected of having PDH, but which do not respond to the conventional dose of dexamethasone. This test would be used in dogs in which PDH was suspected, could not be confirmed with the above test, and evidence of an adrenal tumour could not be found
Endogenous ACTH plasma concentrations	In theory, this test discriminates normal dogs and dogs with adrenal tumours and PDH. There is some overlap of values and to be most useful the dog should be tested after being hospitalised overnight and at least two different samples should be analysed. Very low values are consistent with an adrenal tumour and dogs with PDH should have very high levels
Corticotrophin stimulation test	This test measures pre- and post-cortisol concentrations of plasma ACTH after corticotrophin has been administered. This test is very costly and is not indicated in most clinical situations

Fig. 6.13 Diagnostic tests for hyperadrenocorticism (adapted from course notes of Dr Valerie Fadok).

Adrenal sex hormone dysfunction

Description. Adrenal sex hormonal synthesis alopecia is a rare cause of alopecia in the dog and has strong breed predilections. In the past, this syndrome was referred to as 'growth hormone responsive alopecia' because affected dogs had an abnormal growth hormone response tests and some responded to the exogenous administration of growth hormone. Recent studies have shown that this syndrome is more likely to be caused by a dysregulation of adrenal sex hormone synthesis resulting in excess production of progesterone and androgens of adrenal origin. Affected dogs may have a partial or total adult-onset deficiency in 21-hydroxylase that leads to progestin and androgen excess. This disease syndrome is most common in Pomeranians, Keeshonds, Chow Chows, Miniature Poodles, and Samoyeds. It is most often seen in males and it begins between 9 months and 2 years of age, but may be seen in elderly dogs.

Clinical signs. Bilaterally symmetrical alopecia begins on the trunk and tends to spare the head and extremities. Friction areas may be affected first. The primary hairs are often lost first but both primary and secondary hairs will eventually be lost. The hair coat may be described as 'fuzzy' or 'woolly' by the owner. Hair-loss will eventually progress to involve the entire trunk, although there may be patches of hair growth scattered throughout the trunk. Hyperpigmentation of the skin is common. Interestingly, hair may regrow in areas that have been traumatised via skin scrapings, skin biopsy or wounds. Alternatively, the author has seen a few dogs with abnormal hormone tests where the hair has regrown spontaneously without treatment. This observation raises questions about the proposed pathogenesis of the disease.

Diagnosis. Definitive diagnosis may be difficult to achieve without response to therapy, i.e. castration. A skin biopsy should be performed to rule out follicular dysplasia. Histological changes are suggestive but not diagnostic for this disease, as it may be impossible to differentiate this syndrome from post-clipping alopecia, follicular dysplasia, hyperoestrogenism and hyperadrenocorticism. Classic histological findings include hair follicle arrest in catagen, flame follicles and follicular atrophy.

Endocrine function tests to rule in or out hypothyroidism and hyperadrenocorticism should be performed. Sex hormone assays are difficult to obtain and normal values for each breed are not available. Furthermore, these tests are expensive and have not been very helpful in the author's experience.

Treatment. If the dog is sexually intact the first treatment is surgical neutering. Some dogs will respond temporarily to the exogenous administration of human growth hormone (0.15 IU/kg SC twice weekly for 6 weeks). Side-effects of this therapy include sudden death from acute anaphylaxis and transient or permanent diabetes mellitus. Response to therapy usually occurs within 3 months and hair regrowth is often temporary. Another novel therapy is the administration of mitotane after documenting abnormal adrenal sex hormone production via an ACTH-stimulation test, reproductive hormone panel and endogenous ACTH serum concentrations. Considering the heritable nature of this disease and the fact that the clinical abnormalities are limited to the skin, it seems highly questionable to use any other therapy than surgical neutering.

Prognosis. The prognosis for a normal quality of life is excellent.

Canine testicular tumours (Sertoli cell tumour, interstitial tumours and seminomas)

Description. Alopecia in these conditions is caused by the excess production of oestrogens or testosterones from a tumour in the testes. It is most often seen in cryptorchid dogs.

Clinical signs. This disease is relatively rare. Dermatological signs usually begin with mild hair-loss and seborrhoea in the flanks. Marked hair-loss and seborrhoea then develop in the flanks, caudal thighs, perineal, genital and ventral abdominal areas. As the disease progresses, hyperpigmentation and lichenification develop. Gynaecomastia, pendulous prepuce and attraction to other male dogs develops in the later stages. In some dogs with Sertoli cell tumours, a red linear area develops just proximal to the prepuce. This is a cutaneous marker for Sertoli cell tumours. Boxers, Shetland Sheepdogs, Pekingese, Weimaraners, and Cairn Terriers are predisposed. Clinical signs develop most commonly in middle-aged dogs.

Diagnosis. These tumours may or may not be palpable in the abdomen or testes. Definitive diagnosis requires castration and documentation of a testicular tumour. Skin biopsy may be helpful in establishing that an endocrine dermatopathy is present but it is not diagnostic. Follicular atrophy is present, along with histological changes consistent with chronic inflammatory skin disease. If biopsies are submitted, they should be from the centre of areas with maximal alopecia and from areas of hyperpigmentation and lichenification.

Treatment. Castration or laparotomy to remove the testes is the treatment of choice. It may take several months before clinical signs resolve and hair begins to regrow.

Prognosis. Most testicular tumours are benign and do not metastasize. Sertoli cell tumours are rarely malignant and metastasis is uncommon.

Hyperoestrogenism in female dogs

Description. This is a rare syndrome in intact female dogs. The exact cause is unknown but the condition is believed to be due to elevated oestrogen levels. It may occur in bitches with ovarian tumours or cysts. A clinically indistinguishable form of this disease may occur in bitches receiving exogenous oestrogens for the treatment of urinary incontinence.

Clinical signs. Bilaterally symmetrical alopecia begins in the genital and perineal regions. It will gradually progress to involve the abdomen, caudal and medial thighs, chest, trunk and neck. Hyperpigmentation, lichenification and seborrhoea may also be seen. Gynaecomastia and vulvar enlargement may also be present. Some bitches may have abnormal oestrous cycles, while others may show signs of nymphomania. This syndrome is most common in older intact female dogs.

Diagnosis. Diagnosis is made most often on the basis of history, clinical signs and response to surgical neutering. Measurement of serum concentrations of oestradiol, progesterone and testosterone during dioestrus may be helpful in documenting this disease, however, the diagnosis is most efficiently and cost-effectively made by response to surgical neutering.

Treatment. Ovariohysterectomy is the treatment of choice. Resolution of clinical signs and hair regrowth will take 3 to 4 months in most bitches.

Prognosis. The prognosis is excellent.

Hypoestrogenism in female dogs

Description. This syndrome has been reported in female dogs that have supposedly been neutered at an early age. There is a deficiency of sex hormones. In most neutered bitches, the adrenal glands produce enough sex hormones for day-to-day maintenance of normal cell function. It has been suggested that in affected bitches there is an adrenal sex hormone synthesis dysfunction. Although oestrogen is the hormone most commonly believed to be deficient, some bitches have responded to testosterone supplementation. Sex hormone metabolism occurs in the skin and it is possible that there is a receptor defect in the skin. The exact pathogenesis is controversial and essentially unknown.

Clinical signs. The earliest clinical sign of this syndrome is bilaterally symmetrical alopecia in the perineal and genital area. The alopecia gradually progresses to the medial thighs, ventral abdomen and neck. Alopecia may also occur on the ears. Hyperpigmentation of the skin may occur. Genitalia may be infantile. Some bitches may show urinary incontinence. This syndrome may be clinically indistinguishable from pattern alopecia of dogs.

Diagnosis. Definitive diagnosis is made most commonly via history of early surgical neutering, physical examination and response to sex hormone replacement. Skin biopsies will be supportive but not diagnostic of a suspected endocrine disorder.

Treatment. Most animals will respond to diethylstilbestrol (0.1–1 mg *per os* once daily for 3 to 4 weeks). If hair growth is evident, a maintenance dose once or twice weekly is recommended. Diethylstilbestrol may cause bone marrow suppression:

pretreatment complete blood count and platelet counts are recommended and these parameters should be monitored every 2 weeks for the first month of therapy and then 3–4 times per year. Reactions are idiosyncratic. Alternatively, methyltestosterone at 1 mg/kg *per os* (do not exceed 30 mg total) every other day for 1–3 months has also been reported to be effective. Once hair regrowth is noted, the dosage frequency is decreased to twice weekly. Exogenous testosterones can cause hepatotoxicity; serum liver enzymes should be monitored monthly during the first 4 to 6 months of therapy and then twice a year. Behavioural changes are rarely noted with either drug but if they occur the dosage should be decreased.

Prognosis. The prognosis is excellent for a good quality of life.

Hypoandrogenism of male dogs

Description. This is a rare syndrome of castrated dogs and is most common in male dogs that have been neutered at a young age. The exact pathogenesis is unknown; the condition may be caused either by inadequate adrenal gland synthesis of sex hormones or by defective metabolism of sex hormones in the skin at the receptor sites.

Clinical signs. This syndrome is most common in middle-aged or older dogs that have been castrated when young. Anecdotal reports exist of clinically similar syndromes occurring in adult male dogs with soft atrophic testicles. Bilaterally symmetrical alopecia begins in the perineal and genital region. The alopecia progresses to the medial thighs and ventral trunk and neck. Occasionally, dogs have a history of urinary incontinence that is responsive to testosterone.

Diagnosis. Definitive diagnosis is made most often via the history, physical findings and response to replacement hormone therapy. It is essential to eliminate hypothyroidism, hyperadrenocorticism and exogenous glucocorticoid use from the differential diagnosis list. Skin biopsies may support the diagnosis of an endocrinopathy, but are not diagnostic.

Treatment. Treatment consists of methyltestosterone at 1 mg/kg *per os* (do not exceed 30 mg total)

every other day for 1 to 3 months. Once hair regrowth is noted, the dosage frequency is decreased to twice weekly. Exogenous testosterones can cause hepatotoxicity; serum liver enzymes should be monitored monthly during the first 4 to 6 months of therapy and then twice a year. Behavioural changes are rarely noted with drug therapy but if they occur the dosage should be decreased to 0.5 mg/kg or less, if necessary.

Prognosis. The prognosis for a good quality of life is excellent.

Congenital alopecia (Fig. 6.14)

Description. Congenital alopecia or congenital hypotrichosis is a rare disease of dogs that is characterised by varying degrees of hair-loss from birth. Affected dogs are born with less than the normal

(a)

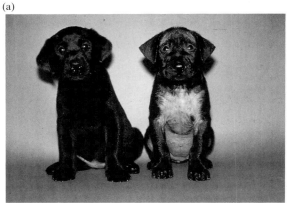

(b)

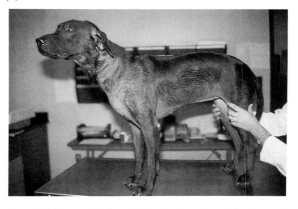

Fig. 6.14 Congenital hypotrichosis in a dog. (a) shows the puppy at approximately 8 weeks of age with a litter mate. (b) shows the dog as an adult. Courtesy of Dr Gail Kunkle, University of Florida.

number of hair follicles in their skin. This disease may be present with other ectodermal defects, such as abnormal dentition. A male sex-linked inheritance is believed to be the mode of transmission .

Clinical signs. Affected puppies have clearly demarcated areas of alopecia that are evident at birth. The alopecia may be complete or partial. The head is most commonly affected. Males are predisposed. Affected breeds include Labrador Retrievers, Poodle, Basset Hounds, Beagles, Bichon Frise, and Rottweilers.

Diagnosis. Definitive diagnosis is made via skin biopsy. The most alopecic area should be sampled. Additionally, a normally haired area should be biopsied for comparison. Histologically, there is a marked decrease in the number and density of hair follicles. Follicles may be small, but are not abnormal in structure. Complete absence of adnexal glands may be found in some cases.

Treatment. There is no treatment.

Prognosis. This is not a life-threatening disease. Affected dogs should not be bred and should be protected from prolonged exposure to sunlight.

Acquired pattern alopecia

Description. This relatively common skin disease is characterised by bilaterally symmetrical hair-loss that develops in adult dogs. The hair-loss is gradual and may be genetic in origin.

Clinical signs. The hair-loss usually begins on the pinnae and extends to involve the ventral neck, ventral chest and perineal area. The hairs gradually diminish in size and eventually there are no hairs or only very small secondary hairs. The skin may be hyperpigmented and mild scaling may be present. There is a breed predilection for Dachshunds and Boston Terriers; however, it has also been seen in Whippets, Chihuahuas, Manchester Terriers, and Italian Greyhounds. There is no sex predilection and most dogs are at least 1 year or older before clinical signs become evident.

Diagnosis. This is a diagnosis of exclusion; more common endocrinopathies should be ruled out

before making a tentative diagnosis. Skin biopsy may be helpful in differentiating acquired pattern alopecia from endocrine alopecias. In acquired pattern alopecia the hair follicles are very small, but not predominantly in the telogen phase. In endocrine dermatoses, diminutive hair bulbs are not a feature and most hairs are in catagen or telogen phase.

Treatment. Treatment is not necessary as this is not a life-threatening disease. In a few cases, the author has observed hair regrowth in dogs treated with mibolerone (2.0 µg/kg *per os* daily).

Prognosis. The prognosis for a good quality of life is excellent. Owners should be told that the hair-loss is permanent.

Telogen effluvium and anagen defluxion

Description. Telogen effluvium is a rare syndrome in dogs characterised by the widespread loss of hair. This occurs in response to a major metabolic stress such as fever, illness, pregnancy, lactation or shock. All of the hair follicles are prematurely stopped in their growth and synchronised in the telogen phase. When new hairs begin to grow behind the old hairs, there is a massive shedding of the hair coat. This massive shed usually occurs weeks after the stressful episode.

Anagen defluxion is less severe than telogen effluvium and is limited to the growing hairs. A stressful metabolic event causes damage to the shaft of the growing hairs. The affected hairs tend to break easily and are characterised by an abnormally shaped shaft with a constriction or other obvious structural defect. This syndrome is analogous to 'wool break' in sheep. It has been seen most commonly by this author in dogs receiving chemotherapy and may occur within days of the event. This tends to occur in dogs in which most hairs are in anagen for prolonged periods, e.g. Poodles, Bichon Frise.

Clinical signs. In telogen effluvium there is a widespread loss of hair that rapidly occurs over days or a week. In most cases the head is spared. There is no inflammation present and the skin appears normal. In anagen defluxion, there is a less dramatic loss of hair and the animal tends to shed excessively. Close examination of the skin may show that the hairs are broken midshaft and that part of the hair is still retained in the hair follicle.

Diagnosis. Definitive diagnosis is made most often on the basis of history and clinical signs. Skin biopsy may help support the diagnosis. A biopsy should be taken, preferably as soon as possible after the shedding is noted to be most useful. Histologically, hairs are diffusely in telogen for telogen effluvium. In anagen defluxion, longitudinal sections of skin may show hair shaft damage as evidenced by a marked decrease in shaft diameter or distortion of the shaft.

Treatment. No treatment is required. Both conditions will spontaneously resolve when the new hair coat grows.

Prognosis. The prognosis is excellent.

Colour dilute alopecia

Description. Colour dilute alopecia is a hereditary canine skin disease seen in colour-dilute dogs, e.g. 'blue' coats. It is not known if the colour-dilute gene is directly responsible for the skin changes or if it is associated with follicular changes. This disease is considered to be a disorder of keratinisation. However, some authors consider it to be a manifestation of follicular dysplasia/dystrophy.

Clinical signs. Affected dogs are born with a normal hair coat and over several years gradually develop hair-loss. Most dogs are affected by 5 to 6 years of life. Early signs of the disease begin as a drying and dullness of the hair coat. The hairs are brittle and coat quality is poor. Affected hairs fragment and a 'moth-eaten' alopecia develops. The hair-loss becomes progressively worse and comedones and small papules develop in the more severely affected areas. Hyperpigmentation and seborrhoea are common. Most dogs are plagued by recurrent secondary pyodermas. This disease is most common in blue Dobermann Pinschers and other blue breeds such as Dachshunds, Great Danes, Whippets, Italian Greyhounds, Chow Chows, Miniature Pinschers, Chihuahua, Shetland Sheepdogs, Schipperkes, Irish Setters, Standard Poodles and Yorkshire Terriers. In addition, it has been seen in Irish Setters and fawn and red Dobermann Pinscher.

Diagnosis. Definitive diagnosis requires a skin biopsy and a history of the patient being from a colour-dilute breed. Histologically, there is clumping of the melanin in the hair follicles and epidermis. Hair follicles are dystrophic and atrophied. Most follicles are plugged with keratin and contain short, thin irregular hairs.

Treatment. Affected dogs may respond to once-daily isotretinoin (1–2 mg/kg) or etretinate (1 mg/kg). Response to therapy may take 2 to 3 months and treatment is lifelong.

Prognosis. Clients should be told that the hair-loss is permanent. These dogs require lifelong therapy for recurrent pyodermas and seborrhoea. At the time of writing it is unknown how effective long-term isotretinoin is in maintaining long-term hair regrowth.

Cutaneous neoplasia/epitheliotropic lymphoma

The most common skin neoplasia to result in diffuse alopecia is cutaneous lymphoma or epitheliotropic lymphoma. This is a T-cell lymphoma that invades the follicular and non-follicular epithelium. Hair-loss is caused by the destruction of hair follicles. Definitive diagnosis is made by skin biopsy. This is discussed in detail elsewhere in the text.

7

Scaling and Crusting

IAN MASON

Disorders associated with scaling and crusting are frequently encountered in canine dermatology. Scaling and crusting can be considered as distinct entities, but they often occur simultaneously and so will be considered together.

Scale is an accumulation of rafts of cells from the stratum corneum on the skin and within the coat. Scaling may be associated with apparent oiliness of the skin and hairs. Disorders associated with scaling, with or without oil and crust formation, have been referred to as **seborrhoea**. This term has been applied to skin diseases associated with qualitative and quantitative defects in cutaneous lipid (sebum) production (i.e. greasiness and scaling with odour, or dryness with scaling); strictly speaking, however, seborrhoea should be reserved as a term for conditions where there is an increase in sebum production. The pathogenesis of the skin diseases formerly classified as seborrhoea is much more complex than the name implies and nowadays it is accepted that seborrhoea is a misnomer. The preferred name for this group of diseases is **disorders of keratinisation**. Currently, in only one of these disorders (primary idiopathic seborrhoea) has a defect in keratinisation been demonstrated and so it is possible that the new name for this complex group of disorders will also be shown to be inappropriate.

Excessive scaling in dogs may be due to a primary defect in keratinisation or, much more commonly, may be secondary to another disease process. Almost any inflammatory skin disease can lead to secondary scaling. In many instances scaling does not occur alone; concomitant pruritus, crust formation, alopecia, greasiness and odour of the skin and coat may also be present (Fig. 7.1). There are important parallels between scaling disorders and pyoderma. In both, there is usually an underlying cause and it is essential that a thorough diagnostic approach is implemented before a diagnosis of a primary keratinisation disorder (or idiopathic pyoderma) can be made. Often pyoderma and scaling co-exist. In some instances, one underlying cause may lead to both clinical presentations. In other cases, the pyoderma occurs because scaling skin is more susceptible to infection.

The diagnosis and treatment of scaling disorders may be complex, prolonged, time-consuming and extremely costly. This should be clearly explained to the owner at the outset. The prognosis for primary scaling disorders is reasonably good, but lifelong topical and systemic therapy will be required. In secondary cases, the prognosis varies depending on the cause; the prognosis is excellent if the underlying cause is diagnosed and successfully treated.

Crusts form when exudates (serum, pus or blood) dry on the skin surface (Fig. 7.2). Surface squames, topical medicaments and hairs may also be involved within crusts. Crusts are usually associated with pustular disease (*Chapter 10*) or ulcerative and erosive dermatoses (*Chapter 8*). Fluid exudes on to the surface of erosions and ulcers and may be released following rupture of pustules and vesicles (for example, in superficial pyoderma or pemphigus foliaceus, Fig. 7.3). In either case, crusts form when such

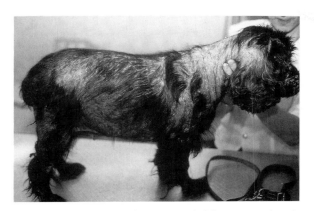

FIG. 7.1 Extensive alopecia accompanied by crust and scale formation with areas of erosion and erythema due to a drug eruption affecting the neck of a Cocker Spaniel. Slide courtesy of Richard Harvey.

fluids become associated with hair and scale and then dry (Fig. 7.4). The approach to such scaling disorders is described in *Chapters 8* and *10*. Crusts may also be present in keratinisation disorders, especially those diseases associated with excessive grease formation; these are considered in this chapter.

Keratinisation Disorders

The first step in the diagnostic approach is to determine whether the scaling disorder is primary or secondary. Primary disorders are much less prevalent and it is prudent, during the investigation of these disorders, to regard the problem as secondary until proved wrong. Dermatoses leading to secondary keratinisation defects may be classified as pruritic or non-pruritic. Primary disorders are often hereditary and are assumed to arise from abnormalities of epidermal or glandular function. Primary scaling disorders are often diagnosed by the elimination of all possible underlying causes from the differential diagnosis.

Examples of conditions leading to secondary scaling are shown in Fig. 7.5. Figure 7.6 lists the primary scaling disorders. The secondary disorders have been classified according to the presence or absence of pruritus; however, it should be remembered that many disorders of keratinisation are susceptible to secondary pyoderma which may induce or worsen pruritus. Trial therapy with antimicrobial agents (*Chapter 32*) will enable the distinction between those cases where pruritus is due to secondary pyoderma, and those cases where the disorder is inherently pruritic. Superficial pyoderma is often associated with fine scaling; for an approach to superficial pyoderma, refer to *Chapter 10*.

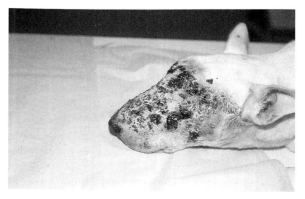

FIG. 7.2 English Bull Terrier with well demarcated, erythematous, pruritic facial dermatitis due to *Trichophyton mentagrophytes*. Note the alopecia and crusting. Slide courtesy of Richard Harvey.

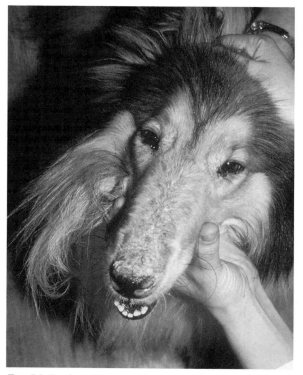

FIG. 7.3 Erythematous crusting area on the nose of a Rough Collie. Note that the nasal planum is affected. Inflammation which affects the planum nasale as well as the haired skin is suggestive of an immune-mediated condition, in this case pemphigus foliaceus. Slide courtesy of Richard Harvey.

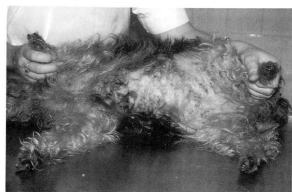

FIG. 7.4 Elderly Yorkshire Terrier with pruritic, erythematous crusted erosions on the ventrum and flanks due to epitheliotropic lymphoma (mycosis fungoides). Slide courtesy of Richard Harvey.

Fig. 7.5 Examples of secondary disorders of keratinisation in dogs.

EXAMPLES OF SECONDARY DISORDERS OF KERATINISATION IN DOGS	
Pruritic	
Hypersensitivity	Flea allergy dermatitis Atopy Food allergy/intolerance
Ectoparasitism	Sarcoptic mange Cheyletiellosis
Malassezia dermatosis	
Non-pruritic	

Metabolic	Endocrine
	   Hypothyroidism
	   Hyperadrenocorticism
	   Sex hormone-related
	Nutritionally deficient diet, inadequate absorption/utilisation
	   of dietary fat or zinc
	Other
	   Hepatocutaneous syndrome (superficial necrolytic
	   dermatitis)

Demodicosis	
Dermatophytosis	
Immune-mediated	Pemphigus foliaceus, pemphigus erythematosus
Neoplasia	Epitheliotropic lymphoma, actinic keratosis, squamous cell carcinoma
Other	Low environmental humidity

The Diagnostic Approach

History (Fig. 7.7) and physical examination will yield important clues to the type of keratinisation disorder present. This will narrow the differential diagnosis from the list presented in Figs 7.5 and 7.6 and will indicate which diagnostic tests are likely to lead to a specific diagnosis. Failure to find an underlying cause should lead the clinician to consider the possibility that a primary disorder of keratinisation is present.

Physical examination

A full physical and dermatological examination may indicate that metabolic or endocrine disease is present. The presence or absence of ectoparasites may be noted on examination. The nature and distribution of the scale and other lesions may also give important diagnostic clues and so narrow the differential diagnosis. The list of further reading gives sources for more detail.

The diagnostic plan

The diagnostic plan is summarised in Fig. 7.8. Once a history has been taken and the animal thoroughly examined, a list of the most likely causes can

be drawn up. At that stage a diagnostic plan can be formulated. Clearly, this will vary depending on which diseases are suspected. For example, if an endocrine disorder is likely to be involved, then evaluation of thyroid function and tests for hyperadrenocorticism are indicated (*Chapter 6*). Similarly, the approach to pruritic disorders (allergic or ectoparasitic) is covered in *Chapter 5*.

Irrespective of any of the information gleaned from the history and physical examination, all dogs with scaling disorders should have skin scrapings, coat brushings, hair plucks and adhesive tape samples taken for microscopy. The author's approach is to rule out ectoparasitism, dermatophytosis and *Malassezia* dermatitis from the differential diagnosis at the first opportunity. More specific tests such as blood assays and biopsy should be undertaken

EXAMPLES OF PRIMARY SCALING DISORDERS IN DOGS
Primary idiopathic seborrhoea Follicular dystrophy/dysplasia Epidermal dysplasia Ichthyosis Vitamin A-responsive dermatosis Sebaceous adenitis Nasodigital hyperkeratosis Lichenoid psoriasiform dermatosis Schnauzer comedo syndrome Ear margin dermatosis

Fig. 7.6 Examples of primary scaling disorders in dogs.

later where indicated. Details of these tests and their indications are given in *Chapter 3*.

Adherence to the diagnostic approach detailed throughout this book should enable the clinician to identify the underlying cause in almost all cases of secondary defects of keratinisation. However, in some instances no diagnosis will have been achieved. This may indicate that a primary keratinisation disorder is present. In some instances these are diagnosed by elimination of all other causes. In others, the diagnosis is made by histopathology.

The principles of the clinical management of keratinisation disorders are detailed in *Chapter 33*.

Selected Keratinisation Disorders

Primary idiopathic seborrhoea

Description. The term primary idiopathic seborrhoea is applied to any generalised scaling disease of unknown cause. Not surprisingly, this is the most common of the primary disorders. No research has

been performed on this disorder in any breed except American Cocker Spaniels and, to a lesser extent, Irish Setters. In Cocker Spaniels it has been shown that the epidermis, hair follicle and sebaceous gland are hyperproliferative, with cell renewal time for the living epidermis being decreased from 22 to 8 days. This results in overproduction of squames and in scaling. There is evidence that these abnormalities are not due to humoral influences but arise as a result of a primary epidermal cell defect.

Clinical signs. The clinical picture varies. The disorder is usually encountered in young dogs. Primary seborrhoea in Dobermann Pinschers, Irish Setters and German Shepherd Dogs is usually associated with a dull dry coat and focal to diffuse accumulations of white to grey non-adherent scale (formerly known as **seborrhoea sicca**). In Spaniels, Basset Hounds, Shar Peis and West Highland White Terriers a more greasy disorder is usually seen (**seborrhoea oleosa**). Characteristically, greasy yellow to brown clumps of lipid and scale adherent to the skin and the hairs are seen. There is often a

APPROACH TO SCALING DISORDERS: HISTORY	
Factor	**Differential diagnosis**
Breed	
American and English Cocker Spaniel	Primary idiopathic seborrhoea; vitamin A-responsive dermatosis; *Malassezia* dermatitis
West Highland White Terrier	Primary idiopathic seborrhoea; epidermal dysplasia; atopy; *Malassezia* dermatitis
Dobermann Pinscher	Primary idiopathic seborrhoea; follicular dysplasia; hypothyroidism
Basset Hound	Primary idiopathic seborrhoea; *Malassezia* dermatitis
Shar Pei	Primary idiopathic dermatitis; atopy; hypothyroidism; follicular dysplasia
Irish Setter	Primary idiopathic seborrhoea; hypothyroidism
Boxer	Hyperadrenocorticism; hypothyroidism; follicular dysplasia
Age of onset	
Less than 2 years	Primary keratinisation disorders. These are hereditary and so occur in young dogs
4–10 years	Secondary scaling due to endocrinopathy, hypersensitivity or immune-mediated disorders
8 years onwards	Neoplastic and metabolic disorders (e.g. epitheliotropic lymphoma or hepatocutaneous syndrome)
Progression of lesions	
Scaling preceded pruritus, crusting, inflammation and odour	Primary keratinisation disorder
Pruritus, inflammation and odour preceded scaling	Secondary keratinisation disorder
Affected in-contact animals	Ectoparasitism or dermatophytosis
Seasonality	Atopy, flea allergic dermatitis or biting insects (ants, flies, mosquitos)
Concurrent signs (e.g. polyuria, polydipsia, polyphagia, thermophilia)	Metabolic/endocrine disease

FIG. 7.7 Approach to scaling disorders: History.

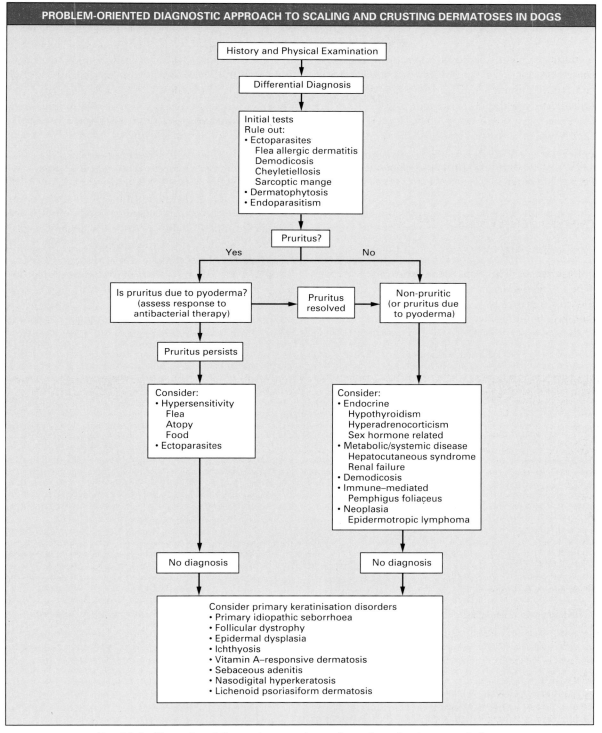

PROBLEM-ORIENTED DIAGNOSTIC APPROACH TO SCALING AND CRUSTING DERMATOSES IN DOGS

History and Physical Examination

Differential Diagnosis

Initial tests
Rule out:
• Ectoparasites
    Flea allergic dermatitis
    Demodicosis
    Cheyletiellosis
    Sarcoptic mange
• Dermatophytosis
• Endoparasitism

Pruritus?

Yes — No

Is pruritus due to pyoderma?
(assess response to
antibacterial therapy)

Pruritus
resolved

Non-pruritic
(or pruritus due
to pyoderma)

Pruritus persists

Consider:
• Hypersensitivity
    Flea
    Atopy
    Food
• Ectoparasites

Consider:
• Endocrine
    Hypothyroidism
    Hyperadrenocorticism
    Sex hormone related
• Metabolic/systemic disease
    Hepatocutaneous syndrome
    Renal failure
• Demodicosis
• Immune–mediated
    Pemphigus foliaceus
• Neoplasia
    Epidermotropic lymphoma

No diagnosis

No diagnosis

Consider primary keratinisation disorders
• Primary idiopathic seborrhoea
• Follicular dystrophy
• Epidermal dysplasia
• Ichthyosis
• Vitamin A–responsive dermatosis
• Sebaceous adenitis
• Nasodigital hyperkeratosis
• Lichenoid psoriasiform dermatosis

Fɪɢ. 7.8 Problem-oriented diagnostic approach to scaling and crusting dermatoses in dogs.

concurrent ceruminous otitis externa. A marked rancid odour is often present. Severe cases have significant secondary pyoderma, inflammation and pruritus (formerly known as **seborrhoeic dermatitis**).

Diagnosis. The diagnosis of primary idiopathic seborrhoea is based on history, physical examination and elimination of primary causes. Histopathology may **support** this diagnosis.

Treatment. The management of scaling disorders is covered in detail in *Chapter 33*. A major part of the treatment of these disorders is topical shampoo therapy to reduce scale, crusts and grease from the skin surface. The selection and use of such shampoos should be tailored to the specific case. Some topical agents facilitate the removal of surface debris, (such as benzoyl peroxide) whereas others (such as coal tar) reduce the epidermal mitotic rate. Some shampoos contain moisturisers (indicated in cases of 'seborrhoea sicca') and some contain antimicrobial agents (to control bacterial or yeast populations).

Oral treatment with synthetic vitamin A derivatives (retinoids) such as etretinate have been shown to be effective in idiopathic seborrhoea of American Cocker Spaniels. Other beneficial treatments include systemic antimicrobial agents, oral essential fatty acid supplements and, if used cautiously, glucocorticoids.

Prognosis. The prognosis varies with the severity of the condition. However, primary idiopathic seborrhoea is incurable and life-long therapy is required. In some cases an intensive, costly and time-consuming treatment protocol is needed to keep the animal comfortable and odour-free. Dedicated owners are needed!

Follicular dystrophy

Description. This term encompasses a group of diseases in which hair-loss and abnormalities of hair pigmentation occur. Several breeds are affected although Dobermann Pinschers appear to be most prone. The pathogenesis of these disorders is poorly understood. Although these defects are associated with hair-loss, they are discussed here as they are associated with metabolic defects of the follicular epidermis. They are also discussed in *Chapter 6*.

Follicular dystrophy has been divided into two forms: **colour dilute** (formerly known as **colour mutant**) **alopecia** and **follicular dysplasia**. The distinction between these disorders is based on the colour of the original coat. If the coat was originally dilute, as is seen in blue and fawn Dobermann Pinschers, then colour dilute alopecia is present. If normal non-dilute, usually black, hairs are affected then the disorder is referred to as follicular dysplasia. It is not yet clear whether these are two distinct syndromes or the same syndrome affecting different coloured hairs.

Clinical signs. Colour dilute alopecia is a hereditary tardive alopecia seen in blue and fawn individuals of a number of breeds including Dobermann Pinschers, Great Danes, Whippets, Italian Greyhounds, Yorkshire Terriers, Miniature Pinschers, Irish Setters, Dachshunds, Chow Chows, Poodles, Chihuahuas, Salukis and Newfoundlands. The incidence of colour dilute alopecia in blue and fawn Dobermann Pinschers is high: 58% and 90%, respectively. Follicular dysplasia is less common than colour dilute alopecia but has been reported in non-dilute coloured (i.e. red/tan and black/tan) Dobermann Pinschers, Bearded Collies, cross-breeds and sporadically within other breeds.

The disorder starts gradually as a partial 'motheaten' alopecia of the appropriately coloured hairs; for example, in blue and fawn Dobermann Pinschers, the tan points are spared. The onset is usually before 3 years of age. Hair-loss is usually complicated by dry scaling and secondary folliculitis. Eventually extensive alopecia and severe scaling are seen. Pruritus is only a feature if secondary pyoderma is not controlled.

Diagnosis. History (coat colour, breed and age of onset) may indicate that follicular dystrophy is present. A tentative diagnosis may be made by microscopic examination of plucked hairs. Large black clumps of disorganised melanin (macromelanosomes) will be present within the hairs and there is often distortion and breakage of the hairs associated with these structures. Definitive diagnosis is based on histopathology.

Treatment. The hair-loss is irreversible and the condition is incurable. The aim of therapy is to minimise secondary bacterial infection and scaling.

Frequent bathing with antibacterial shampoos may be of value (*Chapter 33*). Suitable products contain ethyl lactate or benzoyl peroxide. However, one consequence of frequent bathing, particularly using benzoyl peroxide, is that the skin will become even more dry and scaly. Humectant and emollient rinses may counteract this effect. Secondary pyodermas should be treated with systemic antimicrobial agents.

There are reports that the retinoid isotretinoin is of value in the management of this disorder. Retinoids are expensive, difficult to acquire and not licensed for use in animals.

Prognosis. Although the disorder is incurable, the prognosis for a good quality of life is favourable and most owners are able to cope with their dog's disorder.

Vitamin A-responsive dermatosis

Description. Vitamin A-responsive dermatosis is relatively uncommon but is included here as it can easily be misdiagnosed as primary idiopathic seborrhoea. The disorder is mostly encountered in American or English Cocker Spaniels less than 3 years old. It is not a disease of nutritional deficiency but may be due to a defect in the metabolism or utilisation of vitamin A. Alternatively, response to vitamin A supplementation may simply be pharmacological due to a direct effect of this nutrient on epidermal metabolism.

Clinical signs. Scaling, follicular plugs (**comedones**), a dry easily epilated coat and hyperkeratotic plaques with 'fronds' of keratinaceous material protruding from the hair follicle ostia are the usual lesions. Pruritus, otitis and odour may be present.

Diagnosis. Diagnosis is based on history, clinical signs and elimination of other keratinisation disorders from the differential diagnosis. Generalised scaling with hyperkeratotic plaques in a young adult American or English Cocker Spaniel is suggestive of this diagnosis. Histopathology is helpful but a definitive diagnosis can only be made following a beneficial response to oral vitamin A supplementation.

Prognosis. The disorder is incurable but will remain in remission whilst oral vitamin A therapy is administered.

Epidermal dysplasia (see Plate 5)

Description. This disorder has been reported only in West Highland White Terriers. It appears to be a genetic abnormality of keratinisation, although there is some controversy regarding its pathogenesis. It is an extremely severe disorder which usually starts within the first year of life (Plate 5).

Clinical signs. Epidermal dysplasia occurs in young dogs and is associated with ventral erythema and pruritus. The disorder rapidly generalises and leads to what has been termed **'armadillo disease'**. Severely affected dogs have erythema, alopecia, pruritus, hyperpigmentation, lichenification, greasy skin, odour, otitis, pyoderma and lymphadenopathy. Secondary *Malassezia* infection is seen in some cases.

Diagnosis. The diagnosis is said to be based on finding characteristic histopathological epidermal lesions (dysplasia); however, the author has investigated a number of cases of 'armadillo disease' in West Highland White Terriers and has yet to find one with these reported changes. It may be that epidermal dysplasia is a misnomer. It is the author's opinion that this diagnosis should be made on the basis of history and clinical signs along with elimination of all other possible causes and that histopathology should not be relied upon.

Treatment. Epidermal dysplasia is generally nonresponsive to topical therapy and systemic antimicrobial, glucocorticoid, retinoid or essential fatty acid treatments. Two forms of therapy have been suggested.

In early cases, immunosuppressive doses of glucocorticoids may be of value. Oral prednisolone, at 1–2 mg/kg daily, is the drug of choice, but treatment must be implemented before chronic irreversible changes occur within the skin. Once a response is seen the treatment is tapered to find the lowest effective alternate-day maintenance dose.

In animals with secondary *Malassezia* infection, the yeast may be playing a significant role in the pathogenesis of the disorder, particularly in the development of pruritus. In such cases, there may be a significant improvement in the condition following antifungal therapy. Oral ketoconazole at 10 mg/kg daily for up to 14 days has been recommended. This drug is not licensed for use in small animals. Topical antifungal agents such as ketoconazole shampoo, selenium sulphide shampoo and chlorhexidine are often ineffective in inducing a remission but can be used regularly for maintenance after ketoconazole has been administered. Ketoconazole has a number of other effects including immunosuppression and so improvement following the use of this medicament does not necessarily imply that the disorder was induced by yeast.

Prognosis. The prognosis is poor and euthanasia is often requested.

Sebaceous adenitis

Description. This is an inflammation of and around the sebaceous glands leading to loss of these structures and consequent dry skin, scaling and hair-loss. The majority of cases have been seen in young adult to middle-aged Standard Poodles, Hungarian Vizslas, Akitas and Samoyeds. It has also been documented sporadically in a number of other breeds. The aetiology and pathogenesis are unknown. Four hypotheses concerning the aetiology and pathogenesis of this disorder have been proposed:

- Damage to the sebaceous glands is immune-mediated or autoimmune.
- Loss of the sebaceous glands is genetic or developmental.
- There is a primary keratinisation defect in the sebaceous gland ducts leading to blockage with keratin and lipid, destroying the sebaceous gland by 'back-pressure'.
- Lipid metabolism is defective, leading to abnormal epidermal keratinisation and sebaceous gland function.

It is possible that more than one of these factors is involved.

Clinical signs. There appear to be two forms of sebaceous adenitis. The first form is seen in long-coated breeds (Standard Poodles, Akitas and Samoyeds). Initial clinical signs are scaling, partial alopecia and a dull, brittle coat. Affected areas include the dorsal mid-line, the dorsum of the muzzle, the top of the head and the neck. There is usually no pruritus or odour in the early stages. However, in some individuals the disease progresses and larger quantities of tightly adherent scale and follicular plugs develop. Secondary pyoderma is a common sequel leading to pruritus and odour.

The second form of sebaceous adenitis is less severe and affects short-coated breeds such as the Vizsla. The clinical signs are 'moth-eaten' alopecia and scaling, affecting the trunk, ears and head. Clinically, this may be indistinguishable from pyoderma. Pruritus and secondary pyoderma are rare.

Diagnosis. The diagnosis is based on history (especially breed) and clinical findings. Elimination of other causes will narrow the differential diagnosis. Confirmation of the diagnosis is achieved by histopathology, and several sites should be sampled. Typically pathology will reveal inflammation around the sebaceous glands. In advanced cases, the sebaceous glands are absent and are replaced by fibrous tissue.

Treatment. Antiseborrhoeic shampoos, conditioners and humectants, along with essential fatty acids, may help early or mildly affected cases. Chronic and more severe cases may be helped by the use of high doses of essential fatty acids and the daily topical spray application of a 50–75% mixture of propylene glycol in water. The aim of treatment is to increase the lipid content of the stratum corneum and so to restore normal water vapour function. It has been suggested that immunosuppressive agents such as glucocorticoids and cyclosporin A may prevent further sebaceous gland destruction. Retinoids (isotretinoin or etretinate, 1 mg/kg *per os* daily) have also been used in the management of this disorder with variable results.

Prognosis. The prognosis varies with breed. Although the loss of sebaceous glands is irreversible, the form of sebaceous adenitis affecting short-haired dogs appears to respond well to therapy. Conversely, the disease has a much worse prognosis in long-haired breeds, especially Standard Poodles and Akitas. Secondary bacterial infection, pruritus and odour may become significant and refractory problems and long-term antimicrobial therapy or even euthanasia may be indicated in some Standard Poodles. The prognosis is also dependent on the speed with which a diagnosis is made. In early cases, fewer sebaceous glands will have been lost and so the prognosis is better than in more chronic cases. It has been suggested that the pathogenesis of sebaceous adenitis in the Poodle is more rapid than in other breeds and this may partly explain the worse prognosis.

Ear margin dermatosis

Description. This is a rare idiopathic, bilaterally symmetrical defect of the pinnae of Dachshunds, Dobermann Pinschers and other short-haired breeds.

Clinical signs. In the early stages the dermatosis is characterised by greasy 'plugs' adhering to the skin and hairs of the pinnal margins. Although pruritus is usually absent, alopecia may develop. Some severe untreated cases may progress to ulceration and necrosis of the pinnal margins, which resolves with scarring and fissure formation.

Diagnosis. In early cases, this is a clinical diagnosis (sarcoptic mange should be considered if pruritus is present). In severe cases, the differential diagnosis is quite complex and includes immune-mediated disorders and neoplasia (*Chapter 8*).

Treatment. Mild, early cases can be managed easily with topical therapy. Antiseborrhoeic shampoos used locally to remove scale, crust and oil are usually helpful. Treatment is usually repeated regularly to maintain remission. More severe cases can be managed with topical glucocorticoid creams. Ulcerated tissue can be removed surgically in severely affected dogs. Tissue should be resected well into normal tissue.

Prognosis. The outcome depends on the severity of the condition. It is incurable but usually can be managed successfully using the measures detailed above. In general, it is a cosmetic problem.

Idiopathic nasodigital hyperkeratosis

Description. This idiopathic disorder is characterised by accumulation of keratin and crusts on the planum nasale, footpads or both. It is usually seen in Spaniels. In other breeds, nasodigital hyperkeratosis may develop physiologically with age.

Clinical signs. The lesions are tight, thick, dry accumulations of keratin which are often cracked, fissured, eroded or ulcerated. Severe footpad lesions may lead to lameness.

Diagnosis. If the disease is confined to the nose and feet and the dog is otherwise healthy, the diagnosis is made on clinical grounds. Sudden onset apparently idiopathic nasodigital hyperkeratosis in old dogs, should have biopsy material submitted to histopathology as the lesion may be neoplastic.

Treatment. The hyperkeratotic tissue can be encouraged to slough by hydration. Wet dressings followed by an application of a barrier such as petroleum jelly will seal water in the stratum corneum. In more severe cases, keratolytic substances such as salicylic acid may be of value. A gel containing this substance along with lactic acid and urea is available and is of value in such cases. Topical retinoid gel (tretinoin) is also useful in the management of this disorder but may be irritant. In cases where secondary infection is a feature, antimicrobial gels and ointments are indicated. Inflammation may be controlled with topical glucocorticoids. Occasionally, very pronounced hyperkeratosis is present and this may lead to lameness. Hyperkeratotic areas can be carefully debrided under anaesthesia.

Prognosis. The problem is usually simply cosmetic. In cases where pain and lameness are present, the prognosis is less favourable, although most respond to the benign treatments listed above.

Ichthyosis

Description. Ichthyosis is an extremely rare congenital disorder affecting terriers, particularly West Highland White Terriers, and their crosses. It is characterised by the presence, from birth, of severe scaling of the body and footpads. It has been assumed that this is a genetically determined disorder although the genetic background of affected dogs has not been investigated.

Clinical signs. This disorder is characterised by tightly adherent fine white scales covering the entire body. These may be waxy and rather more crusted in the intertriginous regions. The ventral surface is often most severely affected and feathered or frond-like projections of keratin may be seen. Alopecia, hyperpigmentation and lichenification are sometimes associated with this disorder. Severe hyperkeratosis of the footpads is a consistent feature of canine ichthyosis.

Diagnosis. A history of congenital scaling as described above in a young terrier is highly suggestive that this disorder is present. The diagnosis is confirmed by histopathology.

Treatment. Lifelong therapy to control scaling is required. The regular use of antiseborrhoeic shampoos is of great value in removing the scale and reducing odour. Humectant and emollient sprays are also useful in the management of this disorder. Retinoids (both etretinate and isotretinoin) have produced excellent results, with remission seen within 2 to 3 months of the onset of treatment.

Prognosis. The prognosis is guarded, as life-long therapy is required for this incurable condition. However, with committed and diligent owners, good results can be achieved.

Schnauzer comedone syndrome

Description. This keratinisation disorder affects Miniature Schnauzers exclusively and is thought to be genetic in origin. It is characterised clinically by comedone formation along the dorsal mid-line. It has been suggested that it arises as a result of a developmental defect in keratinisation of the follicular epidermis, leading to follicular plugging, comedone formation and secondary bacterial folliculitis.

Clinical signs. The clinical presentation is one of crusted, papular comedones along the dorsal mid-line from the neck to the tail. It usually occurs in young adults of either sex. In early and mild cases, the lesions are difficult to see but are readily palpated. In advanced cases, the lesions are more easily visible and pruritus or discomfort is evident, especially if secondary bacterial infection is present.

Diagnosis. The history of comedone formation on the dorsal mid-line of a young Miniature Schnauzer is highly suggestive that Schnauzer comedone syndrome is present. Diagnosis is confirmed by histopathology.

Treatment. Benzoyl peroxide shampoos are indicated, as they remove follicular plugs and debris as well as having an antimicrobial effect. Such shampoo therapy is required regularly for life. Systemic antibiotics may be needed intermittently to control secondary bacterial infection. Glucocorticoids are contraindicated as they encourage comedone formation. Intractable cases have been shown to benefit from systemic retinoid therapy (isotretinoin).

Prognosis. The prognosis is favourable although most cases need life-long topical therapy.

Lichenoid-psoriasiform dermatosis

Description. Lichenoid-psoriasiform dermatosis is an extremely rare keratinisation defect which predominantly affects English Springer Spaniels.

Clinical signs. Dogs of both sexes, under 2 years of age, are affected. The lesions are non-pruritic, erythematous, lichenoid papules and plaques affecting the medial aspect of the pinnae, the external ear canal, the preauricular and periorbital skin, the lips, prepuce and inguinal region. In chronic cases, crusts, greasy scale and papillomatous-like lesions may develop.

Diagnosis. History and physical examination along with elimination of other disorders from the differential diagnosis will enable a tentative diagnosis to be made. Histopathology confirms the diagnosis.

Treatment. This disorder is rather refractory to treatment. Medicaments which have been used include antimicrobial agents, glucocorticoids, vitamin A and topical antiseborrhoeic agents. If secondary pyoderma is present, then some improvement is seen after antimicrobial therapy. Improvement, but not total resolution of lesions, has been seen following immunosuppressive doses of oral prednisolone (2 mg/kg).

Prognosis. Prognosis is guarded to poor, depending on the severity of the lesions.

Lethal acrodermatitis

Description. Lethal acrodermatitis is recognised exclusively in English Bull Terrier puppies. Affected animals have subnormal plasma zinc concentrations despite being fed a diet that is balanced. Poor growth, weakness, lethargy and death occur in all cases. It is thought that the disease arises due to a metabolic defect in the utilisation of zinc as oral and parenteral administration of this mineral fails to ameliorate the problem.

Clinical signs. Affected puppies have paler hairs than unaffected litter-mates and are weak, reluctant to suckle and grow poorly. They have difficulty in eating and have a somewhat arched or vaulted hard palate in which food lodges. There are behavioural abnormalities, often aggression, and the posture is unusual with the front legs abducted and the digits splayed. Affected individuals are prone to the development of diarrhoea and pneumonia. The skin lesions include hyperkeratosis between the toes and footpads, and a papular, pustular and hyperkeratotic dermatosis affecting the body orifices, especially those of the head. This may develop into furunculosis. Ceruminous otitis externa and deep pyoderma of the elbows and hocks are seen.

Diagnosis. History and clinical signs are helpful. Histopathology of affected skin reveals signs compatible with zinc-responsive dermatosis, namely parakeratosis, hyperkeratosis and pyoderma.

Treatment. There is no effective treatment.

Prognosis. Death is inevitable, with the mean survival time being 6 months. Euthanasia of affected puppies is recommended.

Pemphigus foliaceus and erythematosus

Description. Pemphigus foliaceus (**PF**) is the most common immune-mediated disease in the dog. The aetiology and pathogenesis are somewhat unclear. In the dog, three main forms of the disease are recognised:

- Spontaneous pemphigus foliaceus (**SPF**)
- Drug-induced pemphigus foliaceus (**DPF**)
- Chronic disease associated pemphigus foliaceus (**CDPF**)

The distinction between these three forms is made on the basis of history and response to therapy. DPF cases usually have a history of the administration of a drug, including vaccines or anthelmintics, and usually remain in remission after treatment provided that exposure to the precipitating medicament is not repeated. Cases of CDPF occur more frequently in older animals which have had chronic dermatoses. Treatment is usually lifelong in cases of SPF and CDPF.

Pemphigus erythematosus is much less common than PF. Lesions are usually confined to the head. Some features of the disease are compatible with discoid lupus erythematosus (**DLE**, *Chapter 8*).

Two other forms of pemphigus — pemphigus vulgaris and vegetans — have been reported in the dog but these disorders are exceptionally rare and there is some doubt about the existence of pemphigus vegetans in this species. Pemphigus vulgaris is discussed fully in *Chapter 8*.

The pathogenesis of pemphigus involves immune-mediated destruction of the intercellular material of the epidermis, a process that is termed **acantholysis**. The precise mechanism by which this process is initiated and the actual mechanism of acantholysis are poorly understood although it is known to be auto-antibody-induced. It is probable that the antigen involved is desmoglein, a glycoprotein part of the desmosome. Factors such as exposure to ultraviolet light or viruses are said to be involved in some cases. Genetic factors may be involved. Chronic disease and drug therapy are implicated in the pathogenesis of CDPF and DPF respectively.

Breakdown of intercellular bonding leads to clefting within the epidermis and the release of free keratinocytes (acantholytic cells) into the clefts. These clefts are filled with fluid, polymorphonuclear cells (neutrophils and eosinophils) and acantholytic cells.

Clinical signs. All forms of PF and PE are clinically similar. There is usually scaling and crusting overlying an erythematous macular to pustular dermatosis. Physical removal of crusts will often reveal alopecia and erosions. Lesions typically affect the dorsum of the muzzle (this is often the first site to be affected), the dorsal medial canthus of the eyes and the pinnae. Pemphigus foliaceus may also affect the foot pads and nail folds. The primary lesion is an epidermal vesicle. However, because of the fragile and thin nature of the canine epidermis, such lesions are transient and often hard to find. More typically this is a disease of crusting (Plate 9).

Diagnosis. History and clinical findings are helpful in establishing a diagnosis of pemphigus foliaceus. Microscopical examination of stained impression smears made from the undersurface of crusts of the exposed surface of erosions after crust removal may reveal large numbers of acantholytic cells and associated polymorphonuclear cells. Usually, there are no or few bacteria present in these specimens. The presence of large numbers of bacteria should lead to the suspicion that pyoderma is present. Such results should be regarded with caution as bacterial toxins may cause acantholysis. Acantholysis induced by bacteria is usually less marked than that seen in pemphigus. However, it is possible to misdiagnose pemphigus for pyoderma. If immunosuppressive therapy is used, the results can be disastrous for the animal. If in doubt as to whether the problem is pyoderma or pemphigus, it is prudent to treat with antibiotics to evaluate response before using immunosuppressive therapy.

A further complication exists: pyoderma can occur secondary to pemphigus. The differentiation of these two disorders may be exceptionally difficult in such cases. *If in doubt, treat with antibiotics first.*

Histopathological examination may be helpful if intact vesicles are sampled. However, such lesions are rare as they are very fragile and so are only present for a short period. In the author's experience it can be difficult to find suitable lesions for biopsy and so the histopathological diagnosis of pemphigus can be hard to make. A 'bulla watch' (observation of the hospitalised animal for the eruption of a lesion suitable for biopsy) is recommended but this is a very time-consuming procedure.

Immunocytochemistry using direct antibody techniques is a costly and time-consuming procedure. Such testing detects antibody, usually IgG, in the intercellular spaces of the stratum corneum, but its reliability has been questioned. Few laboratories are able to offer this service.

Treatment. The treatment of these disorders is covered in detail in *Chapter 31*. Immunosuppressive doses of glucocorticoids (usually prednisolone) are employed. Often, glucocorticoid therapy is augmented with azathioprine therapy.

Prognosis. The prognosis varies. Cases of DPF will remain in remission following withdrawal of immunosuppressive therapy. Other cases require lifelong treatment. The prognosis depends on the dose and types of medication required to keep the disease in remission. Azathioprine and prednisolone are associated with well documented side-effects and patients on such therapy need to be carefully monitored as described in *Chapter 31*. Long-term therapy may be associated with demodicosis, dermatophytosis, liver disease and bone marrow suppression.

8

Ulcerative Skin Lesions

KAREN MORIELLO

The terms **ulcer** and **erosion** refer to defects in the skin caused by inflammation, self-trauma or auto-immune or infectious processes. These defects may or may not contain serum, blood, or inflammatory cells/exudate. Clinically, the appearance of ulcers and erosions may be indistinguishable. **Technically, an ulcer is a defect in the skin that involves a break in the basement membrane. An erosion is a superficial defect in the skin that only involves the epidermis.** For simplicity, the term 'ulcerative' in this chapter will refer to both erosive and true ulcerative skin diseases.

Ulcerative skin diseases may be subtle or dramatic in clinical appearance. Obvious ulcers are usually noticed by clients. Ulcerative diseases of the mucous membranes, especially in the mouth, are often maloderous. A foul smell 'may be the only client complaint.' When presented with a patient with ulcerative skin lesions it is important to determine rapidly if the cause is self-trauma (ulcers/excoriations due to pruritus), infectious (bacteria, yeast or deep fungal organisms), neoplasia, metabolic (uraemia), or autoimmune/immunological.

In this chapter, the diseases in which ulceration is a part of the pathogenesis and therefore nearly always a feature will be discussed in detail.

Selected Skin Diseases Characterised by Ulceration

Lipfold pyoderma

Description. Lipfold pyoderma is a common skin disease of dogs with abundant skin around the mouth. The folds of skin are constantly moist and exposed to large numbers of bacteria. This results in large amounts of tissue maceration and ulceration. Although there are breed predispositions, lipfold pyoderma can occur in any dog with predisposing facial anatomy. Also, it is important to recognise

that this condition may be present in dogs with facial pruritus.

Clinical signs. Lipfold pyoderma is most common in dog breeds with pendulous lips, e.g. Cocker Spaniels, Springer Spaniels, Bulldogs. Owners often complain about a foul odour around the

DIFFERENTIAL DIAGNOSIS OF ULCERATIVE SKIN LESIONS IN DOGS	
Focal lesions	Demodicosis Staphylococcal infection/pyotraumatic dermatitis Intertriginous or frictional infection Systemic fungal infection Fungal kerion Neoplasia Calcinosis cutis
Face and/or nasal lesions	Solar thermal damage Squamous cell carcinoma Uveodermatological syndrome Discoid lupus erythematosus Epitheliotropic lymphoma and other neoplastic diseases Systemic fungal infection Deep bacterial pyoderma Dermatomyositis Pemphigus foliaceus/erythematosus
Mucocutaneous lesions	Uraemia/renal failure Aerobic and anaerobic infection Systemic lupus erythematosus Bullous pemphigoid Pemphigus vulgaris Toxic epidermal necrolysis Erythema multiforme Drug reaction Candidiasis
Generalised or large regional lesions	Thermal injury Systemic drug reaction Systemic lupus erythematosus Toxic epidermal necrolysis Erythema multiforme Generalised demodicosis Generalised deep bacterial pyoderma Systemic fungal infection
Axillary and inguinal lesions	Intertriginous or frictional lesions *Malassezia* spp. or candidiasis Urine scald Demodicosis Bullous pemphigoid Systemic lupus erythematosus Toxic epidermal necrolysis Erythema multiforme Drug reaction

FIG. 8.1 Differential diagnosis of ulcerative skin lesions in dogs.

FIG. 8.2 Approach to patients with ulcerative skin disease: History.

APPROACH TO PATIENTS WITH ULCERATIVE SKIN DISEASE: HISTORY	
Factor	**Differential diagnosis**
Breed	
Dachshunds	Intertriginous/frictional pyoderma
Huskies, Samoyeds, Alaskan Malumutes	Uveodermatological syndrome
Collies, Shetland Sheepdogs	Dermatomyositis; bullous pemphigoid; systemic lupus erythematosus (SLE); ulcerative disease of Shetland Sheepdogs
Age of onset	
More than 5 years	Neoplasia
Pruritus before development of lesion	Pyoderma; pyotraumatic dermatitis
History of 'sunbathing' in area of lesion development	Solar damage; squamous cell carcinoma
History of drug exposure	Drug reaction; toxic epidermal necrolysis (TEN); erythema multiforme; candidiasis
Complaint of anorexia, depression, fever, weight-loss, lameness, or other signs of systemic illness	Systemic lupus erythematosus; uraemia/renal failure
History of slow onset	Neoplasia; deep pyoderma; systemic fungal; autoimmune skin diseases
History of acute/abrupt onset	Drug reactions; toxic epidermal necrolysis; fungal kerion

dog's mouth or head. The lipfold pyoderma may or may not be painful or pruritic and exudation and secondary crusting is common. Depending upon the duration of the pyoderma and the depth of the fold, ulceration may be mild or severe. Lesions develop slowly and are limited to the area of the skin involved in, or immediately surrounding, the fold. Ulceration involving the lips, commissures and mouth is suggestive of other diseases (see Fig. 8.1). Some dogs may develop a *Malassezia* infection in their facial folds and this is characterised by intense facial pruritus.

Diagnosis. Diagnosis is most often made via clinical signs. Skin scrapings and impression smears are useful to determine if demodicosis or a secondary bacterial agent is present.

Treatment. Medical management of lipfold pyoderma requires lifelong maintenance therapy. The owner will need to wash the affected area daily with an antibacterial shampoo such as benzoyl peroxide or chlorhexidine and thoroughly dry the area. It is important to keep facial folds as dry and clean as possible. Astringent agents (e.g. witch hazel) should

APPROACH TO PATIENTS WITH ULCERATIVE SKIN DISEASE: PHYSICAL EXAMINATION	
Physical finding	**Differential diagnosis**
Obesity and/or short legs	Intertriginous pyoderma; urine scald
Lesions in white or sun-exposed areas	Squamous cell carcinoma; thermal injury
Fever, weight-loss; muscle atrophy; lameness; or other systemic signs	Systemic lupus erythematosus; uraemia
Lesions exudative or covered with a crust	Bacterial or fungal infection; kerion; demodicosis; pyotraumatic dermatitis
Lesions associated with hair-loss	Demodicosis; bacterial pyoderma; deep fungal; pyotraumatic dermatitis; underlying pruritic skin disease
Ulceration associated with sloughing of skin or Nikolsky sign	TEN; thermal burn; SLE; generalised demodicosis; deep pyoderma; systemic drug reaction; anaerobic infection
Mucocutaneous ulceration limited to mouth	Uraemia; lipfold pyoderma; combined anaerobic/aerobic infection; bullous pemphigoid

FIG. 8.3 Approach to patients with ulcerative skin disease: Physical examination.

DIAGNOSTIC PLAN FOR ULCERATIVE SKIN LESIONS

At the initial visit:

1. **Determine if the patient is pruritic.** If pruritus is a strong component of the history, see *Chapter 5*
2. **Consider the possibility of trauma, exposure to caustic agents, or thermal injuries**
3. **Consider the possibility of a systemic drug reaction.** Patients may have reactions to parenteral drugs, oral drugs and topical agents. Drug reactions can occur in dogs that are currently receiving drugs or have received them recently (days or weeks); they can also occur suddenly in dogs that have been receiving a drug (e.g. heartworm preventive) for a long period without adverse affects

> **Focused diagnostic tests:** Impression smears to determine if there is an infectious agent present or if there is suspicion of neoplasia. Skin scrapings should be performed to determine if demodicosis is present. If there is a recent drug history, discontinue any systemic or topical drugs for 3 – 7 days and re-examine the patient

Focal Area of Ulceration

1. *If there is a focal area of ulceration with or without marked hair-loss,* consider demodicosis, fungal kerion, bacterial infection (including pyotraumatic dermatitis), a fold pyoderma and possible neoplasia. **Fungal kerions** are acute, inflammatory and exudative; they are most common on the nose and feet. Areas of **pyotraumatic dermatitis** are also acute and inflammatory and are usually pruritic/painful and exudative

> **Focused diagnostic tests:** Skin scrapings should be performed to determine if demodicosis is present. Impression smears should be examined to determine if the predominant cell population is inflammatory, if an infectious agent can be identified or if the lesion is possibly neoplastic. Ulcerative neoplastic lesions are difficult to diagnose via impression smears because inflammatory cells are often so predominant. Superficial fungal cultures are not cost-effective in the diagnosis of a fungal kerion because cultures are often negative due to the inflammatory nature of the lesion

2. *If skin scrapings are negative, and there is no immediate suspicion of neoplasia and the impression smear is supportive of a bacterial infection,* treat appropriately
3. *If there is no response to antibiotic therapy,* consider the possibility of an unidentified infectious agent, neoplastic skin disease or other cause of a non-healing wound

> **Focused diagnostic tests:** Perform a skin biopsy using a long elliptical excision. Histological examination of an ulcer is rarely diagnostic and examination of the margin or periphery is most helpful. If the lesion is exudative, impression smears for Gram stain and routine cytological examination should be obtained. A wedge of tissue should be submitted for aerobic and anaerobic bacterial culture and deep fungal culture if the lesion(s) worsen or if the results of the Gram stain suggest that an infectious agent is present

Ulcerations on the Face and Nose

If ulcerations are present on the face or nose, consider the possibility of neoplasia, autoimmune skin disease, and infectious agents

> **Focused diagnostic tests:** Skin scrapings should be performed to determine if demodicosis is present. Facial demodicosis causing ulceration is uncommon in adult dogs but is a cause of ulceration in young dogs. Impression smears from the surface of the ulcer should be examined for the presence or absence of inflammatory cells, bacteria or acantholytic cells. If skin scrapings and impression smears are non-diagnostic, skin biopsies from several representative areas should be collected and examined

Mucocutaneous Ulcerations

1. **A careful examination of the mucocutaneous junctions should be performed.** *If ulcerations are limited to the oral mucosa and the mouth and the breath are fetid,* consider uraemia/renal failure

> **Focused diagnostic tests:** Serum urea nitrogen and creatinine concentrations should be determined to confirm the presence of uraemia and secondary ulceration

2. *If the patient is not uraemic or if uraemia is not suspected,* consider anaerobic or aerobic bacterial infections, drug reactions, caustic agents and mucocutaneous candidiasis

> **Focused diagnostic tests:** Perform impression smears of the lesion, scrape smears of the margin of the lesion and routine skin scrapings to look for bacteria, candidiasis and demodicosis. If the lesions are exudative and large numbers of degenerate neutrophils are present, perform an anaerobic and aerobic bacterial culture

3. *If cytology and cultures do not identify an infectious agent,* strongly consider an autoimmune or immune-mediated skin disease

> **Focused diagnostic tests:** Skin biopsies will be required for definitive diagnosis. The patient should be carefully examined for the presence of vesicles and bullae. If possible, intact vesicles/bullae should be biopsied via elliptical excision. If these are not available for biopsy, a wide elliptical excision including the ulcer and its margin should be submitted for routine histopathology. If the patient is showing signs of systemic illness or if the mucocutaneous ulceration is severe or multifocal, submit fluid sample for haematology, antinuclear antibody test, urinalysis and serum biochemistry panel for evidence of systemic lupus erythematosus. If the initial biopsies are non-diagnostic, the patient should be hospitalised and observed every few hours for the development of vesicles/bullae. These lesions are very transient and should be harvested immediately

Continued

DIAGNOSTIC PLAN FOR ULCERATIVE SKIN LESIONS

Generalised or Multifocal Areas of Ulceration

If there is generalised ulceration or multifocal areas of ulceration, consider the possibility of severe life-threatening skin diseases. Thermal burns, drug reactions, autoimmune/immune-mediated disease and generalised deep pyoderma due to demodicosis or systemic fungal are all likely possibilities

> **Focused diagnostic tests:** Because these lesions are severe and the underlying causes are possibly life-threatening, the following tests should be performed at the initial visit: skin scrapings for demodicosis; impression smears; Gram stain of exudate; and aerobic and anaerobic bacterial and fungal cultures. Skin biopsies from several representative areas should be submitted for routine histopathology. Serum biochemistry panel, urinalysis, haematology and an antinuclear antibody test should also be undertaken

Axillary and Inguinal Ulceration

1. If ulceration is present in the axillary or inguinal region, consider fold pyoderma and superficial pyoderma, yeast infections, urine scald and demodicosis

> **Focused diagnostic tests:** Skin scrapings should be performed to determine if demodicosis is present. Impression smears of exudate and scrape smears from the margin of the lesion should be collected to look for bacteria, *Malassezia* spp. and *Candida* spp.

2. *If skin scrapings and cytology are non-diagnostic,* consider a therapeutic trial of oral antibiotics for 21 – 30 days. If the skin lesions are not suggestive of a bacterial skin disease, proceed to step 3
3. *If the skin scrapings and cytology are non-diagnostic and there is no response to oral antibiotics,* strongly consider autoimmune/immune-mediated skin diseases as the most likely cause

> **Focused diagnostic tests:** Collect numerous long elliptical skin biopsies from the margin of the lesion for routine histopathology; biopsy of the ulcer itself is rarely diagnostic. Repeat impression smears looking for infectious agents. Submit blood for haematology, serum biochemistry panel and antinuclear antibody test. Urine should be submitted for a complete urinalysis

Fig. 8.4 Diagnostic plan for ulcerative skin lesions.

be avoided because they can sting; they decrease wound healing and cannot be used on a long-term basis. Topical antibacterial creams that do not contain glucocorticoids (e.g. mupiricin cream) may be helpful in some patients. Many dogs will benefit from a 3–4 week course of oral antibiotic therapy; however, signs readily occur when oral antibiotics are stopped. If the dog is pruritic, diseases such as food allergy, atopy or *Malassezia* dermatitis should be pursued.

Prognosis. This is not a life-threatening disease but it can be very frustrating for both owner and veterinarian; clients must be very committed to daily cleaning. Surgical ablation may be curative in some cases but in many cases the lipfolds recur in time.

Cutaneous neoplasia

It is beyond the scope of this chapter to describe all of the cutaneous neoplasias that can present as focal areas of ulceration. Squamous cell carcinomas, mast cell tumours and apocrine cell carcinomas are just a few of the more common skin tumours that can present as areas of ulceration. Cytology and skin biopsy are required for a final diagnosis.

Calcinosis cutis

Description. Calcinosis cutis is caused by the deposition of calcium in the skin. The most common cause is canine hyperadrenocorticism (spontaneous or iatrogenic). Calcium deposition in the skin may occur secondary to percutaneous penetration of calcium salts. In some cases the cause is unknown.

Clinical signs. Calcinosis cutis usually presents as hard plaques in the skin. In some dogs, the areas may be very inflamed; pruritic and focal areas of ulceration may develop. In rare instances of calcinosis cutis, a focal area of ulceration that resembles an area of pyotraumatic dermatitis may be seen (G.A. Kunkle, University of Florida, personal communication).

Diagnosis. Skin biopsy is diagnostic for calcinosis cutis.

Treatment. There is no specific treatment. The cause of the dystrophic mineralisation must be identified and treated. In most cases, calcinosis cutis in dogs is due to canine hyperadrenocorticism or iatrogenic hyperglucocorticoidism.

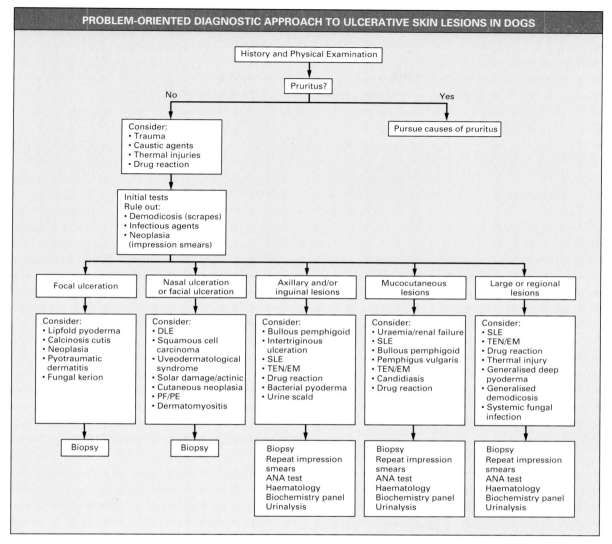

PROBLEM-ORIENTED DIAGNOSTIC APPROACH TO ULCERATIVE SKIN LESIONS IN DOGS

History and Physical Examination

Pruritus?

No → Yes

Pursue causes of pruritus

Consider:
• Trauma
• Caustic agents
• Thermal injuries
• Drug reaction

Initial tests
Rule out:
• Demodicosis (scrapes)
• Infectious agents
• Neoplasia
  (impression smears)

| Focal ulceration | Nasal ulceration or facial ulceration | Axillary and/or inguinal lesions | Mucocutaneous lesions | Large or regional lesions |

Consider:
• Lipfold pyoderma
• Calcinosis cutis
• Neoplasia
• Pyotraumatic dermatitis
• Fungal kerion

Consider:
• DLE
• Squamous cell carcinoma
• Uveodermatological syndrome
• Solar damage/actinic
• Cutaneous neoplasia
• PF/PE
• Dermatomyositis

Consider:
• Bullous pemphigoid
• Intertriginous ulceration
• SLE
• TEN/EM
• Drug reaction
• Bacterial pyoderma
• Urine scald

Consider:
• Uraemia/renal failure
• SLE
• Bullous pemphigoid
• Pemphigus vulgaris
• TEN/EM
• Candidiasis
• Drug reaction

Consider:
• SLE
• TEN/EM
• Drug reaction
• Thermal injury
• Generalised deep pyoderma
• Generalised demodicosis
• Systemic fungal infection

Biopsy

Biopsy

Biopsy
Repeat impression smears
ANA test
Haematology
Biochemistry panel
Urinalysis

Biopsy
Repeat impression smears
ANA test
Haematology
Biochemistry panel
Urinalysis

Biopsy
Repeat impression smears
ANA test
Haematology
Biochemistry panel
Urinalysis

FIG. 8.5 Problem-oriented diagnostic approach to ulcerative skin lesions in dogs.

Prognosis. Dystrophic mineralisation is usually reversible if it is caused by **hypercortisolaemia**, presuming the underlying cause is treated.

Discoid lupus erythematosus

Description. Discoid lupus erythematosus (DLE) is an autoimmune skin disease and is believed to be a benign variant of systemic lupus erythematosus. The exact pathogenesis of canine DLE is unknown but it is believed that sunlight, genetics and viruses may all be involved.

Clinical signs. DLE is believed to be more common in female dogs. Although there is no age predilection, several breeds appear to be predisposed including Collies, German Shepherd Dogs, Siberian Huskies, and Shetland Sheepdogs. The most commonly recognised form of canine DLE is localised to the face; however, the author has seen several cases of DLE-like disease sparing the nose and involving only the face and/or trunk of the dog, in a group of dogs that presented with hairloss and exfoliation. Multifocal areas of ulceration were present in some areas. The clinical signs of classic nasal DLE usually begin slowly. There are areas of macular nasal depigmentation that gradually coalesce. The cobblestone appearance of the planum nasale disappears. Ulceration and 'melting away' of the nasal folds occurs, in addition to moderate to severe nasal crusting. The cartilage of the nose is lost and haemorrhage can occur if the process continues.

Diagnosis. Definitive diagnosis is based upon the clinical signs, skin biopsy and antinuclear antibody test. The best skin biopsy sites are non-ulcerated depigmented areas. Skin biopsies for routine histopathology are the most cost-effective diagnostic tool. Biopsies consistent with DLE show vacuolar degeneration of the basal cell layer, secondary ulceration/erosion and a lichenoid infiltrate in the dermis. Direct immunofluorescence may only be diagnostic (positive deposition of antibody at the basement membrane) in 66% of cases. An antinuclear antibody test is recommended in dogs in which the differential diagnosis may include systemic lupus erythematosus. ANA tests are negative in dogs with discoid lupus erythematosus.

Treatment. All dogs affected with DLE should be kept out of strong sunlight; there is anecdotal evidence that sunlight will cause exacerbations of DLE. The initial treatment of choice is a combination of tetracycline and niacinamide, vitamin E therapy and/or topical glucocorticoids. Dogs weighing 10 kg or less receive 250 mg each of tetracycline and niacinamide t.i.d. Dogs weighing over 10 kg should receive 500 mg of each drug t.i.d. Response to therapy may take up to 3 months and if this drug combination is successful, treatment is lifelong. Oral vitamin E (400 to 800 IU *per os* b.i.d.) has been reported to be useful alone or in combination with other drugs in the management of DLE. Response to therapy may take several months, but this drug is relatively inexpensive and safe.

Topical glucocorticoid therapy alone may control some cases of DLE. Initial therapy requires that a potent fluorinated steroid be used daily for 10 to 15 days. When the disease is in remission, topical glucocorticoid therapy can be decreased to alternate day applications and often or less potent glucocorticoid can be used. The use of topical glucocorticoids can induce systemic and biochemical changes commonly associated with the use of systemic glucocorticoids; clients should be warned of potential adverse affects. If severe disfiguration, ulceration or haemorrhage are present, more aggressive therapy is indicated. Systemic glucocorticoids (1 mg/kg *per os* b.i.d.) for 14 to 30 days should be used until the disease is in remission. Concurrent vitamin E therapy may be used and may hasten recovery and minimise glucocorticoid dependence. Once the lesions are in remission, oral glucocorticoids should be gradually tapered to alternate-day use. Topical glucocorticoids can be introduced gradually and may control these more severe cases once the severe lesion is in remission.

In cases where DLE cannot be controlled with systemic glucocorticoids, azathioprine (1 to 2 mg/kg *per os* once daily) may be used. Once the lesion is in remission, a maintenance dose of azathioprine every 48 to 72 hours can be used. This disease has a tendency to wax and wane and it is common for dogs to experience frequent relapses throughout the course of their life. When relapses occur, the lesion should be treated aggressively with either oral or potent topical glucocorticoids.

Prognosis. This is not a life-threatening disease and is the milder autoimmune skin disease.

Actinic keratosis/solar damage/squamous cell carcinoma

Description. Actinic keratosis and solar damage are caused by intense exposure to excessive ultraviolet light. Lesions occur in lightly haired areas. Many affected dogs are known to be sunbathers.

Clinical signs. Lesions may have any combination of erythema, scaling, papules and focal ulcers. In some dogs, lesions may be raised, ulcerated nodules. The skin may feel abnormally thickened and hard. Squamous cell carcinomas and actinic keratoses are most common on the inner thigh of dogs but they may also occur on the nose, face and eyelids.

Diagnosis. A skin biopsy is required for a definitive diagnosis.

Treatment. Excision is the treatment of choice. There is preliminary clinical evidence that some of these lesions may respond to etretinate therapy (1 mg/kg b.i.d.).

Prognosis. Actinic lesions are considered to be precancerous.

Epitheliotropic lymphoma

Description. Epitheliotropic lymphoma is a cutaneous T-cell lymphoma.

Clinical signs. The earliest clinical signs are erythema and scaling. As the disease progresses, cutaneous plaques, ulcers, and nodules develop. Lesions are most often seen on the trunk; however, several cases of epitheliotropic lymphoma have been seen by the author and others that were clinically indistinguishable from DLE.

Diagnosis. A skin biopsy is required for definitive diagnosis.

Treatment. There is no effective treatment, though isotretinoin 3–4 mg/kg b.i.d. may slow the progression of lesions.

Prognosis. Most dogs die or are euthanased within 6 months to 3 years of the diagnosis. However, many dogs can live for a long time without discomfort.

Uveodermatological syndrome (See Chapter 9)

Pemphigus complex (See Chapter 7)

Uraemic stomatitis

Description. The accumulation of excessive amounts of urea in the blood, along with other waste substances, leads to the constellation of clinical signs and biochemical abnormalities resulting from renal failure (Plate 6).

Clinical signs. Mucocutaneous ulceration of the gum, gingiva, hard palate and tongue may be caused by uraemia. In uraemic patients, the breath is fetid, the animal is depressed and usually has signs of systemic illness. The fetid breath is caused in part by bacterial overgrowth due to decreased saliva production.

Diagnosis. Refer to a textbook of internal medicine for a detailed discussion of this condition, including its treatment. Minimally, urinalysis should be performed on plasma creatinine and urea concentrations measured for any patient being evaluated with the complaint of mucocutaneous ulceration.

Candidiasis

Description. This is a **rare** disease caused by the yeast *Candida* spp. This organism is a normal commensal of the gastrointestinal and genital tracts of most mammals. Mucocutaneous candidiasis occurs in animals that are debilitated by systemic diseases, are immunosuppressed, or are receiving immunosuppressive drugs (Plate 7).

Clinical signs. Ulcers and erosions coated with thick, foul-smelling crusts and exudate are seen most commonly. Any mucocutaneous junction may be affected. In addition, lesions may be seen in the nail bed, nares, vulva, scrotum, external ear, perineum, and glabrous skin. Affected areas are almost always secondarily affected with aerobes and anaerobes. Lesions are very painful and the animal is usually systemically ill. Candidiasis may complicate any of the mucocutaneous skin diseases. Local candidiasis may be seen in female dogs with vulvar fold pyodermas or moist dermatitis. These areas are chronically ulcerated, exudative, moist and erythematous.

Diagnosis. Because mucocutaneous candidiasis can mimic autoimmune skin diseases and the treatment is vastly different, it is important to rule this disease out when presented with a patient with mucocutaneous ulceration. Definitive diagnosis can be made via skin biopsy and cytology (*Chapter 3*). Skin biopsies should be obtained with care and intact crusted lesions need to be sampled. The reference laboratory should be specifically instructed to process any separated crusts. Ulcerated lesions should not be biopsied because it is unlikely that the organism will be found in these sections. Candidiasis is usually associated with a superficial epidermal pustular pattern of inflammation. Yeast or pseudohypha can be seen in crusts or pustules.

Treatment. Mucocutaneous candidiasis responds best to systemic antifungal drugs such as itraconazole (10 mg/kg *per os* once daily), fluconazole (5–10 mg/kg *per os* once daily) or ketoconazole (5–10 mg/kg *per os* once daily). Treatment should be continued for at least 1–2 weeks after clinical cure; the author initially prescribes a 14-day treatment course and then re-examines the patient. Daily maintenance therapy may be indicated to prevent relapses if an underlying immunosuppressive disease is identified and/or immunosuppressive drugs are required for treatment of another disease.

Systemic antifungal drugs may be used in the localised treatment of candidiasis, e.g. fold pyoderma, in addition to appropriate topical treatment. Localised areas of candidiasis due to folds are difficult to treat and cure because the dog's anatomy usually predisposes the dog to reinfection/recolonisation. Topical application of human products containing miconazole or clotrimazole (e.g. vaginal cream) are cost-effect for the chronic treatment of localised lesions. Lesions of cutaneous candidiasis that do not show a response to antifungal therapy in 3–5 days should be cultured for aerobic and anaerobic bacteria.

Prognosis. The prognosis is guarded. The presence of mucocutaneous candidiasis should be considered a serious illness. Many of these dogs develop these lesions because they are immunosuppressed. The prognosis is better in dogs with localised candidiasis due to excessive moisture (e.g. in vulvar folds).

Systemic lupus erythematosus

Description. Systemic lupus erythematosus (SLE) is a rare autoimmune disease that affects multiple organs including the skin. The disease is caused by presence of circulating autoantibodies against a wide range of tissue antigens. The deposition of antigen–antibody complexes in tissues is responsible for the constellation of clinical signs. The aetiology of the disease syndrome is multifactorial and viruses, genetics and immune dysfunctions have all been cited as possible causes. The clinical signs are usually due to an idiopathic cause but they can be triggered by drugs, vaccinations and sunlight.

Clinical signs. There is no age or sex predilection for this disease; however, there are anecdotal reports that female dogs may be predisposed. Collies, German Shepherd Dog, Shetland Sheepdog,

Poodle and Spitz breeds are predisposed. Animals with SLE are usually systemically ill (fever, depression, and/or anorexia). One or more body systems are usually involved and patients may have anaemia, thrombocytopenia, proteinuria, polyarthritis, polymyositis, diffuse lymphadenopathy, splenomegaly and dermatological signs. Cutaneous signs of SLE are extremely variable and include vesicles/bullae, erosive dermatitis, footpad ulceration, paronychia, pododermatitis, erythema, exfoliative dermatitis, alopecia, panniculitis and depigmentation. Lesions are usually symmetrical and have a predilection for the face, ears, and distal extremities. Purpura can also be seen due to thrombocytopenia.

Diagnosis. Definitive diagnosis can be very difficult since this disease can mimic several other skin diseases and systemic diseases. In most cases it is difficult to make a definitive diagnosis because it is rare to have a case that meets all the criteria. A presumptive diagnosis can be made by excluding other skin diseases. A complete blood count and thrombocyte count, urinalysis, serum chemistry profile panel, ANA test and skin biopsy are recommended. Joint taps, Coombs' tests and kidney biopsy may be needed to make a diagnosis, depending upon the dog's signs. Anaemia, thrombocytopenia, alterations in kidney function and a positive ANA test may be seen. In some cases, laboratory tests are essentially normal. Several representative skin biopsy samples should be collected. Erythematous areas adjacent to ulcers/erosions are good choices, in addition to intact vesicles/bullae. Frank ulcers are not usually very helpful to examine histologically. If panniculitis is present, a full-thickness skin biopsy should be submitted. The classic histological findings are basal cell vacuolation, necrosis of basal cells, vesiculation and a lichenoid or interface dermatitis. These changes are particularly convincing if they involve the outer root sheath of hair follicles. Unfortunately, skin biopsies may be non-diagnostic in many cases of SLE. Direct immunofluorescence should be positive at the basement membrane zone but this is an inconsistent finding; lack of positive DIF does not preclude the diagnosis.

Treatment. Treatment of this disease can be very difficult depending upon the patient's presenting signs and referral to a specialty clinic may be necessary in some cases (see *Section VI*).

Prognosis. The prognosis is guarded. This disease is difficult and complicated to manage.

Bullous pemphigoid

Description. This is an autoimmune skin disease caused by autoantibodies directed against the bullous pemphigoid antigen at the dermal–epidermal junction (Plate 8).

Clinical signs. There is no age or sex predilection. Collies, Shetland Sheepdog and Dobermann Pinscher may be predisposed. The hallmark lesion of this autoimmune skin disease is a turgid subepidermal vesicle. Vesicles are often quite large and irregular in shape and they eventually ulcerate. Unlike the vesicles of other autoimmune skin diseases, these are relatively 'tough' and do not rupture easily. There are several clinical variations of this disease described in the literature. It is unknown if these clinical presentations are truly variants of the disease or rather reflect the stage at which the disease was diagnosed. In one form, ulcerations and vesicles/bullae are limited to the mucocutaneous junctions and the oral mucosa. In another form, mucocutaneous ulceration and inguinal and axillary ulceration are found. Other reports describe symmetrical lesions in the periocular, perioral, oral, nailbed, ears and intertriginous areas. Lesions may be chronic or acute (Fig. 8.6) Additionally, it is common for secondary bacterial infections to be present.

Diagnosis. Definitive diagnosis is made by cytological examination of the contents of a vesicle (no acantholytic cells should be present), a negative ANA test, normal urinalysis, complete blood count, and serum chemistry panel and compatible skin biopsies. Skin biopsies should be from intact vesicles. These vesicles should be taken by excisional elliptical biopsy to maximise the opportunity to obtain a diagnostic specimen. Classic histological changes include a subepidermal vesicle/bulla, a mild dermal infiltrate of eosinophils and neutrophils, oedema and possible ulceration of the epidermis depending upon where the biopsy is taken from. Ideally, direct immunofluorescence is positive at the basement membrane zone.

Treatment. Treatment is described in *Section VI*.

Prognosis. The prognosis is guarded. This disease is not usually immediately life-threatening unless there is a secondary infection that overwhelms the body or is enhanced by the use of immunosuppressive drugs. Many dogs are euthanased because lesions are not satisfactorily controlled/eliminated with immunosuppressive drugs.

Pemphigus vulgaris

Description. Pemphigus vulgaris is a very rare autoimmune skin disease caused by autoantibodies binding to desmosomes in the intercellular spaces. The pathogenesis of pemphigus vulgaris is essentially identical to that of the outer pemphigus diseases (foliaceus, erythematosus and vegetans).

Clinical signs. There is no age, sex or known breed predilection for this disease. It is characterised by ulceration of the mucosae. The oral mucosa, lips, eyelids, nostrils, anus, prepuce and genitalia are most commonly affected. Secondary bacterial infections are common and may result in widespread ulceration. Rare reports of cutaneous involvement (groin, axilla, nailbed) are present in the literature and their validity is unknown. Affected dogs are anorexic, depressed, and febrile. Saliva may be very thick and a fetid odour to the breath is common. Bullous pemphigoid and pemphigus vulgaris can be clinically indistinguishable.

Diagnosis. Definitive diagnosis is made by cytological examination of the contents of a vesicle and noting the presence of acantholytic cells, a negative

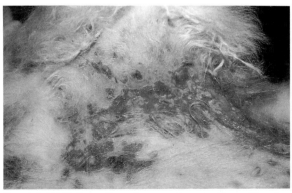

FIG. 8.6 Multiple erythematous erosions in the axilla of a dog cross with bullous pemphigoid. Slide courtesy of Richard Harvey.

ANA test, normal urinalysis, complete blood count, and serum chemistry panel and compatible skin biopsies. Skin biopsies should be from intact vesicles, which should be taken by excisional elliptical biopsy to maximise the opportunity to obtain a diagnostic specimen. Classic histological findings include a suprabasilar cleft leading to the formation of a bulla/vesicle, rounded up basilar cells (row of 'tombstones'), acantholysis, and secondary ulceration, exudation and crust formation. Ideally, direct immunofluorescence shows positive intercellular fluorescence.

Treatment. Treatment is described in *Section VI*.

Prognosis. Guarded. This disease is extremely rare and may be difficult to control. If lesions can be satisfactorily controlled, the quality of the dog's life is generally good provided that there are no life-threatening side-effects from the immunosuppressive drugs.

Erythema multiforme (EM)

Description. Erythema multiforme is a rare ulcerative skin disease that is caused by cell-mediated death or idiopathic death of epidermal cells. It is more common than toxic epidermal necrolysis (TEN). The inciting cause may be a drug, infection, neoplasia or unknown.

Clinical signs. The disease usually has an acute onset of erythematosus macules and papules that spread peripherally and clear centrally. Urticarial plaques, vesicles and bullae may also occur. These lesions are most common at the mucocutaneous junctions, nasal mucosa, pinnae, axillae and inguinal regions. Widespread ulceration may occur. Affected animals are usually systemically ill with fever, depression and anorexia. Mild lesions may mimic bacterial pyodermas, spreading pyoderma and bullous autoimmune skin diseases. Some cases may be severe enough that TEN develops.

Diagnosis. Definitive diagnosis requires a skin biopsy. The most classic finding is widespread death of individual keratinocytes.

Treatment. Identification and treatment of an inciting cause, particularly a drug reaction, is critical. Treatment is primarily supportive (see treatment of TEN below).

Prognosis. Good to guarded. The author is aware of several cases of erythema multiforme that waxed and waned for 6 months before resolving.

Toxic epidermal necrolysis (TEN)

Description. Toxic epidermal necrolysis is a rare, severe, life-threatening skin disease of dogs. It is believed to be caused by a lymphocyte and macrophage-mediated mechanism of immunological injury. Drug reactions are the most common known inciting cause; however, visceral neoplasia and infections have also been documented.

Clinical signs. The first signs of TEN are widespread erythema of the skin. The skin may be painful upon palpation. Rapid (2–48 hours) and widespread full-thickness necrosis of the epidermis occurs. Ulceration is evident as the epidermis sloughs. The epidermis may shed in sheets of skin resembling tissue paper. The most common sites are the oral mucosa, footpad, face and skin of the trunk.

Diagnosis. Definitive diagnosis is made by a skin biopsy. Several representative skin biopsies from areas of erythema without ulceration should be examined. Histologically, widespread epidermal necrolysis and acute coagulation necrosis are seen. Because of the acute nature of the disease, there is little inflammation present in the epidermis until ulceration develops.

Treatment. **TEN is one of the few dermatological emergencies.** Treatment should be initiated as soon as biopsies are obtained. These patients are treated as if they had severe thermal burns. It is critical to maintain appropriate hydration and nutrition. If there is severe oral ulceration, total parenteral nutrition may be necessary. These patients require frequent whirlpool baths daily to remove exudate and debris from the hair and skin. Chlorhexidine is the antibacterial agent of choice for whirlpool baths. Clipping of the hair coat is recommended but this may need to be done under general anaesthesia because of the extreme pain involved. The affected sites may require frequent debridement.

Aerobic and anaerobic bacterial cultures and sensitivities are very useful to guide systemic antibiotic therapy. Systemic antibiotics **will not** shorten the course of the event, but may minimise life-threatening secondary bacterial infections. Combination therapy with cephalexin (20 mg/kg t.i.d.) and an aminoglycoside should be used initially until culture results are available. Wet–dry bandages and/or silver sulphadiazine ointment are recommended on the lesions.

Glucocorticoids are not indicated in the treatment of TEN unless the patient is in shock or is rapidly deteriorating. There is some evidence to suggest that glucocorticoids may be more harmful than beneficial. One of the major causes of death is the extensive fluid, electrolyte and colloid losses through the skin. **Aggressive fluid therapy is indicated**. Refer to internal medicine textbooks for discussions on burn therapy management and total parenteral nutrition.

Prognosis. The prognosis is poor and most dogs with TEN die from complications of the disease or the owner elects euthanasia due to the cost of treatments.

Cutaneous drug reactions

Description. Cutaneous drug reactions are caused by an idiopathic reaction to a topical, parenteral or oral drug. Type 1–4 hypersensitivity reactions have been implicated.

Clinical signs. The clinical signs of a cutaneous drug reaction are extremely variable. Drug reactions may present as urticaria, maculopapular eruptions, local areas of erythema, erythroderma, exfoliations, purpura, mucocutaneous ulceration, suppurative necrosis, TEN, EM and injection site reactions.

Diagnosis. Definitive diagnosis is difficult and requires a careful history and physical examination. Any combination of the following observations may suggest a cutaneous drug reaction:

- The reaction does not resemble a pharmacological action of the drug.
- The reaction results from a small amount of the drug, the reaction occurs within several days following initial administration of the drug.

- The reaction is characterised by one or more of the typical hypersensitivity reactions.
- The reaction recurs with challenge.
- The causative agent cross-reacts with similar drugs.
- Resolution occurs within days of discontinuing the drug.

In most cases of cutaneous drug reactions, laboratory work is not very helpful. A thorough drug history and skin biopsy are most helpful.

Treatment. Treatment requires identification of the causative agent and discontinuation of the drug. Supportive care may be necessary in some patients.

Prognosis. The prognosis is variable, from very good to guarded depending upon the clinical signs.

Generalised ulceration

Description. Generalised ulceration is a sign of a severe, potentially life-threatening injury. The causes are numerous and include generalised demodicosis and secondary pyoderma, deep bacterial and fungal infections, systemic drug reactions, TEN and EM, systemic lupus erythematosus and thermal burns.

Clinical signs. Dogs with generalised ulceration are usually systemically ill (fever, anorexia, depression). The skin is often painful to the touch. The hair coat is matted with blood and/or exudate and is odorous. Large areas of the skin are sloughed and the underlying dermis is visible.

Diagnosis. Definitive diagnosis *minimally* requires skin scrapings for demodicosis, cytological examination of exudate for bacteria and fungi, aerobic and anaerobic cultures for bacteria, and skin biopsies at the **initial visit**. Depending upon the other clinical signs and severity of the lesions, a complete blood count, serum chemistry panel, deep fungal culture or titres and ANA may be indicated.

Treatment. Pending the results of the laboratory tests, the dog must be treated symptomatically. The patient should be sedated, if necessary, and the entire hair coat clipped to see the extent of the lesions. The dog should receive several whirlpool baths per day in a chlorhexidine or benzoyl peroxide shampoo. If a sepsis is present, systemic antibiotics are indicated.

Prognosis. Variable, depending upon the cause of the lesions.

Intertriginous pyoderma/ulceration

Description. Intertriginous ulceration/maceration is caused by the repeated friction of two skin surfaces rubbing against one another. The two most common sites for this are the axillary and inguinal regions. This is most common in short-legged or obese dogs. Intertriginous ulceration/maceration may also occur in vulvar folds and facial folds. These areas may be colonised secondarily by yeasts such as *Candida* and *Malassezia*.

Clinical signs. The affected area is hairless, moist, erythematous and exudative. In most cases, there is a strong offensive odour. If *Malassezia* is present, there is often a thick waxy exudate. Candidiasis or secondary bacterial infections are more ulcerative and usually have a thinner exudate.

Diagnosis. Definitive diagnosis is usually obvious. Clinical lesions are present in areas of folds and are exudative. The major challenge is to determine whether or not a secondary infection is present. Skin scrapings, impression smears and skin biopsies may be required to determine the aetiology of the secondary infection.

Treatment. The most important step in treatment is to convince the owner that this is a lifelong problem that can be managed, but not cured. If the animal is obese, weight-loss may be helpful in minimising the severity of the lesions. Systemic antibiotics or antifungals are very helpful in treating acute cases aggravated by bacteria or yeast infections. Frequent baths (2–3 per week) with an antibacterial or antiseborrhoeic shampoo are very useful. Some owners have reported that moisturising lotions help to reduce frictional rubs and increase the interval between re-exacerbations.

Prognosis. This is not a life-threatening disease.

Urine scald

Description. Urine scald is essentially an irritant reaction to the presence of urine on the skin. This occurs most commonly in recumbent dogs, but may be seen in those with urinary incontinence and perineal fold pyoderma. Secondary infections with bacteria or *Candida* may occur.

Clinical signs. Urine scald is characterised by moist ulcerative dermatitis in the area where urine is present. In recumbent dogs, the urine scald may extend down the medial thigh. The skin and/or hair coat is usually urine-soaked or smells of urine, unless the owner has washed the dog just prior to presentation. Depending upon the severity, a secondary infection may be present.

Diagnosis. Diagnosis is usually made by clinical signs and the history of exposure to urine.

Treatment. The most important step in the treatment of urine scald is prevention. Animals at risk should have good nursing care to prevent urine leakage from the bladder. Affected animals should have frequent whirlpool baths per day until healing is evident. The area should be covered in an antibiotic cream and the surrounding skin covered in a thick layer of white petroleum jelly. The latter will allow any urine to drain off of the skin and not puddle.

Prognosis. Prognosis is good. However, animals with urine scald that are recumbent are also at risk from decubital ulcers.

Ulcerative dermatosis of Shetland Sheepdogs and Collies

Description. This is a newly recognised skin disease that resembles bullous pemphigoid, but is believed to be a variant of canine familial dermatomyositis.

Clinical signs. This disease of adult dogs has only been recognised in Shetland Sheepdogs and Collies. The intertriginous areas of the groin and axillae are most often affected; the mucocutaneous junctions of the eyes, mouth, genitalia and anus may also be affected. Lesions are usually symmetrical. Concurrent myositis has been documented in several dogs. Clinically, the disease is indistinguishable from bullous pemphigoid.

Diagnosis. Definitive diagnosis requires muscle conduction studies, muscle biopsies and skin biopsies. Histological changes are very similar to those in dermatomyositis except that they are more severe. Numerous necrotic keratinocytes are present in the basement membrane. Dermal–epidermal vesiculation is noted and it may extend into the outer hair follicle sheath. Follicular atrophy, common in dermatomyositis, is not seen. This disease may be difficult for the pathologist to differentiate from EM and lupus.

Treatment. Treatment is described in *Section VI*.

Prognosis. The prognosis is guarded.

9

Pigmentary Disorders

KAREN MORIELLO

Changes in the colour of the skin or hair coat are often first noticed by the owner. Most changes in pigmentation are of cosmetic concern but there are pigmentary disorders that are markers for systemic disease.

Several terms are used in the veterinary literature to describe depigmentation of the skin and hair coat. In human medicine **vitiligo** describes idiopathic depigmentation of the hair or skin characterised by destruction of melanocytes. It is presumed to be an autoimmune skin disease. **Poliosis** specifically refers to premature greyness of the hair in humans. **Leucoderma** is an acquired type of localised loss of melanin pigmentation in the skin; it differs from vitiligo in that it includes not just autoimmune but all potential causes of depigmentation. **Leucotrichia** is an acquired type of localised whiteness (depigmentation) of the hair. For simplicity, only the terms **leucoderma** and **leucotrichia** will be used in this chapter to describe depigmentation of the skin and of the hair, respectively. The term vitiligo will be reserved for depigmenting disease of immune-mediated origin.

The most important reason for pursuing the underlying cause of changes in pigmentation of the skin or hair is to determine whether or not the change is a manifestation of a generalised skin disease or, more seriously, a manifestation of a systemic disease.

Selected Diseases of Altered Pigmentation

Albinism

Description. Albinism is a very rare permanent skin condition caused by a hereditary lack of pigmentation. It is transmitted by a recessive gene. Albinos have melanocytes in their skin, but lack the enzyme tyrosinase needed for melanin synthesis.

Clinical signs. Albinos have white skin and hair, in addition to unpigmented irises.

Diagnosis. Definitive diagnosis is usually made by the history and clinical signs. These animals are born with the condition. Biopsy specimens will show a lack of melanin granules in the skin and hair follicles.

Treatment. There is no treatment.

DIFFERENTIAL DIAGNOSIS OF INCREASED PIGMENT IN THE SKIN OR HAIR OF DOGS	
Post-inflammatory hyperpigmentation due to chronic skin diseases	Flea allergy dermatitis Atopy and food allergy Friction Seborrhoeic dermatitis
Multifocal post inflammatory hyperpigmentation	Syperficial pyoderma Dermatophytosis
Parasitic	Demodicosis
Endocrinopathies	Hyperadrenocorticism Hypothyroidism Sex hormone dermatoses
Neoplasia and other causes	Melanoma Lentigo or melanoplakia

FIG. 9.1 Differential diagnosis of increased pigment in the skin or hair of dogs.

DIFFERENTIAL DIAGNOSIS OF DECREASED PIGMENT IN THE SKIN OR HAIR OF DOGS	
Diffuse pigmentation	Albinism Hereditary or idiopathic leucotrichia or leucoderma
Nasal or facial depigmentation	Discoid lupus erythematosus Epitheliotropic lymphoma Seasonal depigmentation Uveodermatological syndrome Metabolic depigmentation Hereditary or idiopathic leucotrichia or leucoderma Leishmaniasis
Focal depigmentation	Previous site of injury, trauma, vaccination, clipping, etc. Idiopathic leucoderma or leucotrichia

FIG. 9.2 Differential diagnosis of decreased pigment in the skin or hair of dogs.

FIG. 9.3 Approach to changes in pigmentation: History.

APPROACH TO CHANGES IN PIGMENTATION: HISTORY	
Factor	**Differential diagnosis**
Breed 　Collie 　Chow Chow 　Rottweiler, Dobermann Pinscher, Belgian 　　Tervueren, Newfoundland, Afghan Hound, 　　Samoyed, Siberian Huskie, Golden 　　Retriever, Irish Setter, Pointer 　Akita, Samoyed, Siberian Huskie	Canine cyclic haematopoiesis Tyrosinase deficiency Hereditary depigmentation of face and nose Uveodermatological syndrome
Age of onset 　At birth or within the first few months of life	Congenital defects
Seasonality	Seasonal nasal depigmentation
Location	Post-traumatic depigmentation
Pruritus	Post-inflammatory hyperpigmentation 　secondary to chronic dermatitis
Concurrent skin diseases	Post-inflammatory hyperpigmentation 　secondary to chronic dermatitis
Changes in dietary or elimination habits	Hyperadrenocorticism; hypothyroidism
Concurrent organ dysfunctions	Systemic lupus erythematosus; 　uveodermatological syndrome

FIG. 9.4 Approach to changes in pigmentation: Physical examination.

APPROACH TO CHANGES IN PIGMENTATION: PHYSICAL EXAMINATION	
Physical finding	**Differential diagnosis**
Ulceration and crusting of nose and face	Discoid lupus erythematosus; pemphigus; 　epitheliotropic lymphoma; sunburn
Concurrent ocular disease or changes	Uveodermatological syndrome; albinism
Focal depigmentation	Idiopathic leucoderma or leucotrichia; post- 　trauma depigmentation
Multifocal hyperpigmented areas of hair-loss	Pyoderma; demodicosis; dermatophytosis
Diffuse hyperpigmentation with hair-loss	Hyperadrenocorticism; hypothyroidism; 　adrenal sex hormone dysfunction
Macule or patch of hyperpigmentation 　without inflammation or hair-loss	Lentigo/melanoplakia; melanoma
Raised hyperpigmented nodule or tumour	Naevus, melanoma

Prognosis. Albinism in animals is not known to be associated with any lethal traits. These animals are more susceptible to sun-induced damage and should have restricted exposure to strong sunlight. Affected individuals should not be bred.

Hereditary and idiopathic leucoderma and leucotrichia

Description. These conditions are clinically indistinguishable entities. They usually occur in adult animals of any age and are acquired. The leucoderma/leucotrichia is referred to as hereditary if there is a known breed predisposition or if related dogs have shown similar depigmentation of hair or skin. If no cause for the leucoderma or leucotrichia is found, the condition is called idiopathic.

Clinical signs. Most cases of leucoderma and leucotrichia occur in young adults, although they may occur at any age. The depigmentation may be symmetrical or asymmetrical and it most often occurs on the nose, face, lips, buccal mucosa and footpads. In severe cases, depigmentation may affect the trunk (Fig. 9.7).

Diagnosis. Definitive diagnosis is made by the history, clinical signs and skin biopsy. Histologically, there is a lack of melanocytes and melanin pigment in the affected areas. In rare situations, an underlying metabolic disease may be the cause of

DIAGNOSTIC PLAN FOR CHANGES IN PIGMENTATION

Hypopigmentation or Acquired Loss of Pigmentation

Localised lesions

1. *If the lesion is localised,* consider the possibility of depigmentation due to previous injury at the site. 'Injury' may include clipping of the hair, vaccination, thermal injury or physical trauma
2. *If there is no history of previous injury,* consider idiopathic leucotrichia/leucoderma

> **Focused diagnostic test:** A skin biopsy is needed to confirm the loss of melanocytes in a specific area and absence of inflammatory cells or changes consistent with lupus erythematosus

Facial/nasal

1. *If the depigmentation is limited to the planum nasale and the nose is otherwise normal,* consider the possibility of idiopathic leucoderma or vitiligo, seasonal nasal depigmentation or contact dermatitis
2. *If the depigmentation involves the planum nasale and if erythema, crusting and/or ulceration are present,* consider the possibility of discoid lupus erythematosus, epitheliotropic lymphoma, uveodermatological syndrome or metabolic depigmentation
3. *If the depigmentation involves the planum nasale, mucous membranes, lips, eyelids and facial hair,* consider uveodermatological syndrome

> **Focused diagnostic tests:** Perform a careful ophthalmological examination to rule out concurrent uveitis (uveodermatological syndrome), a serum biochemistry profile (metabolic depigmentation) and a skin biopsy (discoid lupus erythematosus, epitheliotropic lymphoma, uveodermatological syndrome)

Diffuse depigmentation

1. *If the depigmentation has been present since birth or developed shortly thereafter,* consider a congenital defect of depigmentation, i.e. albinism. These animals usually lack pigmentation in the iris
2. *If the depigmentation is acquired,* consider hereditary or idiopathic leucotrichia/leucoderma

> **Focused diagnostic test:** Perform a skin biopsy to confirm the absence of melanocytes

Hyperpigmentation of Skin

At the initial visit, consider the possibility that the hyperpigmentation may be due to a chronic inflammatory dermatosis. *If pruritus is present,* it is advisable to pursue the causes of pruritus first (*Chapter 5*)

Focal area of hyperpigmentation

1. *If the hyperpigmented area is focal and associated with scale and/or hair-loss,* consider localised demodicosis
2. *If the hyperpigmented area is raised or indurated,* consider malignant melanoma or melanocytoma

> **Focused diagnostic test:** Skin biopsy and skin scrapings

Multifocal and diffuse hyperpigmentation

1. *If multifocal areas of hyperpigmentation are present,* consider demodicosis or superficial pyoderma. Patchy hair-loss surrounding areas of hyperpigmentation increases the probability of these two diseases

> **Focused diagnostic test:** Numerous deep skin scrapings to rule out demodicosis. If skin scrapings are negative, initiate a trial of oral antibiotics for 3–4 weeks to rule out a bacterial pyoderma

2. *If there is no response to oral antibiotic therapy,* consider the possibility of dermatophytosis, especially if lesions continue to develop and hair-loss persists

> **Focused diagnostic tests:** Perform a dermatophyte culture. If the culture is negative and lesions continue to develop, perform a skin biopsy

3. *If diffuse hyperpigmentation is present, alone or with any combination of hair-loss, lichenification, or seborrhoea,* consider the possibility of an endocrinopathy

> **Focused diagnostic tests:** Perform the endocrine function test that is most supported by the history and physical examination. If the history and physical findings are non-specific, evaluation of a serum biochemistry panel, urinalysis and haematology may be helpful. Thyroid function can be evaluated by a TSH response test or basal T4 concentrations evaluated in conjunction with a serum cholesterol concentration. Adrenal dysfunction can be evaluated by either an ACTH response test or low-dose dexamethasone response test. Adrenal sex hormone abnormalities can be evaluated by surgical neutering and determination of sex hormone concentrations. If these tests are normal, perform a skin biopsy

FIG. 9.5 Diagnostic plan for changes in pigmentation.

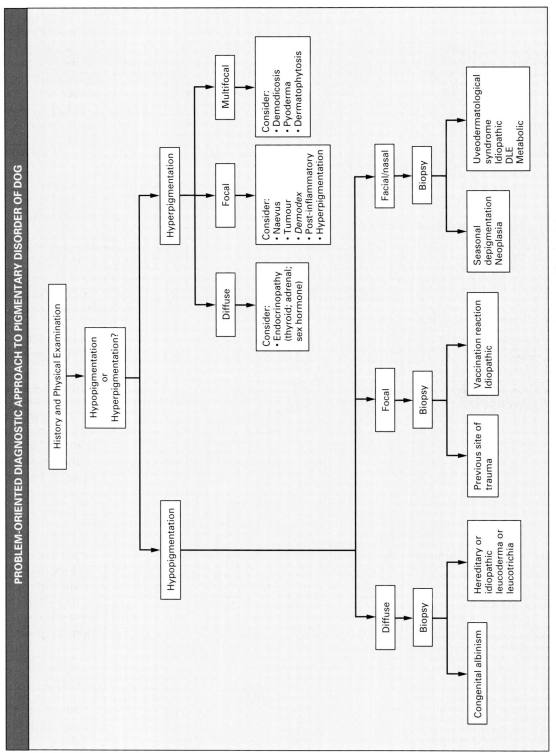

FIG. 9.6 Problem-oriented diagnostic approach to pigmentary disorder of dogs.

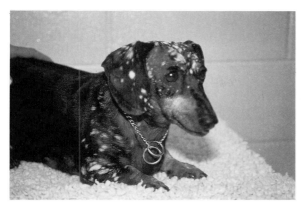

FIG. 9.7 Idiopathic leucoderma and leucotrichia in a dog.

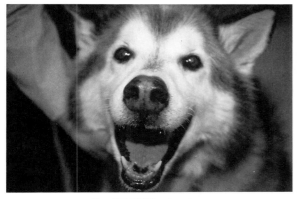

FIG. 9.8 Vitiligo in a dog.

the depigmentation (see Metabolic depigmentation, below).

Treatment. There is no treatment.

Prognosis. The prognosis for repigmentation is guarded. Some depigmented areas may spontaneously repigment, although this is rare. The author has seen several Shar Pei dogs with leucoderma and leucotrichia on the face that spontaneously resolved (repigmented) over a period of several months. Except for cosmetic appearances, these dogs are otherwise healthy. Affected individuals should not be bred.

Vitiligo (see Fig. 9.8)

Description. This term, borrowed from human medicine, is used occasionally in veterinary medicine to describe acquired focal depigmentation of the skin of dogs. In humans, vitiligo is believed to be

caused by antimelanocyte antibodies and is considered to have an autoimmune basis. Other potential causes include a lack of normal protective mechanisms that eliminate toxic melanin precursors and neurochemical mediators that inhibit melanogenesis or destroy melanocytes. Antimelanocyte antibodies have only been documented in Belgian Tervuerens. In dogs, there appears to be a strong hereditary predisposition. In reality, vitiligo and idiopathic or hereditary leucoderma and leucotrichia may all be the same disease.

Clinical signs. Vitiligo is a rare acquired condition that is characterised by progressive depigmentation of the skin. Lesions are usually well circumscribed. Depigmentation may progress to the planum nasale, lips, muzzle, buccal mucosa and footpads. Inflammation is usually absent. Complete or partial symmetry is common (Fig. 9.8). Lesions may wax and wane. The full extent of the depigmentation usually occurs within 3 to 6 months after the onset.

Diagnosis. Definitive diagnosis may be difficult to document. The best diagnostic tool is a wedge/elliptical skin biopsy from the edge of a newly developing lesion. Histologically, there is a lack of or marked reduction in melanocytes. In very early lesions, a mild interface dermatitis consisting of lymphocytes and macrophages may be seen. Dogs presenting with depigmented lesions should be screened for metabolic diseases that have been associated anecdotally with rare cases of depigmentation (see Metabolic depigmentation).

Treatment. There is no treatment.

Prognosis. The prognosis for repigmentation is guarded. The clinical signs may wax and wane and there are anecdotal reports of permanent repigmentation. Clients should be told that the depigmentation is probably permanent. With the exception of a metabolic cause for depigmentation, the prognosis for overall health is excellent.

Non-inflammatory nasal depigmentation

Description. Nasal depigmentation is a relatively common and benign condition that affects only the planum nasale. It is characterised by a loss of pigmentation of the non-haired nose. There is no associated inflammation, crusting, erythema or ulceration. The condition may be seasonal, with repigmentation occurring in the spring or summer, or it may be permanent. There may be hereditary predisposition. Some textbooks have referred to this condition as 'Dudley nose'.

Clinical signs. The depigmentation usually occurs in a young adult dog with normally black planum nasale. It is limited to the non-haired nose and may start as a focal area of depigmentation or may be generalised. The black planum nasale may depigment in a multifocal or mottled pattern. Depigmentation of the nose may be white, pink, grey or brown. Owners may report some cyclicity to the depigmentation suggesting that there is a seasonal pattern. There is no associated inflammation.

Diagnosis. Definitive diagnosis is usually made by history and clinical signs. The absence of subsequent development of inflammation, erythema, crusting and ulceration often helps to distinguish this syndrome from discoid lupus erythematosus, epitheliotropic lymphoma or other more serious causes of nasal depigmentation.

Treatment. There is no treatment. If the depigmentation is severe enough to predispose the dog to sunburn, restricted activity during the day is recommended. Sunscreens labelled as safe for infants may be applied to the nose but their use is of limited benefit as most dogs simply lick off the sunscreen.

Prognosis. The prognosis is good and spontaneous repigmentation may occur, but owners should be told that the condition may be permanent.

Uveodermatological syndrome

Description. Uveodermatological syndrome in dogs is similar to the disease in people referred to as Vogt–Koyanagi–Harada (VKH) syndrome. Some of the veterinary literature refers to cases of uveodermatologic syndrome as canine VKH. Uveodermatological syndrome is characterised by depigmentation of the skin and mucous membranes that is associated with ocular disease (uveitis). This is a rare but important disease. The cutaneous depigmentation is not hazardous to the dog's health; however, early recognition is important in controlling or minimising the ocular disease changes, which may lead to blindness.

Clinical signs. There is a breed predilection for Akitas, Samoyeds and Siberian Huskies, although any dog can be affected. Most affected individuals are between the ages of 6 months and 6 years. In most cases, the disease begins with mild ocular changes. Owners may complain of opacity of the cornea (corneal oedema), blepharospasm, conjunctivitis and serous ocular discharge. Owners may or may not note subtle depigmentation of the eyelid margins and they may complain of premature greying of the haircoat.

Ocular changes, which usually precede cutaneous changes, include blepharospasm, conjunctival inflammation, corneal oedema, serous discharge, aqueous flare, iris swelling and miosis. Retinal haemorrhage or degeneration, retinal detachment, optic disc hyperaemia and haemorrhage may be seen. If left untreated, glaucoma, cataracts and blindness may occur. Significant ocular changes usually occur before cutaneous signs are noted. Dermatologically, depigmentation of the eyelid margins, planum nasale, buccal mucosa, tongue and leucotrichia are most commonly noted. Oral and nasal erosions may occur in advanced cases. Rarely, footpad hyperkeratosis has been seen. Neurological signs have not been reported in dogs with ocular or cutaneous changes.

Diagnosis. The dermatological signs of uveodermatological syndrome may mimic discoid lupus erythematosus, pemphigus, idiopathic leucoderma/leucotrichia or epitheliotropic lymphoma. Diseases due to infectious agents, particularly *Blastomyces dermatitidis*, may also mimic this disease, specifically the ocular component. Definitive diagnosis may be delayed or difficult if the presence of concurrent eye disease is missed in either the history or physical examination. Any dog presenting with depigmentation of the face should receive a complete and careful ophthalmic examination. Skin biopsies should be obtained from numerous representative areas.

Histological findings compatible with this disease include an interface dermatitis consisting of histiocytic-type cells, decreased numbers of melanocytes and 'melanin dropout' or loss of melanin from melanocytes in the epidermis and accumulation of melanin in the dermis. It is critical to eliminate the possibility of infectious causes of uveitis before making a definitive diagnosis. Fungal serum titres, conjunctival scrapings and cytological analysis of aspirates of fluid from the anterior chamber are recommended for this purpose. The latter procedure should be performed by a veterinary ophthalmology clinic.

Treatment. It is imperative that infectious causes of uveitis be eliminated before initiating treatment. Treatment is directed at minimising the inflammation associated with the disease, specifically the ocular inflammation. In general, systemic glucocorticoids (prednisolone, 2.2 mg/kg *per os* daily) for several weeks are used. Over the course of several months, the dosage can be gradually reduced if the dog responds. If there is a lack of response or a worsening of the ocular and/or skin changes, azathioprine (1–2 mg/kg *per os* daily) may be included in the treatment regimen. Cutaneous depigmentation may resolve. Other sources can give more specific information on the treatment of the concurrent eye disease. Referral to a veterinary ophthalmologist for management is strongly suggested. Briefly, topical glucocorticoids are used to decrease the inflammation associated with the anterior uveitis. Subconjunctival injections of triamcinolone acetate may be needed. Miosis or hyphaema may benefit from topical atropine or phenylephrine.

Prognosis. Guarded. The most serious consequence of the disease is permanent blindness. Affected dogs will require lifelong monitoring at 4–6 month intervals. Affected dogs should not be bred.

Epitheliotropic lymphoma

Description. Epitheliotropic lymphoma is a cutaneous T-cell lymphoma that affects the epidermis and follicular epithelium (*Chapter 11*). It is also commonly referred to as **mycosis fungoides**.

Clinical signs. This disease most commonly presents as an exfoliative disease but in rare instances it may begin (or first be noticed) with nasal or facial depigmentation. Erythema, scaling, crusting and ulceration are almost always present. It is not uncommon for epitheliotropic lymphoma to mimic discoid lupus erythematosus or pemphigus when it presents with facial lesions.

Diagnosis. Skin biopsy.

Treatment. There is no effective treatment.

Prognosis. The prognosis is guarded, however dogs may live for many months without discomfort.

Discoid lupus erythematosus

Description. Discoid lupus erythematosus is an autoimmune skin disease that has a predilection for the face and nose of dogs.

Clinical signs. This disease most commonly presents as nasal depigmentation with associated nasal crusting, ulceration and erythema.

Diagnosis. Skin biopsy.

Treatment and prognosis. The disease is discussed in *Chapter 8*.

Metabolic depigmentation

Description. Metabolic depigmentation describes causes of depigmentation due to systemic diseases, such as diabetes mellitus, or lack of pigmentary enzyme pathways. Metabolic depigmentation is very rare and most reports are anecdotal.

Clinical signs. Metabolic depigmentation can cause leucoderma, leucotrichia or any change in the normal pigment of the patient. Black-coated dogs may develop rust or red-coloured hair coats. Metabolic depigmentation should be considered in any young dog with sudden depigmentation of hair or skin or in older animals with depigmentation and concurrent systemic illness. Depigmentation of the hair coat can also occur with iatrogenic hypercortisolaemia.

Diagnosis. Definitive diagnosis is difficult for several reasons. The causes of metabolic depigmentation involving enzyme pathways of canine pigmentation are poorly understood and difficult to test. There are only a few documented cases of tyrosinase enzyme deficiencies in the veterinary literature and these assays are not readily available for the veterinary practitioner. Reports of depigmentation associated with diabetes mellitus, hypothyroidism, and mineral or nutrient deficiencies are extremely rare and anecdotal. It is clinically cost effective to screen patients for common metabolic diseases via serum chemistry profile panels when the history and physical examination suggests systemic illness.

Treatment. Specific treatment depends upon identification of the specific disease. There is no known treatment for individuals with tyrosinase deficiencies. Additionally, there is no conclusive clinical evidence to support recommending dietary vitamin and mineral supplements in animals with depigmentation disorders.

Melanocytoma, lentigo, melanoplakia

Description. Melanocytoma, lentigo and melanoplakia are terms used to describe the benign accumulation of melanocytes in the skin and mucous membranes.

Clinical signs. The benign accumulation of increased numbers of melanocytes in the skin appears as an area of dark pigmentation. Almost exclusively, the area of melanocytic accumulation is flat and appears as a darkly pigmented macule or patch.

Diagnosis. If the darkly pigmented lesion is acquired, it is important to rule out malignant melanoma via a skin biopsy. In most instances, the lesion is static and has been present for years with little or no change.

Treatment. No treatment is required.

Prognosis. The prognosis is excellent.

For further discussion elsewhere in the text (see *Demodicosis, Hypothyroidism, Adrenal Sex Hormone Dysfunction, Hyperadrenocorticism, Chapter 6; Superficial Pyoderma, Chapter 10*).

10

Pyoderma and Pustular Lesions

IAN MASON

Pyoderma, or bacterial skin disease, is commonly encountered in canine practice. The micro-organism involved is usually *Staphylococcus intermedius*. Other staphylococcal species and other bacteria have occasionally been associated with this disorder. *Staphylococcus intermedius* is a normal inhabitant of the skin surface and mucous membranes. It has been suggested that the skin in dogs has less well developed innate resistance and anatomical barriers than that of other species and so is particularly prone to bacterial disease. Pyoderma is a secondary phenomenon; normal skin is resistant to bacterial disease. Virtually any primary canine skin disorder can lead to secondary pyoderma.

The precise pathogenesis of canine pyoderma is unclear. Coagulase-positive staphylococci are members of the skin microflora. It has therefore been assumed that some factor or factors must affect cutaneous defence mechanisms, thereby allowing these normally harmless bacteria and their toxins to penetrate into the skin, causing inflammation and tissue damage and/or affect the cutaneous microenvironment, so promoting multiplication of staphylococci to exceed a threshold or 'critical mass' for disease.

Primary diseases leading to pyoderma include hypersensitivity, ectoparasitism and metabolic/endocrine disease (Fig. 10.7). It is possible that inflammation of skin as a result of ectoparasitism or allergy may increase skin surface temperature and humidity. The self-trauma associated with such disorders will degrade skin barriers. Serum and blood may ooze on to the skin surface and provide a source of nutrients for staphylococci. These substances may further contribute to the high surface humidity.

Metabolic disease is often associated with immunosuppression and may have an effect on physical barriers within the skin (e.g. defective lipid metabolism may affect epidermal permeability barriers). Alternatively, there may be a more general effect on humoral and cellular immunity.

Confusion exists regarding the terminology and classification of pyoderma. This probably arises from our incomplete understanding of the mechanisms by which pyoderma develops. **Primary pyoderma** is used to describe cases where no underlying disease is identified. However, the author suggests that the term **idiopathic pyoderma** be used to refer to such cases. It is probable that primary pyoderma does not exist. *Staphylococcus intermedius* is not sufficiently virulent to cause skin disease in a normal host. It is the author's opinion that some host factor must be present which allows proliferation and penetration of this bacterium and the development of pyoderma.

There is debate regarding the recurrent nature of pyoderma. Again, it is the author's opinion that all pyodermas will recur unless the underlying cause is identified and treated. In general, cases of idiopathic pyoderma will require lifelong antimicrobial therapy as described in *Chapter 32*. However, occasionally cases of idiopathic pyoderma are apparently cured following antimicrobial therapy. These cures are said to persist indefinitely even after antimicrobial therapy is discontinued. It is probable that permanent resolution of pyoderma following antimicrobial therapy is due to some other factor in the animal's management being altered. Examples include the institution of good flea and ectoparasite control, the use of good grooming measures such as regular clipping, combing and bathing, or an improvement in the plane of nutrition. Many cases of non-recurrent pyoderma have been previously treated with glucocorticoids: discontinuation of such therapy along with appropriate antimicrobial treatment will lead to an apparent cure.

Pustules are one of the hallmarks of pyoderma. Paradoxically, pustules are quite rare in the dog despite the high incidence of pyoderma. This apparent discrepancy is explained by the fact that pustules are only present in canine skin for a short while before they rupture. Instead of pustules, a range of

DIFFERENTIAL DIAGNOSIS OF PYODERMA AND PUSTULES IN DOGS	
Staphylococcal pyoderma	Superficial pyoderma Impetigo Folliculitis Deep pyoderma Acne (muzzle/chin pyoderma) Interdigital pyoderma Pressure point pyoderma Anal furunculosis Nasal pyoderma
Immune-mediated/ autoimmune disorders	Pemphigus foliaceus Pemphigus erythematosus Pemphigus vegetans Drug eruptions (including erythema multiforme/toxic epidermal necrolysis)
Other diseases	Contact irritant dermatitis Sub-corneal pustular dermatosis Sterile eosinophilic pustular dermatitis Linear IgA dermatosis Bullous impetigo Acral lick dermatitis (See Chapter 34)

FIG. 10.1 Differential diagnosis of pyoderma and pustules in dogs.

primary and secondary lesions may be present ranging from papules and vesicles to crust formation, scaling, epidermal collarettes, hyperpigmentation and ulceration, depending on the aetiology and other factors. It should be recognised that these lesions represent a chronological sequence of lesion development. The absence of pustules does not rule out a diagnosis of pyoderma or other pustular disease. Disorders other than pyoderma may lead to pustule formation (Fig. 10.1). Typically these belong to the immune-mediated or autoimmune group. They are rather uncommon. Again, in these disorders, pustules are transient.

Bacterial skin disease is often pruritic. This may be due to production of inflammatory toxins and enzymes by the bacteria, or because the primary disease is pruritic. For example, pruritus occurs in hypothyroidism or demodicosis when secondary pyoderma supervenes. *Chapter 5* gives an account of pruritic skin disease in dogs, including the rather complex approach to pruritic pustular disease (Fig. 5.6).

In essence, the initial aim is to establish whether the pruritus is due to the pyoderma or the primary disease. If the underlying disease is pruritic, then the approach outlined in *Chapter 5* needs to be adopted along with antimicrobial therapy. If the pruritus is solely due to the secondary bacterial infection, then the list of possible underlying diseases is completely different to that for the primary pruritic case. This topic will be discussed in more detail later in this chapter.

With the exception of pyoderma, the diseases listed in Fig. 10.1 are uncommon or even rare. The immune-mediated and autoimmune diseases are included even though they more typically present with bullae, vesicles, crusts and ulcers rather than pustules. They are discussed in more detail in *Chapter 8*. Sub-corneal pustular dermatosis is a rare disorder in which sterile pustules form within the interfollicular living epidermis. It may be pruritic, although the degree of pruritus varies. It has been a number of years since a case was reported in the veterinary literature. Sterile eosinophilic pustular dermatitis is an uncommon and highly pruritic disorder.

In order to identify the cause of a pustular dermatosis, the methodical approach detailed in *Chapter 2* must be applied. Important diagnostic clues may be obtained from the history and physical examination, so narrowing the differential diagnosis and enabling the clinician to rank the likely causes. Figures 10.2 and 10.3 show examples of aspects of

APPROACH TO CANINE PYODERMA AND PUSTULAR DISEASE: HISTORY	
Factor	**Differential diagnosis**

Breed
  Boxer, Great Dane, Dobermann Pinscher
  German Shepherd Dog
  Bull Terrier
  Akita, Bearded Collie, Newfoundland
  Rough and Smooth Collies, Shetland Sheepdog
	Acne
	Generalised deep pyoderma
	Pedal pyoderma
	Pemphigus foliaceus
	Bullous pemphigoid

Age of onset 3 months to a year	Acne, impetigo
Medication	Drug eruption
Severe pruritus	Sterile eosinophilic pustular dermatitis

FIG. 10.2 Approach to canine pyoderma and pustular disease: History.

APPROACH TO PYODERMA AND PUSTULAR DISEASE: PHYSICAL EXAMINATION	
Physical finding	**Differential diagnosis**
Distribution of lesions	
Symmetrical, affecting dorsum of muzzle, pinnae, feet	Immune-mediated disorders
Chin and lips	Acne
Nature of lesions	
Ulcers	Pemphigus vulgaris; bullous pemphigoid

FIG. 10.3 Approach to pyoderma and pustular disease: Physical examination.

the history and physical examination which may eliminate possible causes or increase the index of suspicion that a certain disease is involved. The contents of these tables should be regarded as guidelines as exceptions will occur. **Pyoderma** is common and the other disorders shown in Figs 10.2 and 10.3 are rare.

Skin Diseases Associated Primarily with Pustules

Classification of Staphylococcal Pyoderma

Pyodermas may be classified according to depth of infection (surface, superficial and deep) or by aetiology.

Although **surface pyoderma** does not lead to papule and pustule formation, it will be considered in this chapter for convenience. Surface pyoderma is characterised by superficial erosion of the stratum corneum with associated erythema, alopecia, exudation, pruritus and secondary bacterial colonisation. Two major subgroups are recognised:

acute moist dermatitis ('wet' or 'summer' eczema, pyotraumatic dermatitis or 'hot spot') and intertrigo (skin fold dermatitis).

Superficial pyoderma is defined as bacterial disease involving the superficial portion of the hair follicle (superficial folliculitis) or the epidermis immediately below the stratum corneum (impetigo).

Deep pyodermas are serious, potentially life-endangering conditions where bacterial infection involves not only the hair follicle but also the dermal and subcuticular tissues.

Classification by depth of infection is useful as antimicrobial therapy needs to be more aggressive and prolonged in deeper cases (*Chapter 32*). Recognition of the depth of infection also influences the diagnostic approach. Deep pyoderma usually requires more detailed investigation. Bacterial culture and sensitivity and histopathology are usually indicated in deep pyoderma but may not be necessary in the more superficial forms of this disease.

It is also valuable to classify pyoderma disorders according to the underlying aetiology as this will help in formulating a diagnostic plan (Fig. 10.7).

DIAGNOSTIC PLAN FOR PYODERMA AND PUSTULAR DISEASE
1. If pustules are present
Focused diagnostic test: Examine stained smears from pustules (*Chapter 3*). This may identify staphylococci, immune cells and, in pemphigus, acantholytic cells
2. Rule out ectoparasitism
Focused diagnostic test: Microscopy of skin scrapings, hair pluckings and coat brushings (*Chapter 3*) and trial therapy and flea eradication (*Chapter 9*)
3. If pruritus is present
Focused diagnostic test: Use antibacterial therapy (*Chapter 31*) to determine whether this is due to the primary disorder or due to secondary bacterial infection (*Chapter 5*, Fig. 5.6)
If pruritus is due to the primary disease, correction of this disorder along with antimicrobial therapy may resolve the pyoderma (*Chapter 5*)
If pruritus is resolved by antimicrobial therapy, then suspect hypothyroidism, demodicosis or idiopathic pyoderma
If lesions are not resolved by antimicrobial therapy, suspect immune-mediated disease and the other non-bacterial causes of pustular disease
4. If no diagnosis is achieved
Further tests: Undertake specific tests, e.g. analysis of blood samples for endocrine disease (*Chapter 3*), histopathology for the other non-bacterial disorders

FIG. 10.4 Diagnostic plan for pyoderma and pustular disease.

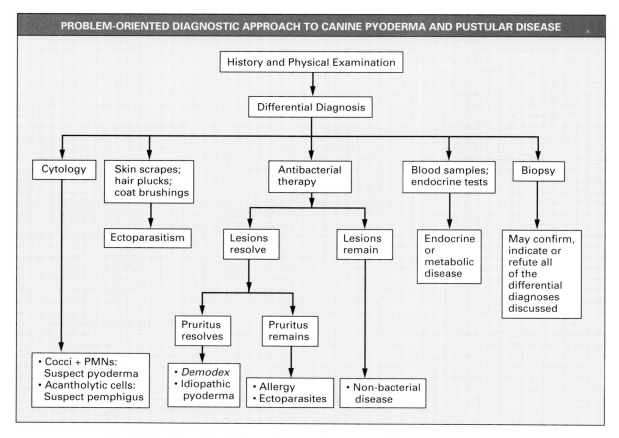

FIG. 10.5 Problem-oriented diagnostic approach to canine pyoderma and pustular disease.

Surface Pyoderma

Acute moist dermatitis

Description. Although this condition is common and is familiar to every clinician, its pathogenesis is poorly understood. The problem is worse during warm, humid weather. Underlying factors are listed in Fig. 10.7. It has been suggested that local irritation from the primary problem leads to self-trauma which initiates an itch–scratch cycle and can rapidly lead to quite extensive areas of cutaneous damage. The condition is extremely pruritic and may be painful on palpation.

Clinical signs. Acute moist dermatitis is characterised by the rapid development of highly pruritic to painful erosions of the skin surface associated with alopecia, exudation and erythema. Lesions typically affect the trunk, neck, face, tail base area

and the lateral aspects of the hind limbs (Fig. 10.6). Lesions are often solitary, although multiple lesions can occur. The site affected may be related to the underlying cause. For example, lesions associated with flea allergic dermatitis often affect the dorsal rump and proximal dorsal tail area, whereas cases associated with otitis externa may have lesions on the face or the side of the neck.

Diagnosis. Acute moist dermatitis is a clinical diagnosis. Demodicosis, neoplasia, early cases of calcinosis cutis and deeper forms of pyoderma may present with similar signs and need to be eliminated from the differential diagnosis. Skin scrapings should be taken for microscopy from all cases. Biopsy specimens should be taken for histopathology in cases which do not respond rapidly to therapy. A careful investigation of the possible underlying cause should be made.

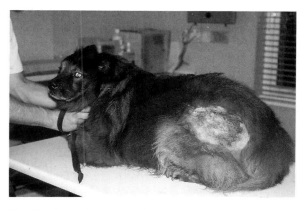

FIG. 10.6 Large, highly pruritic patch of erythema and alopecia on the rump of a cross bred dog. Acute moist dermatitis is commonly seen in dogs with thick coats. Every effort should be taken to identify the underlying cause in this case anal sacculitis. Slide courtesy of Richard Harvey.

Treatment.

1. Identify underlying cause and treat. Flea eradication is mandatory as fleas are a common cause of this disorder.
2. Restore ventilation to the area by clipping the affected area and adjacent hair. This may be painful and chemical restraint may be necessary.
3. Remove surface debris by gentle cleansing with a dilute antimicrobial solution such as saline, povidone-iodine or chlorhexidine. Occasionally systemic antimicrobial agents are needed (*Chapter 32*).
4. The use of topical and systemic glucocorticoids should be avoided. Although they may be of value in the initial management of self-trauma, they may mask an inaccurate diagnosis of the underlying cause of the condition.

5. Further self-trauma should be prevented by the use of an Elizabethan collar.

Prognosis. Most cases resolve rapidly following appropriate treatment although recurrence is common if the underlying cause cannot be found or corrected.

Intertrigo (skinfold pyoderma)

Description. Anatomical defects at certain body sites may, in some breeds, cause adjacent areas of skin to impinge, leading to poor ventilation and creating frictional trauma. Furthermore, such sites are often close to areas of saliva, tear and urine release. Hence, a relatively warm and humid microenvironment rich in tissue fluids develops, facilitating secondary bacterial colonisation. Examples of intertrigo include facial fold dermatitis (Pekingese, Pugs and other brachycephalic breeds); lipfold dermatitis (Spaniels); bodyfold dermatitis (Shar Peis and obese individuals of other breeds), tailfold dermatitis (breeds with 'corkscrew' tails such as English Bulldogs and Pugs) and vulvar fold dermatitis (usually seen in bitches which were spayed young and have an infantile vulva, Plate 10).

Clinical signs. Pruritus, odour, erythema, exudation associated with body or skin folds are present in intertrigo.

Diagnosis. The diagnosis is clinical.

Treatment. Ideally, the anatomical defect should be corrected surgically. Facial and labial folds may be treated by fold resection, tailfolds by amputation

PYODERMA: EXAMPLES OF UNDERLYING FACTORS	
Surface pyoderma	
Acute moist dermatitis	Flea allergy, otitis externa, anal sacculitis, inadequate grooming, poor coat ventilation, painful musculo-skeletal conditions, decubital sores
Intertrigo	Anatomical defects (facial, lip, tail, vulvar and body folds), obesity
Superficial pyoderma	
Impetigo	May be associated with poor management of pups (dirty housing, poor nutrition, ecto- or endoparasitism, viral infection). May be idiopathic
Folliculitis	Hypersensitivity, ectoparasitism, endocrinopathy, anatomical/immunological factors, idiopathic
Deep pyoderma	Cause may determine site affected. Consider demodicosis, hypothyroidism, hypersensitivity, foreign body, anatomical/immunological factors. May be idiopathic

FIG. 10.7 Pyoderma: Examples of underlying factors.

of the tail, and vulvar folds by episioplasty. In the case of show animals, it is important that clients are fully informed of the implications of these procedures, as removal of facial folds and corkscrew tails will debar these animals from the showring.

Bodyfolds of obese individuals may be corrected by restriction of caloric intake. This is ineffective in Shar Peis, however, as the presence of cutaneous folds is genetically determined, and so palliative measures involving long-term antimicrobial and antiseborrhoeic shampoos are indicated.

Prognosis. The prognosis is excellent provided that the anatomical defect can be corrected; otherwise, long-term palliative medical treatment is needed.

Superficial Pyoderma

Impetigo

Description. Impetigo or juvenile pustular dermatitis is a relatively benign pustular dermatosis affecting the inguinal and axillary regions of sexually immature dogs, usually puppies 3 to 9 months of age. It is not contagious and is often associated with poor management of puppies. However, well managed litters may also develop this condition.

Clinical signs. The disease is characterised by subcorneal pustules (i.e. pustules not involving the hair follicle) affecting the relatively glabrous areas (principally the groin and axillae). Occasionally mild pruritus may be present. The pustules rupture easily and a dried, yellowish exudate may be present.

Diagnosis. Clinical history and physical examination are usually sufficient to indicate that impetigo is present. In some instances, biopsy and histopathology, along with culture of pustule contents, may be necessary.

Treatment. Most cases recover spontaneously once the underlying management problem has been resolved or at sexual maturity. Topical antimicrobial therapy with an antimicrobial shampoo (*Chapter 32*) may be of value. Occasionally short-term systemic antimicrobial therapy is required. Glucocorticoids are contra-indicated as they encourage deepening and worsening of the infection.

Prognosis. Prognosis is excellent, with spontaneous recovery being observed in the majority of cases.

Folliculitis

Description. Superficial staphylococcal folliculitis is an extremely common canine disorder. Despite this, the aetiology and pathogenesis remain unclear. The primary lesions are papules and pustules affecting the superficial portion of the hair follicle. Most cases are secondary to some other disorder and hypersensitivity, ectoparasitism and internal disorders (especially hypothyroidism) should be considered as possible causes of this condition.

Virtually any breed, sex or age of dog can be affected. In general the clinical history depends on the primary disorder present. For example, a pruritic superficial dermatitis in a young adult terrier with foot chewing and facial lesions is suggestive of atopy. However, a non-pruritic pyoderma in a lethargic Golden Retriever would indicate that thyroid function be evaluated.

Clinical signs. The cardinal lesion of superficial folliculitis, irrespective of the underlying cause, is the follicular pustule. As previously discussed, however, pustules may be absent; and a chronological spectrum of lesions ranging from papules through pustules (if present) to scaling, alopecia, hyperpigmentation and epidermal collarette formation may be evident (Plates 11 and 12). Lesions usually affect the ventral relatively glabrous areas such as the axillae, abdomen and groin, although in some instances the dorsal trunk is affected; this leads to a 'moth-eaten' appearance to the coat of short-coated breeds.

Diagnosis. Identification of the disorder described above as superficial folliculitis is straightforward, based on history, clinical signs and response to antimicrobial therapy. However, because this disorder is invariably secondary, the clinician must investigate and identify the underlying cause. Examples of these causes are listed in Fig. 10.7 and the approach to such cases has been discussed above and in *Chapter 5*. A range of diagnostic tests may be indicated, depending on the clinical context. These may include routine tests such as microscopical examination of skin scrapings and other samples for ectoparasites and microscopy of stained contents of pustules. In other cases, allergy tests, blood analyses and endocrine function tests may be required.

Treatment. Management of superficial folliculitis is based on identification and treatment of the underlying cause in association with systemic and topical antimicrobial therapy (*Chapter 32*).

Prognosis. The prognosis varies with the underlying cause, but it is likely that most cases will require long-term therapy. Such therapy may be directed at the underlying cause or at the secondary bacterial complication, or both.

Deep Pyoderma

Description. Deep pyodermas are serious. In severe pyoderma the follicular walls swell, weaken and rupture, releasing hair-shaft keratin, bacteria and bacterial products into the dermis. This results in a pyogranulomatous perifolliculitis or furunculosis.

The deep pyodermas may be localised or generalised. A particularly severe form of generalised pyoderma is seen in German Shepherd Dogs (German Shepherd Dog pyoderma, Plate 13). This is usually idiopathic.

Demodex is the most common cause of deep pyoderma. Other predisposing causes include hypothyroidism, hyperadrenocorticism and immunosuppression associated with neoplasia or internal disease. Some cases are idiopathic and presumed to arise as a result of some undetermined immunological defect. Prolonged administration of glucocorticoids may lead to deep pyoderma.

Localised deep pyodermas include muzzle and chin pyoderma (acne), interdigital pyoderma, anal furunculosis, pressure-point pyoderma and nasal pyoderma. Factors which may be involved in the pathogenesis of these forms of pyoderma are given in Fig. 10.8.

Virtually any breed, age or sex of dog may be affected. The history depends on the form of deep pyoderma present and the underlying cause.

Clinical signs. Cases of deep pyoderma are characterised by the presence of papules, pustules, furuncles and discharging sinuses. The exudate is usually mucopurulent or haemorrhagic. There may be pain, erythema, oedema, ulceration and a disagreeable odour. The coat overlying the affected area may be matted with dried exudate. Regional lymph nodes are enlarged. In generalised cases there may be lethargy, pyrexia and depression. The distribution of lesions depends on the form of deep pyoderma present.

Diagnosis. The presence of deep pyoderma is usually easily determined clinically. However, in some instances, it may be difficult to recognise deep pyoderma without performing histopathology. The rule is to take biopsy samples from any severe or unusual dermatosis. Bacterial culture should be undertaken and antibiotic sensitivity should be determined as this enables appropriate antimicrobial treatment. It is preferable to submit skin biopsy specimens from the centre of the lesions for bacteriology rather than relying on surface swabs.

The underlying cause should be determined if possible as the disorder is potentially life-endangering (Fig. 10.7).

FACTORS WHICH PREDISPOSE TO DEEP PYODERMA	
Condition	**Underlying cause**
Generalised deep pyoderma	Often idiopathic; demodicosis; hypothyroidism
Interdigital pyoderma	Demodicosis; hypothyroidism; hypersensitivity; foreign bodies; dermatomycosis
Muzzle and chin pyoderma	Idiopathic; demodicosis
Pressure-point pyoderma	Poor bedding; obesity; hypothyroidism
Anal furunculosis	Idiopathic; possibly genetic; anatomical or immunological factors
Nasal pyoderma	Idiopathic; some evidence suggests that this is not a form of pyoderma

FIG. 10.8 Factors which predispose to deep pyoderma.

Treatment. Management of deep pyoderma is based on identification and treatment of the underlying cause in association with systemic and topical antimicrobial therapy (*Chapter 32*).

Prognosis. The prognosis varies with the underlying cause, but it is likely that most cases will require long term therapy. Deep pyoderma secondary to disorders such as hypothyroidism bears the best prognosis as thyroxine supplementation may be sufficient to hold the case in remission after an initial course of antibacterial therapy. Demodicosis may be difficult or even impossible to cure and so recurrence of pyoderma may be expected. Deep pyoderma secondary to neoplasia or profound immunosuppression has a poor prognosis.

Generalised pyoderma has a poor prognosis compared with the localised forms of this disease.

If lifelong therapy is indicated, this may be directed at the underlying cause or at the secondary bacterial complication or, most likely, both.

Other Diseases

Immune-mediated/autoimmune disorders

These disorders are covered in detail in *Chapters 7* (pemphigus foliaceus and erythematosus) and *8* (pemphigus vulgaris, bullous pemphigoid and drug eruptions).

Contact irritant dermatitis

This is covered in more detail in *Chapter 5*.

Sub-corneal pustular dermatosis

Description. Sub-corneal pustular dermatosis (SPD) is an exceptionally rare idiopathic sterile pustular dermatosis of dogs. Very few cases have been reported in the veterinary literature. In recent years, it seems that the disease has disappeared with no new cases being reported. Some authorities have suggested that SPD does not exist as an entity. It is possible that cases of pyoderma, bullous impetigo and the immune-mediated disorders were erroneously called SPD and recent advances in dermatological diagnosis have allowed the true diagnosis to be recognised. Alternatively, the disease may simply have disappeared.

Clinical signs. The clinical picture is that of a multi-focal or generalised, pustular to seborrhoea-like dermatosis affecting the head and trunk. Miniature Schnauzers may be predisposed. The disorder may regress and then recur spontaneously. Pruritus varies from none to severe. SPD is poorly responsive to systemic antimicrobial therapy and glucocorticoids.

Diagnosis. Diagnosis is based on history, clinical examination, response to therapy and the exclusion of other pustular disorders (Fig. 10.1). Histopathology of intact pustules shows that the condition is a sub-corneal, interfollicular pustular dermatitis; acantholysis may be present. As diagnostic techniques improve and a greater understanding of the pathogenesis of the pustular disorders is attained, the number of cases of SPD may continue to decline.

Treatment. Dapsone, at 1 mg/kg three times daily, is the drug of choice. Response usually occurs within a month. In some cases, recovery persists following withdrawal of the drug although some cases relapse and need to be treated intermittently to remain in remission. Dapsone is a sulphonamide which is both anti-inflammatory and antibacterial. The drug is not licensed for use in animals. Side-effects during induction of therapy may be serious and include mild anaemia, leucopenia and elevation of liver enzymes. However, these are usually reversible on discontinuation of therapy and often resolve once maintenance therapy commences.

Prognosis. The prognosis varies depending on response to dapsone.

Sterile eosinophilic pustular dermatitis

Description. Sterile eosinophilic pustular dermatitis (SEPD) is a rare idiopathic disorder. It is thought to be immune-mediated as it responds well to glucocorticoids and because there is cutaneous and blood eosinophilia. There is no breed, age or sex predisposition.

Clinical signs. SEPD has an acute onset with multi-focal or even generalised lesions. Papules and pustules develop, and these may be interfollicular or follicular. As expected in canine pustular disease, epidermal collarettes and scale are present. SEPD is a highly pruritic disorder. Most cases do not show systemic signs although some affected individuals may be depressed or anorexic or both, or may have pyrexia and peripheral lymphadenopathy.

Diagnosis. Diagnosis is based on history, physical examination and elimination of other pustular disorders from the differential diagnosis (Fig. 10.1). Haematology reveals a peripheral eosinophilia and stained smears from lesions show numerous eosinophils, occasional neutrophils and acantholytic cells but no micro-organisms. Cultures are negative and histopathology reveals intra-epidermal eosinophilic pustular dermatitis, folliculitis and furunculosis.

Treatment and prognosis. Most dogs respond well to systemic glucocorticoid therapy (prednisolone at 2–4 mg/kg daily) within a week. Withdrawal of therapy leads to recurrence of the disorder and so long-term alternate-day maintenance therapy is required.

Linear IgA dermatosis

Description. Linear IgA dermatosis is another rare canine idiopathic sterile superficial pustular dermatosis. It has only been reported in adult Dachshunds. There is no sex predisposition.

Clinical signs. Linear IgA dermatosis typically affects the trunk. The lesions are multi-focal to generalised and range from pustules to epidermal collarettes, scaling and crust formation. There may be alopecia, erosion and hyperpigmentation. There are no systemic signs and pruritus is minimal.

Diagnosis. Diagnosis is based on history, physical examination and elimination of other pustular disease from the differential diagnosis. Cultures are negative and histopathology reveals sub-corneal or intra-epidermal pustular dermatitis with neutrophils. Immunofluorescence testing shows that IgA is deposited along the basement membrane area.

Treatment and prognosis. Glucocorticoids (prednisolone at 2–4 mg/kg daily) may lead to remission of signs in most cases. Once the condition is

stabilised, minimal-dose alternate-day maintenance therapy can be introduced. Some cases also respond to dapsone therapy using a similar regimen to that for sub-corneal pustular dermatosis. Response to these drugs is variable between cases. Lifelong maintenance therapy is required.

Acral lick dermatitis

Description. Acral lick dermatitis is often associated with deep pyoderma. It is characterised by persistent licking or chewing of the anterior aspect of the lower anterior portion of a limb (usually a forelimb) resulting in a thickened, firm, raised oval plaque. The aetiology is complex and it is not simply a disease of boredom.

It is typically a disease of large, active and affectionate dogs. Often the licking behaviour is a means of seeking attention. Although it is generally accepted that this is a psychosomatic disorder, occasionally there are organic causes such as hypersensitivity, traumatic wounds or underlying orthopaedic problems. Neoplastic or granulomatous diseases may mimic this disorder and need to be differentiated from it. Acral lick dermatitis is neither neoplastic nor granulomatous. A thorough diagnostic approach is needed before therapy is instituted.

Clinical signs. The disease can occur at almost any age although affected dogs are usually 5 years or older. Dobermanns, Great Danes, Labrador Retrievers and other middle-sized to large breeds are usually affected.

Initially the constant licking leads to alopecia. Erosion of the epidermis follows and eventually ulceration is seen. Constant licking prevents healing and secondary bacterial infection occurs. Epidermal hyperplasia and dermal fibrosis lead to nodule formation. The lesions are usually single although occasionally multiple lesions are seen. They are usually unilateral. The most common site is the anterior aspect of the carpus or, less commonly, the tarsus.

Diagnosis. The diagnosis is clinical, based on history and signs. However, it may be necessary to distinguish acral lick lesions from neoplasms and granulomata. Hypersensitivity disorders and painful underlying orthopaedic conditions should be ruled out of the differential diagnosis. Radiography may indicate whether the problem is orthopaedic. Histopathology may indicate whether the disorder is truly acral lick dermatitis rather than a tumour or granuloma.

Treatment. The treatment of acral lick dermatitis is covered in detail in *Chapter 34*. Antibiotics are a useful early aid to the management of this condition and should be used, along with an Elizabethan collar to control pyoderma and to prevent further self-trauma before any other treatment is given. This will allow the clinician the opportunity to investigate the condition properly.

Prognosis. The prognosis is good insofar as the disease is seldom life-endangering. However, acral lick dermatitis is one of the most intractable and difficult canine diseases to resolve and management is often unsuccessful.

Bullous impetigo

Occasionally impetigo occurs in adult dogs. Large, flat pustules are seen. These are somewhat flaccid, yellow to green in colour and may be up to 1 cm in diameter. They are usually associated with immunosuppression — for example, animals receiving therapy for immune-mediated diseases or in cases of hyperadrenocorticism.

11

Nodular Lesions, Non-Healing Wounds and Common Skin Tumours

KAREN MORIELLO

A **nodular** lesion describes any mass that is present on the skin or in the subcutaneous tissue. Most commonly, nodular lesions may be caused by infectious or parasitic agents, foreign bodies or neoplasia. The most important task for the veterinarian when presented with a nodular lesion in a dog is to determine if the aetiology of the nodule is neoplastic, inflammatory or infectious. **Non-healing wounds** are defined as wounds that do not heal within the expected period after appropriate conventional therapy (medical or surgical). Because the diagnostic approach and aetiologies are similar, the problems of nodular and non-healing wounds will be discussed together. The most useful focused diagnostic tests are cytology, skin biopsy and culture.

Selected Skin Diseases Characterised by Nodular and Non-Healing Wounds

Eosinophilic granuloma

Description. Eosinophilic granulomas are more common in cats but they do occur in dogs. There are two general categories. The first is the oral eosinophilic granuloma. These lesions are most common in young Siberian Huskies, but may be seen in a number of other breeds. The cause is unknown and it is suspected that there may be a hereditary predisposition for development of the lesions. The second group of eosinophilic granulomas tend to be focal and solitary and usually lack recurrence. They are believed to be caused by arthropod-bites and are probably hypersensitivity reactions.

Clinical signs. Oral eosinophilic granulomas occur most commonly on the lateral or ventral surface of the tongue or mouth. The author has seen one dog with generalised mucocutaneous lesions. The lesions are well demarcated, brown, proliferative and plaque-like in appearance. There is usually a strong fetid odour to the mouth and this is often what prompts owners to seek veterinary attention. Lesions may be very painful. Another type of eosinophilic granulomas are most commonly found on the haired skin, particularly ear margins. Pain and pruritus are usually absent.

Diagnosis. Definitive diagnosis is made by skin biopsy. Oral eosinophilic granulomas must be differentiated from tumours and the diagnosis is often unexpected.

DIFFERENTIAL DIAGNOSIS OF NODULAR AND NON-HEALING WOUNDS IN DOGS	
Bacterial	Cutaneous bacterial granuloma Staphylococcal furunculosis Actinomycosis Nocardiosis Opportunistic mycobacterial infections
Fungal	Kerion Mycetoma Phaeohyphomycosis Cryptococcosis Blastomycosis Coccidiomycosis Histoplasmosis Sporotrichosis Pythiosis Miscellaneous opportunistic algae and fungi
Hypersensitivity	Arthropod-bite granuloma Eosinophilic granuloma
Parasitic	Leishmaniasis Rhabditic dermatitis Spider-bite
Immune-mediated	Sterile nodular panniculitis Juvenile cellulitis Sterile nodular granuloma and pyogranuloma Histiocytosis
Neoplasia	Round cell tumours Epithelial tumours Spindle cell tumours

FIG. 11.1 Differential diagnosis of nodular and non-healing wounds in dogs.

FIG. 11.2 Approach to no-
dules and non-healing
wounds: History.

APPROACH TO NODULES AND NON-HEALING WOUNDS: HISTORY	
Factor	**Differential diagnosis**
Breed	Certain types of tumours (See *Appendix*)

Age of onset
  Less than 3 months
  More than 2 years
  6–14 years
	
	Juvenile cellulitis
	Histiocytoma
	Neoplasia

History of trauma	Foreign body; opportunistic fungal organism; opportunistic mycobacterial organism

Travel to regions with endemic
  leishmaniasis, or systemic fungal
  organism
	Leishmaniasis; blastomycosis; histoplasmosis;
	  coccidiomycosis

Respiratory signs, weight-loss, lethargy	Systemic fungal infection; opportunistic algae or Protista; systemic neoplasia

FIG. 11.3 Approach to no-
dules and non-healing
wounds: Physical examina-
tion.

APPROACH TO NODULES AND NON-HEALING WOUNDS: PHYSICAL EXAMINATION	
Physical finding	**Differential diagnosis**

Fever and/or signs of systemic illness,
  (weight-loss; respiratory disease;
  gastrointestinal disease)
	Systemic mycoses; systemic opportunistic
	  fungi or algae; systemic/malignant
	  histiocytic disease; systemic neoplasia with
	  cutaneous manifestations; leishmaniasis

Ocular disease	Lymphosarcoma; systemic mycoses
Solitary lesion	Foreign body; abscess; cutaneous neoplasia; arthropod-bite/granuloma

Multiple lesions with or without draining
  tracts or exudation
	Systemic mycoses; opportunistic fungal
	  organism or algae; panniculitis;
	  actinomycoses; nocardiosis; neoplasia; deep
	  bacterial pyoderma

Acute lesion with marked inflammation	Fungal kerion; foreign body; abscess; neoplasia

Slowly developing lesion with exudation	Fungal mycetoma; opportunistic fungus or
	  Protista; foreign body; atypical
	  mycobacterial infection; neoplasia

Treatment. Solitary eosinophilic granulomas will resolve spontaneously if biopsy is not curative. Oral eosinophilic granulomas are treated with systemic glucocorticoids although some will resolve spontaneously. Oral prednisolone (0.5–2.2 mg/kg/day for 10–20 days) is usually curative.

Prognosis. The prognosis is good.

Arthropod-bite granuloma

Description. Nodular lesions at the site of a bite or sting of various arthropods are relatively common. The most common arthropods to cause these reactions are ticks. The reaction is believed to be due to a Type 4 hypersensitivity reaction to the bite of the arthropod.

Clinical signs. These lesions are not commonly reported by clients because they are not easily found in the skin. The initial lesion usually begins with swelling and erythema at the site of the bite. A firm nodule in the skin forms at the site of the bite. The time course is unknown but the author has seen one dog develop generalised nodular lesions within 10 days of being swarmed by mosquitoes. Site predilections for the lesions depend upon the biting arthropod's predilection or preference.

Diagnosis. Definitive diagnosis requires a skin biopsy. A clinical diagnosis alone may suffice if the history is strongly supportive of a known arthropod-bite at the site.

Treatment. In general, lesions will spontaneously regress and no treatment is required. If necessary, oral prednisolone (0.5–2.2 mg/kg/day for 7–10 days) is curative.

Prognosis. The prognosis is excellent.

DISEASES CHARACTERISED BY MIXED INFLAMMATORY INFILTRATES	
With increased eosinophils	Eosinophilic granuloma Arthropod-bite granuloma Spider-bites Pelodera (rhabditic) dermatitis
With neutrophils predominating	Foreign body reactions Fungal kerion Opportunistic infections with fungi and algae Systemic fungal infections Actinomycosis and nocardiosis Opportunistic mycobacterial infections Cutaneous leishmaniasis Panniculitis Juvenile cellulitis Sterile granuloma and pyogranuloma syndrome

FIG. 11.4 Diseases characterised by mixed inflammatory infiltrates.

Spider-bites

Description. Spider-bites are rarely documented in veterinary medicine. Geographic location will dictate which species of venomous spiders are present. Dogs that frequent woodpiles and vacated buildings are most at risk for being bitten.

Clinical signs. Clinical signs may vary from non-detectable to nodular lesions, to widespread tissue necrosis. The face and forelegs are most commonly affected. Erythema and swelling are present at the site of most bites. Depending upon the species, marked swelling, vesicles and skin necrosis can occur within 6 to 12 hours of the bite. Systemic reactions to spider-bites may include salivation, nausea and diarrhoea, ataxia and convulsions. These signs may occur within 6 to 48 hours of the bite.

Diagnosis. Definitive diagnosis is difficult unless there is a strong supporting history of a known bite in the affected area. Histological findings are non-specific and may be compatible with severe vasculitis, severe bacterial infection, severe foreign body reaction, arthropod-bite granuloma and other infectious diseases.

Treatment. Supportive care and appropriate wound management.

Prognosis. Prognosis depends upon the clinical signs exhibited by the patient. However, if life-threatening signs are not observed the prognosis is good.

Pelodera (rhabditic) dermatitis

Description. *Pelodera* dermatitis is a non-seasonal dermatitis that is caused by cutaneous infestation by the larvae of *Pelodera strongyloides*. This nematode is free-living and is capable of invading the skin of dogs only after pre-existing trauma or tissue maceration is present. The most common source of infestation is contaminated bedding. Dogs with pelodera dermatitis usually have a history of sleeping on damp, soiled bedding that is infested with *Pelodera*. The nematode is commonly found in rice hulls, marsh grass and straw.

Clinical signs. The lesions tend to be localised to areas of the dog's body that are in contact with the damp soiled bedding; a ventral distribution is most common. Hair-loss, lichenification, papules, nodules and diffuse thickening of the skin are most commonly observed. Secondary bacterial pyodermas are common. Pruritus is variable and may be severe.

Diagnosis. Definitive diagnosis is made by skin scraping. In infested dogs, large numbers of small motile nematodes (625–650 μm in length) are easily found. Skin biopsy, although not usually necessary for diagnosis, will show nematodes in hair follicles.

Treatment. The most important aspect of treatment is removal of the contaminated bedding and replacement with more suitable bedding. Although the disease is self-limiting, most dogs benefit from mediated antibacterial baths to remove scale and debris from the skin. Additionally, twice-weekly dips in an insecticide formulated to kill fleas will bring rapid relief to the dog. If necessary, oral prednisolone may be prescribed in cases where pruritus is severe.

Prognosis. The prognosis is good.

Foreign body reactions

Description. Foreign body reactions are caused by the penetration of a variety of foreign material, but most commonly organic and plant matter, cactus spines, porcupine quills, fibreglass, gravel and grass awns. Additionally, a foreign body reaction can occur at the site of retained suture material, ruptured hair follicles (keratin is very inflammatory in the skin) and malicious acts, for example rubber bands placed on extremities.

Clinical signs. The very early stages of foreign body penetration are rarely observed by either the veterinarian or the owner. Mild erythema, a small wound and exudation may be present. As the foreign matter penetrates into the tissue via muscular movement, a host reaction ensues. A nodule, draining tract or non-healing wound at the entry site develops. Secondary bacterial infections are common and furunculosis may develop, especially with interdigital foreign body reactions. Secondary infections with *Staphylococcus*, *Nocardia* and *Actinomyces* spp. are common.

Diagnosis. Definitive diagnosis requires evidence of the foreign material. This may be via exploration of tracts and removal of the material or via skin biopsy. It is critical to inform the pathologist that a foreign body reaction is suspected so that the specimen is examined with special stains and polarised light. The latter helps to identify keratin and fibreglass particles. In some cases, radiographs and fistulograms may be needed to locate the foreign body.

DIAGNOSTIC PLAN FOR NODULES AND NON-HEALING WOUNDS

Because many of the diseases that cause nodular or non-healing lesions are potentially life-threatening, efforts should be directed at rapidly determining whether the aetiology is infectious or neoplastic. The most useful in-house diagnostic screening tool is cytological examination of the nodule or wound
1. Perform a fine needle aspirate, impression smear of exudate, tissue imprint or scraping of the margin of the lesion. Collect at least three or four specimens. The slides should be stained with a quick stain and examined under increasing magnification
2. Determine the predominant cell population of the specimen. Infectious and inflammatory skin diseases are characterised by the presence of obvious numbers of inflammatory cells (neutrophils, macrophages, eosinophils, other cells). Neoplastic skin diseases are characterised by very cellular specimens with homogeneous cell types

Specimen Contains Predominantly Inflammatory Cells

Estimate the approximate percentage of neutrophils and mixed inflammatory cells in the specimen (macrophages, neutrophils, plasma cells, lymphocytes, other cells)
1. *If the specimen contains 80–90% neutrophils*, the most likely causes are infectious diseases. The presence of a large number of degenerate neutrophils strongly suggests a bacterial aetiology

> **Focused diagnostic tests:** Obtain additional cytological specimens, if necessary, for Gram stain and special staining and search for an organism. If no infectious agent is found or suspected, submit an aerobic bacterial culture. If lesions are rapidly progressing, the patient is debilitated, or if clinical impression warrants it, submit a biopsy at the initial examination. In general, however, biopsies are not usually necessary at initial examination unless cultures and cytological examination do not identify a pathogen

2. *If the specimen contains a mixed inflammatory cell population consisting of neutrophils, macrophages and other cells*, determine whether or not eosinophils are prominent in the specimen
3. *If eosinophil numbers are increased in the specimen*, the most likely causes are hypersensitivity or parasitic skin diseases

> **Focused diagnostic tests:** Skin scrapings should be performed to rule out demodicosis and nematode infestations. Skin biopsy is required for a definitive diagnosis

4. *If eosinophil numbers are not increased and neutrophils are prominent with macrophages, bacterial, fungal, parasitic and non-infectious inflammatory causes:*

> **Focused diagnostic tests:** The most cost-effective approach at this point is to submit several representative cytological specimens with a skin biopsy to an appropriate reference laboratory. Ideally, cultures for aerobic and anaerobic bacteria and deep fungal organisms should be submitted at the time the biopsy is collected. If there are cost constraints, it is acceptable to wait for the pathology report before submitting cultures, provided that the dog is not systemically ill or rapidly deteriorating. If a definitive diagnosis is not made or if the histological report indicates a pyogranulomatous pattern of inflammation, tissue should be submitted for culture (aerobic, anaerobic and deep fungal organisms). In some reference laboratories it may be necessary to ask the pathologist to perform special stains

Specimen Does Not Contain an Inflammatory Cell Population

1. *If the specimen is acellular without a marked predominance of tissue cells*, re-aspirate the specimen and/or perform a skin biopsy. Neoplasia or an infectious disease process cannot be ruled out
2. *If the specimen is very cellular and contains a homogeneous tissue cell population*, strongly consider neoplasia. Small to medium-sized individual cells with discrete borders are suggestive of round cell tumours. Large round, oval or caudate cells in sheets or clumps are suggestive of epithelial tumours. Small to medium cells with spindle shapes and tails of cytoplasm are suggestive of spindle cell tumours

> **Focused diagnostic test:** If the cytological diagnosis is less than certain, perform a skin biopsy for a definitive diagnosis

FIG. 11.5 Diagnostic plan for nodules and non-healing wounds.

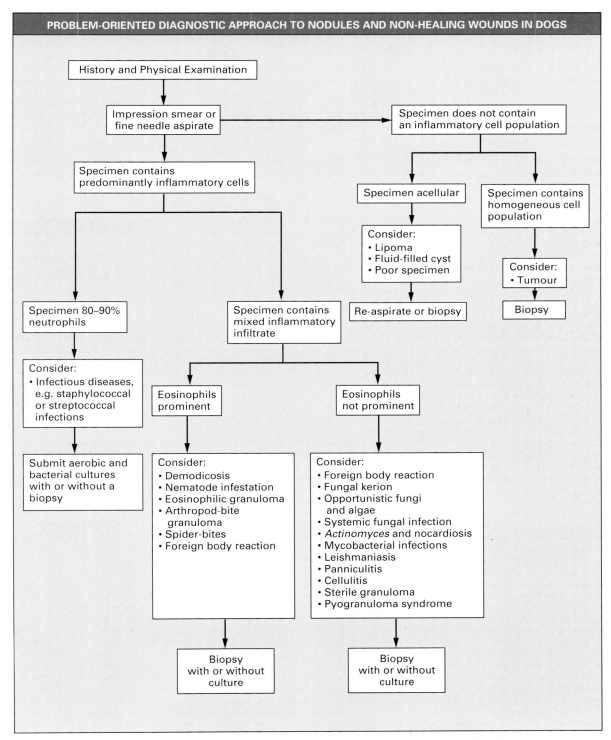

FIG. 11.6 Problem-oriented diagnostic approach to nodules and non-healing wounds in dogs.

Treatment. Effective treatment requires a thorough search for all of the penetrating foreign material and its removal. Because of the risk of secondary infections, the exudate should be cultured and appropriate antibiotic therapy instituted. Foreign body reactions due to keratin are difficult to treat because keratin is so inflammatory in tissue and impossible to remove surgically. Dogs with recurrent interdigital abscesses due to foreign body reactions to keratin or microscopic foreign material may require a combination of surgical curettage and long-term antibiotic therapy. At least 6–8 weeks of oral antibiotics, preferably a bacteriocidal antibiotic, are recommended.

Prognosis. The prognosis is excellent for patients in which a solitary foreign body is found and removed, provided that there are no secondary bacterial infections present. The prognosis for dogs with interdigital furunculosis due to foreign body reactions from keratin or dirt is guarded. These animals usually have an underlying anatomic defect that predisposes them to the problem. Bull Terriers are a classic example. These dogs should be thoroughly screened for complicating pruritic diseases, or diseases which may predispose them to recurrent pyoderma. Some dogs with chronic interdigital furunculosis are atopic or have idiopathic recurrent pyoderma.

Fungal kerion (see Fig. 11.7)

Description. A fungal **kerion** is an acute inflammatory lesion caused by a dermatophyte. The most commonly isolated dermatophyte is *Microsporum gypseum*. Fungal kerions can occur with any of the dermatophytes, but they are most common with the geophilic organisms.

Clinical signs. There is no age, breed or sex predilection; however, dogs that spend a great deal of time outdoors are at increased risk. Fungal kerions are also more common in warm climates. The typical lesion usually occurs on the nose or extremity and is alopecic, exudative and erythematous. Lesions are usually solitary but they may be multiple, especially on the feet. Lesions may be painful or pruritic.

Diagnosis. Definitive diagnosis requires a biopsy. Fungal cultures are usually negative because of the intense inflammation at the lesion site. Most lesions are markedly improved, if not totally resolved, by the time the histopathology report is received.

Treatment. Lesions are self-curing and require no treatment. Severe cases will benefit from warm compresses and antibacterial scrubs to remove debris, and systemic antifungal therapy. Topical antifungal ointments, creams or gels are usually unnecessary.

Opportunistic infections with fungi and algae

Description. There is a wide range of miscellaneous cutaneous infections in the skin with opportunistic fungi and algae. Several terms are used to

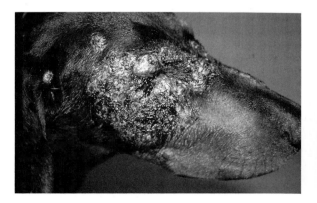

Fig. 11.7 Fungal kerion in a dog.

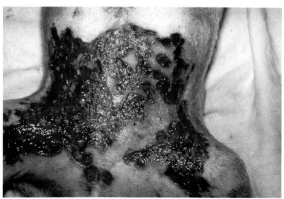

Fig. 11.8 Phaeohyphomycosis in a dog. Slide courtesy of Dr Kenneth Kwochka, The Ohio State University.

subdivide or subclassify these infections, including **mycetoma** and **phaeohyphomycosis** (Fig. 11.8). **Mycetomas** can be caused by either bacteria or fungi and are characterised by swelling, exudation, draining tracts and the presence of tissue granules (usually microscopic). **Phaeohyphomycosis** and **zygomycosis** are clinically indistinguishable from mycetomas. Phaeohyphomycosis is caused by dematiaceous fungi (pigmented fungi) such as *Alternaria*, *Drechslera* and *Curvularia*. These are relatively rare and are most common in tropical and semi-tropicals regions. Almost all of these infections are initiated by a traumatic inoculation of the organism into the skin or exposure of traumatised skin to contaminated soil or water.

Clinical signs. The clinical signs of infection depend upon whether or not the organism has a tendency only to invade the skin and subcutaneous tissues or to spread systemically. Most of the organisms that cause mycetomas and phaeohyphomycosis produce only cutaneous or subcutaneous infections. Infection is most common on the extremities and usually presents as slowly developing nodules with draining tracts. The nodule/tumour is usually cool and painless to the touch, which helps to differentiate it from bacterial abscesses. Occasionally, small granules may be present in the exudate. Animals with systemic opportunistic infections usually present with signs of systemic illness, such as weightloss, lethargy, fever and respiratory signs (coughing, nasal discharge). Concurrent systemic involvement is most common with *Aspergillus*, *Paecilomyces*, *Prototheca* and *Pythium* spp.

Diagnosis. Definitive diagnosis requires a skin biopsy and culture of a wedge of tissue for bacteria and fungi. Definitive identification of the organism is necessary to determine whether or not treatment is possible. In the rare instance of bacterial mycetomas, antibiotic therapy is usually very effective combined with surgical excision. Unfortunately, most of the organisms that cause fungal mycetomas and phaeohyphomycosis are not susceptible to systemic antifungal agents. Effective therapy requires surgical excision or amputation in many instances. No successful therapy is known for systemic opportunistic fungal, algal or pythiosis infections. The development of newer antifungal agents may be promising for potential therapy.

Prognosis. Prognosis for localised opportunistic infections is poor to guarded. The prognosis for systemic opportunistic infections is grave.

Systemic fungal infections

Description. The systemic mycoses are fungal infections that invade internal organs and then disseminate secondarily to the skin. In rare instances, these organisms may involve only the skin. The systemic mycoses include *Blastomyces dermatitidis*, *Coccidioides immitis* and *Histoplasma capsulatum*. Inhalation of spores from contaminated environments is the most common route of infection. *Cryptococcus neoformans*, *Paecilomyces* spp., *Candida albicans* and *Aspergillus* spp. can also cause systemic mycoses in debilitated hosts.

Clinical signs. Systemic signs of illness include fever, weight-loss, lethargy, coughing, nasal discharge, diarrhoea, neurological signs and ocular signs. The cutaneous lesions usually present as nodular to ulcerated lesions that may be solitary or multiple. Early lesions may begin as patches of erythema that quickly develop into nodular lesions, which ulcerate. Regional lymphadenopathy is common and often dramatic.

Diagnosis. Definitive diagnosis can often be made via cytological examination of exudate. Organisms of blastomycosis, coccidioidomycosis, histoplasmosis, and cryptococcosis are very characteristic in appearance. Skin biopsy is also definitive. Culture of infected tissue, skin biopsy and serum fungal titres are the best triad of diagnostic tests when an infective agent is not easily identified on cytological examination of exudate.

Treatment. Systemic antifungal therapy is the treatment of choice for these infections. The reader is referred to the bibliography for a detailed discussion of treatment options. Therapy is time-consuming and expensive and a thorough familiarity with antifungal drugs, complications of use and ancillary therapy is necessary; referral to a specialty clinic may be necessary. Prior to the initiation of therapy, a careful and complete physical examination, including an ophthalmological examination, is necessary to determine the full scope of the infection.

Prognosis. The prognosis is guarded.

Actinomyces and nocardiosis

Description. Infection with *Actinomyces* spp. and *Nocardia* spp. is rare. Infection occurs most commonly via penetrating wounds, especially where foreign bodies such as quills and grass awns are present. Cutaneous nocardiosis may develop secondary to pulmonary nocardiasis in debilitated hosts. Hunting dogs may be predisposed to these diseases.

Clinical signs. Infections of either of these organisms take weeks to months to develop. Systemic signs of fever, weakness, lethargy, pyothorax and dyspnoea plus neurological signs may be present in nocardiosis. Cutaneous lesions begin as granulomas that may progress to subcutaneous abscesses and cellulitis, with ulcerated nodules and draining tracts. Fine granular material may be present in the exudate. The exudate of nocardiosis is brownish red and has been described as 'tomato soup'.

Diagnosis. Definitive diagnosis can be made via cytological examination of exudate, bacterial culture and/or skin biopsy. *Actinomyces* spp. are Gram-positive, non-acid-fast filamentous anaerobic rods. *Nocardia* spp. are Gram-positive, partially acid-fast, branching filamentous aerobes.

Treatment. Effective therapy depends upon locating and removing any penetrating foreign body, if one is present. Actinomycosis can be treated with penicillin (100,000 units/kg/day), sulphonamides (10 mg/kg b.i.d.) or trimethoprim-potentiated sulphonamide (30 mg/kg b.i.d.). Nocardiosis is not particularly responsive to penicillin. Effective therapy requires surgical drainage of the lesion and several months of effective antibiotic therapy based upon culture and sensitivity.

Opportunistic mycobacterial infections

Description. Opportunistic mycobacterial infections refer to several species of atypical mycobacteria that can cause cutaneous infections. These organisms are described as atypical because they grow rapidly on laboratory media when compared with other groups of Mycobacterium organisms. The most commonly isolated atypical mycobacteria are *Mycobacterium fortuitum* and *M. chelonei*. These organisms are free-living and are found in soil and standing water.

Clinical signs. The organisms are inoculated into the skin via a traumatic injury which has subsequently been contaminated with soil or water harbouring the organism. The infection takes weeks to months to develop. The hallmark of this infection is a chronic, non-healing, recurrent abscessing wound with draining tracts and fistulas. Lesions may occur anywhere, but these organisms have a predilection for the inguinal region. Systemic signs are usually absent.

Diagnosis. Definitive diagnosis is made by finding the acid-fast organisms in smears, by culture and/or by skin biopsy. The organisms can be extremely difficult to find because large numbers are not usually present in the skin. The most cost-effective approach is to submit several unstained tissue imprints for acid-fast staining, several large deep wedges of tissue for culture and several large sections of tissue for skin biopsy. It is important to remember that tissue for culture or biopsy should not be collected with a skin biopsy punch, but rather a deep wedge incision using a scalpel blade. The organisms tend to be found in the deep dermis/panniculus and a skin biopsy punch may collect too superficial a sample to be fruitful. The laboratory should be told that organisms are suspected, to ensure that they are cultured appropriately.

Treatment. Lesions usually regress spontaneously but this may take months to years. Wide surgical excision coupled with antimicrobial therapy is the treatment of choice. Antibiotic therapy should be based upon culture and sensitivity. Some newer antimicrobial agents have been very effective in the treatment of this disease. Clofazimine (8–12 mg/kg *per os* once daily), ciprofloxacin (10–15 mg/kg *per os* b.i.d.), and enrofloxacin (5–10 mg/kg b.i.d.) have been reported as effective therapies.

Prognosis. The prognosis is guarded to good depending upon response to therapy.

Cutaneous leishmaniasis

Description. Leishmaniasis is a rare multisystemic disease with cutaneous manifestations. It is caused by the obligate intracellular protozoan *Leishmania* spp. The organism is transmitted by sandflies of the genera *Lutzomyia* and *Phlebotomus*. The infection begins in the skin and then disseminates to internal organs.

Clinical signs. The most common clinical signs are a non-pruritic exfoliative dermatitis. Nodules and ulcers occur as the disease progresses. Symmetrical lesions on the face characterised by periorbital rings of alopecia and scaling are common. Depigmentation of the planum nasale may occur. Peripheral lymphadenopathy is common. Systemic signs of infection include fever, malaise, weight-loss, muscle atrophy, coagulopathy, polyarthritis and renal failure.

Diagnosis. Definitive diagnosis requires identification of the organism in macrophages. Organisms may be found in fine needle aspirates of peripheral lymph nodes, bone marrow or spleen. The organism may also be cultured in specialised diagnostic laboratories. An indirect fluorescent antibody test is available but it is only diagnostic for *Leishmania donovani*. Positive titres indicate exposure to the organism, not active infection.

Treatment. Several agents are available for the treatment of leishmaniasis; it is recommended that the National Centre for Disease Control be contacted before initiating therapy to ensure that the most current therapy is used. All of these agents are expensive and potentially toxic, and there is no guarantee that the protozoan will be eliminated from the body. Sodium stibogluconate 10–50 mg/kg and meglumine antimonate (100 mg/kg) are the two most commonly used drugs. Both agents are administered daily by IV, IM or SC injection. Itraconazole may also be effective against this agent in dogs.

Prognosis. The prognosis is guarded for a complete recovery; relapses are common.

Panniculitis

Description. Panniculitis describes inflammation of the subcutaneous fat. Any of the infectious agents in this chapter can cause infectious panniculitis: there are a large number of potential causes and recognised clinical syndromes. The most important task for a veterinarian when trying to evaluate a patient with a nodule in the subcutaneous fat is to determine the aetiology: infectious, neoplastic or sterile (idiopathic).

Clinical signs. Clinically, panniculitis is most common on the dorsal trunk, although there is a syndrome in German Shepherd Dogs localised to the foot pads. Depending upon the clinical syndrome, lesions may be solitary or multiple and firm to fluctuant. Large nodules may rupture producing a haemorrhagic exudate or a thick, oily discharge. Scarring is common and this may cause the skin to become tightly adhered to the underlying tissue. Hair may or may not regrow in severely affected areas, depending upon the damage to the hair follicles. Systemic signs may include fever, anorexia, depression and lethargy.

Diagnosis. Definitive diagnosis of the cause of panniculitis is expensive and time-consuming. The most cost-effective test to perform initially is a skin biopsy, provided that the results of skin biopsy can be obtained within a few days and the dog is not rapidly deteriorating. This will allow you to determine whether or not neoplasia is present. If you anticipate a delay, or if the dog is showing systemic signs and the nodules are rapidly developing, the nodules should be cultured at the time of first examination. Because lesions are deep in the skin, samples for histopathological examination should be collected via excision of an entire nodule. If the nodule is larger than 0.5 cm in diameter, it should be transected in several planes to allow for adequate fixation in formalin. If it is not possible to submit an intact nodule, then a deep wedge of tissue should be submitted. It is critical to inform the pathologist that you are interested in ruling out infectious agents. Intact nodules should be submitted for aerobic and anaerobic bacterial and deep fungal culture. If neoplasia and infectious agents are ruled out, it is cost-effective to screen the dog for systemic lupus via an ANA test, complete blood count, serum chemistry panel and urinalysis. If these tests are normal or negative, the most likely diagnosis is sterile nodular panniculitis.

Treatment. Treatment depends upon the aetiology. Sterile nodular panniculitis may be treated surgically if there is a solitary lesion or just a few lesions that can be removed surgically. In most cases, however, systemic glucocorticoids are necessary. Prednisolone (2 mg/kg *per os* once daily) is administered until the lesions completely resolve; this usually takes 4–8 weeks. Therapy should be stopped at this point as many dogs will remain in remission. Vitamin E (400 IU *per os* b.i.d.) has been useful as an adjunct or single therapy agent in some dogs.

Prognosis. The prognosis for sterile nodular panniculitis is good but there may be permanent scarring of the skin and permanent hair-loss.

Juvenile cellulitis

Description. Juvenile cellulitis is a form of panniculitis that affects young dogs between the ages of 3 and 16 weeks (Plate 14). It can occur in any breed of dog, but there is a strong hereditary component and breed predilection for Golden Retrievers, Dachshunds, yellow Labrador Retrievers, Lhasa Apsos and Beagles. One or more puppies in a litter may be affected.

Clinical signs. There are several presentations of this disease, varying primarily in severity. There is a local form limited to the eyelid margins that does not progress to generalised lesions. More common, however, is a generalised form that begins on the face. The lips, ears and muzzle swell and thicken. There is a serous to purulent discharge in the ears. Lymphadenopathy is common and often regional lymph nodes will rupture due to abscessation. In severe cases, affected puppies will develop nodular lesions on the dorsal trunk. The puppies are usually depressed, febrile and anorexic. One of the authors (KAM) is aware of several puppies with this disease that were not treated and subsequently died.

Diagnosis. This disease can progress rapidly and a major complication of the disease is severe scarring; therefore diagnostics should be aggressively pursued. Puppies presented with facial swelling may have angioedema from an insect-bite or reaction to a vaccine. Angioedema usually resolves within 6 to 24 hours; it lacks a regional lymphadenopathy and

the exudation that accompanies this disease. The other major differential diagnoses are demodicosis and a secondary deep pyoderma. Deep skin scrapings should be performed to rule out demodicosis. If these are negative and the clinical signs are consistent, a tentative clinical diagnosis of juvenile cellulitis can be made. Impression smears often show a neutrophilic exudate with bacteria and are not very helpful in differentiating this disease from a deep pyoderma. In a deep pyoderma, however, it is unusual for lesions to begin on the face or cause swelling of the lips and exudation of the inner pinnae. Definitive diagnosis requires a skin biopsy but many veterinarians may elect to treat at this stage in the diagnostic plan. Treatment should be initiated pending the biopsy report.

Treatment. This disease does not respond to oral antibiotic therapy even though there is marked exudation and some cocci may be seen on impression smears. The treatment of choice is systemic prednisolone (1–2 mg/kg *per os*) daily until lesions resolve — usually 14–21 days. Prednisolone therapy should be continued on an alternative day basis for an additional 7–10 days before discontinuing therapy. If therapy is stopped prematurely, a relapse of clinical signs may occur. Most puppies benefit greatly from warm-water soaks in a mild antibacterial shampoo, such as chlorhexidine. If there is concern about sepsis, concurrent antibiotic therapy with a bacteriocidal antibiotic may be used. Clinical improvement in attitude is usually seen within 24 to 48 hours after therapy is instituted.

Prognosis. The prognosis is good however the client should be warned that scarring (permanent hair-loss) may occur. Hair-loss on the muzzle, thickening of the muzzle and permanent hyperpigmentation have all been observed in affected puppies. Most puppies, however, respond well to therapy and do not have any permanent cosmetic disfiguration.

Sterile granuloma and pyogranuloma syndrome

Description. This disease syndrome encompasses a relatively common group of diseases all characterised by granulomatous skin lesions that are sterile. Histologically, the disease is manifested by a large histiocytic infiltrate of the skin. It is believed that the cause may be an immune dysfunction associated with persistent antigenic stimulation.

Clinical signs. Lesions may develop in dogs of any age and most commonly are nodules or plaques, ranging in diameter from 0.5 to 2 cm, that are firm, well demarcated and partially alopecic. They usually occur first on the muzzle and spread to the trunk and distal extremities. Lesions may wax and wane, are non-pruritic and do not rupture. Systemic signs are usually absent.

Diagnosis. Refer to comments for panniculitis. It is critical to rule out infectious agents as the cause of the nodules since therapy involves immunosuppressive drugs.

Treatment. The treatment of choice is oral prednisolone (1–2 mg/kg) once daily until lesions completely resolve, usually in 3–4 weeks. Alternate-day prednisone therapy should be continued for an additional 2–3 weeks. It may or may not be possible to discontinue therapy because lesions commonly recur. An alternative therapy for this disease is native or PEG-L-asparaginase. This is a chemotherapeutic agent that is administered via intramuscular injection once weekly. Lesions usually resolve within three to four treatments and the disease can be kept in clinical remission using intermittent therapy (once or twice monthly treatments). The dose is 10,000 IU per treatment. This is an excellent alternative therapy for this disease because the drug has few side-effects and is easy to administer. Unfortunately, the drug is expensive.

Staphylococcal furunculosis with or without haemorrhagic bullae

Description. This is the most common clinical disease encountered in small animal practice in which marked neutrophilic exudation with degenerate neutrophils are seen. This clinical syndrome may occur in any breed of dog at any age.

Clinical signs. Staphylococcal furunculosis is a deep pyoderma of dogs. Clinically, palpable nodules are present in the skin, many of which are large haemorrhagic bullae. These nodules may rupture and ulcers/erosions may be seen. The hair coat is often matted with exudate and the skin is malodorous. The lesions are often painful and affected dogs may resist manipulation of lesions. Depending upon the severity and duration of the condition, the dog may be depressed and febrile.

Diagnosis. Although staphylococcal organisms are most commonly isolated from these lesions, it is critical to perform a thorough diagnostic evaluation of the patient. Definitive diagnosis requires multiple deep skin scrapings to rule out demodicosis (a common cause of deep pyoderma in the dog), Gram staining and cytological examination of exudate to screen for obvious deep fungal organisms, aerobic bacterial culture and skin biopsy.

Treatment. Assuming that skin scrapings are negative for *Demodex* mites and the initial Gram stain and cytological examination of exudate do not identify any unsuspected bacterial or fungal agents, systemic and topical antimicrobial therapy should be initiated. The dog's hair coat should be clipped to allow for a complete assessment of the extent of the lesions and to facilitate therapy. The dog should be bathed in an antibacterial shampoo, e.g. chlorhexidine or benzoyl peroxide, at least twice weekly. Pending the results of the bacterial culture and sensitivity and skin biopsy, a bacteriocidal antibiotic should be prescribed. Deep bacterial pyodermas require aggressive long-term antibiotic therapy for at least 6–8 weeks. See treatment of pyoderma for more information.

Skin tumours

Clinically relevant information on skin tumours can be found in the *Appendix*.

12

Cutaneous Manifestations of Systemic Disease

KAREN MORIELLO

Many skin diseases are either a cutaneous marker of systemic disease or are associated with systemic signs. The following tables summarise these diseases; the text and bibliography offer more detailed information.

CUTANEOUS AND SYSTEMIC SIGNS OF DISEASES CAUSED BY BACTERIAL ORGANISMS		
Disease	**Cutaneous signs**	**Systemic signs**
Deep pyoderma	Pain, exudate, sloughing of skin, odour	Fever, depression, anorexia
Anaerobic infections; clostridia	Oedema, friable skin, dark devitalised skin, pitting oedema, subcutaneous gas	Fever, anorexia, acute death possible
Cutaneous tuberculosis	Nodules on head, neck, legs, yellow to green exudate	Anorexia, weight-loss, fever, lymphadenopathy
Nocardiosis	Non-healing wound, red-brown exudate, draining tracts	Fever, depression, dyspnoea, pyothorax, weakness, neurological signs
Brucellosis	Scrotal dermatitis, draining ulcers on scrotum	Fever, regional lymphadenopathy
Lyme disease	Recurrent areas of pyotraumatic dermatitis	Fever, lameness

FIG. 12.1 Cutaneous and systemic signs of diseases caused by bacterial organisms.

CUTANEOUS AND SYSTEMIC SIGNS OF DISEASES CAUSED BY FUNGAL ORGANISMS		
Disease	**Cutaneous signs**	**Systemic signs**
Candidiasis	Mucocutaneous ulceration, ulceration of the glabrous skin	Associated with immunosuppression, occult neoplasia
Pythiosis	Cutaneous form: Non-healing wound, pruritic nodules, ulcers, fistulas, serosanguinous exudate	Systemic form: Weight-loss, lethargy, diarrhoea, lymphadenopathy
Sporotrichosis	Ulcerated nodules, hair-loss, serosanguinous exudate	Fever, depression, signs associated with organ specific invasion: Bone, respiratory tract, spleen, testes, central nervous system, gastrointestinal tract
Systemic mycoses (blastomycosis, histoplasmosis, coccidioidomycoses, aspergillosis)	Non-healing wounds, draining tracts, papules, nodules, serosanguinous exudate	Fever, weight-loss, depression, cough, nasal discharge, uveitis
Cryptococcosis	Papules and nodules that ulcerate, crusts	Nasal discharge, central nervous system signs, uveitis

FIG. 12.2 Cutaneous and systemic signs of diseases caused by fungal organisms.

CUTANEOUS AND SYSTEMIC SIGNS OF DISEASES CAUSED BY IMMUNE- MEDIATED DISEASES/CONDITIONS		
Disease	**Cutaneous signs**	**Systemic signs**
Atopy	Chronic pruritus, alopecia, excoriations of face, feet, ventrum	In rare cases, associated with chronic respiratory problems: reverse sneezing, rhinitis, asthma
Food hypersensitivity	Chronic pruritus, recurrent pyoderma, papules, pustules	Gastrointestinal signs: diarrhoea
Pemphigus foliaceus	Symmetrical crusting of face, ears, trunk, footpads, pustular eruption	Fever, depression, lameness, anorexia
Pemphigus vulgaris	Mucocutaneous ulceration, oral ulceration, rarely ulceration of groin and axillae	Fever, anorexia, depression, pain at site of ulcers
Bullous pemphigoid	Vesicles and bulla in mouth, at mucocutaneous junctions, groin, axilla, crusts, ulcers	Anorexia, depression, fever, reluctance to walk if axillary and inguinal lesions are severe
Systemic lupus erythematosus	Mucocutaneous ulcers, scaling, footpad ulcers, hyperkeratosis of footpads, nasal depigmentation, marked erythema	Fever, depression, anorexia, anaemia, thrombocytopenia, polymyositis, pericarditis, myocarditis, neurological signs, lymphadenopathy, polyarthritis, glomerulonephritis
Vasculitis	Purpura, haemorrhagic bullae, necrosis of skin, and ulcers on extremities	Fever, depression, anorexia, pitting oedema, polyarthropathy, myopathy
Erythema multiforme	Acute symmetrical macular lesions, urticarial plaques, mucocutaneous ulceration and vesicles of eyelids, conjunctiva, pinnae	Fever, depression, anorexia
Toxic epidermal necrolysis	Acute onset of vesicles, bullae and necrosis of skin. Epidermis will slough. Mucocutaneous junctions, footpads and oral mucosa are most commonly affected	Fever, anorexia, lethargy, cutaneous pain, depression, occult neoplasia
Uveodermatological syndrome	Depigmentation of oral mucosa and eyelids and leucoderma of the face and trunk, depigmentation of nose	Uveitis
Sterile eosinophilic pustulosis	Pruritic, erythematous, follicular and nonfollicular papules and pustules, target lesions	Fever, anorexia, depression, peripheral lymphadenopathy

Fig. 12.3 Cutaneous and systemic signs of diseases caused by immune-mediated diseases/conditions.

CUTANEOUS AND SYSTEMIC SIGNS OF DISEASES CAUSED BY PARASITIC DISEASES		
Disease	**Cutaneous signs**	**Systemic signs**
Dirofilariasis	Chronic, ulcerated nodules on the head, neck, and trunk	Exercise intolerance, cough, depression, weight-loss, fever, jugular pulse
Ticks	Cutaneous nodules at site of bite	Tick-bite paralysis
Demodicosis	Hair-loss, pruritus, scaling, deep pyoderma	Fever, depression, sepsis in demodicosis with deep pyoderma. Demodicosis in an adult dog may be an indicator of occult neoplasia or other systemic disease, e.g. diabetes mellitus
Lice	Pruritus, scaling, alopecia	Anaemia in severe infestations with sucking lice
Fleas	Pruritus, scaling, alopecia, secondary pyoderma	Anaemia in severe infestations

Fig. 12.4 Cutaneous and systemic signs of diseases caused by parasitic diseases.

CUTANEOUS AND SYSTEMIC SIGNS OF DISEASES CAUSED BY ENDOCRINE DISORDERS		
Disease	**Cutaneous signs**	**Systemic signs**
Hypothyroidism	Symmetrical alopecia, hair-loss in frictional areas, dry brittle hair, increased pigmentation, recurrent pyoderma	Dull mental attitude, weight gain, peripheral neuropathies, constipation, vomiting, bradycardia, thrombosis, ataxia, vestibular disease, seizures, poor reproduction, corneal ulceration, corneal lipidosis, uveitis, KCS, retinopathy
Hyperadrenocorticism	Symmetrical alopecia, hair-loss in frictional areas, thin skin, comedones, calcinosis cutis, hyperpigmentation	Polyuria, polydipsia, pendulous abdomen, lethargy, polyphagia, muscle weakness, obesity, anoestrus, panting, testicular atrophy, facial nerve neuropathy
Acromegaly	Thickened skin, excessive folds, hypertrichosis, hard nails	Inspiratory stidor, increased body size, abdominal enlargement, polyuria, polydipsia, polyphagia, fatigue, frequent panting, prognathism, galactorrhoea
Hyperoestrogenism	Bilaterally symmetrical alopecia, enlarged nipples and genitalia	Abnormal oestrus cycles, endometritis/pyometra, nymphomania, anaemia
Oestrogen-responsive alopecia	Bilaterally symmetrical alopecia, infantile genitalia	Urinary incontinence
Sertoli cell tumour	Bilaterally symmetrical alopecia, gynaecomastia, pendulous prepuce, seborrhoea, linear preputial erythema	Palpable or non-palpable tumour of the testes, abdominal mass, cryptorchid

FIG. 12.5 Cutaneous and systemic signs of diseases caused by endocrine disorders.

CUTANEOUS AND SYSTEMIC SIGNS OF DISEASES WITH ENVIRONMENTAL CAUSES		
Disease	**Cutaneous signs**	**Systemic signs**
Burns	Superficial: erythema, oedema, pain Deep: hard skin, sloughing, necrosis, purulent discharge, odour	If > 25% of body is involved systemic signs may include: shock, renal failure, anaemia, respiratory infection, sepsis
Snake-bite	Rapid and progressive oedema, pain, local haemorrhage, sloughing of the skin	Shock, coagulation problems, sepsis, respiratory compromise, cardiac abnormalities, neurological signs
Thallium toxicosis (rotenticide and cockroach poison)	Ulceration, hyperaemia of mucous membranes, alopecia and erythema and necrosis of skin especially in intertriginous areas, ears, genitalia and mucous membranes	Early signs: vomiting, diarrhoea, depression Later signs: nephrosis, polyneuritis, necrosis of skeletal muscle and myocardial muscles. Inflammation of liver, tongue, pancreas
Arsenic poisoning (herbicides, rodenticides, pesticides and arsenical medications)	Necrosis and ulceration of ears, feet, lips and prepuce; rough coat, swollen muzzle	Listlessness, anorexia, weight-loss

FIG. 12.6 Cutaneous and systemic signs of diseases with environmental causes.

CUTANEOUS AND SYSTEMIC SIGNS OF DISEASES CAUSED BY NUTRITIONALLY RELATED DISEASES		
Disease	**Cutaneous signs**	**Systemic signs**
Fatty acid deficiency	Alopecia, erythema, scaling, increased sebum production, pruritus, skin thickening	Associated with intestinal malabsorption, pancreatic disease, chronic liver disease
Protein deficiency	Scaling, pigment-loss, patchy hair-loss, thin hairs, rough dry hair, brittle hairs, delayed wound healing	Intestinal malabsorption, liver disease, starvation
Zinc deficiency or zinc-responsive diseases	Scaling and crusting of the skin especially over pressure point areas. Footpads and nose become crusted and fissured	Anorexia, depression, stunted growth, lymphadenopathy

FIG. 12.7 Cutaneous and systemic signs caused by nutritionally related diseases.

CUTANEOUS AND SYSTEMIC SIGNS OF DISEASES CAUSED BY VIRAL, RICKETTSIAL AND PROTOZOAL DISEASES		
Disease	**Cutaneous signs**	**Systemic signs**
Canine distemper	Hyperkeratosis of footpads and nose	Upper respiratory signs and neurological signs
Rocky Mountain spotted fever (*Rickettsia rickettsia*)	Oedema of legs, erythema, petechiation, necrosis and ulceration of oral mucosa, genitalia and ear margins	Fever, anorexia, lethargy, peripheral lymphadenopathy, neurological signs
Leishmaniasis	Scaling, periocular alopecia, nasal depigmentation, erosions and ulceration of nose, long brittle nails, cutaneous nodules	Fever, weight-loss, lethargy, hepatosplenomegaly, keratoconjunctivitis, lameness, muscle wasting

FIG. 12.8 Cutaneous and systemic signs of diseases caused by viral, rickettsial and protozoal diseases.

MISCELLANEOUS CAUSES OF CUTANEOUS AND SYSTEMIC SIGNS		
Disease	**Cutaneous signs**	**Systemic signs**
Hepatocutaneous syndrome	Erosions, ulcerations, exudation, crusts around the face, legs, junctions of footpads, elbows, ventral thorax and scrotum	Associated with internal disease of liver, pancreas, and idiopathic causes
Panniculitis	Single or multiple subcutaneous nodules in the trunk. Lesions may drain a serosanguinous to yellow-brown oily fluid	Fever, pain, depression, arthralgia — depending upon the underlying cause
Calcinosis cutis	Hard plaques in the skin	Signs associated with hypercortisolaemia (iatrogenic or organic)
Collagenous nevi; nodular dermatofibrosis	Hard nodules on the paws, extremities and trunk of dogs, particular German Shepherd Dogs. Nodules may ulcerate	Weight-loss, polyuria, polydipsia, uterine leiomyomas; these dogs often develop bilateral renal cystadenocarcinomas
Canine cyclic haematopoiesis (Grey Collie syndrome)	Affected dogs have a silver coat, light coloured nose	Affected dogs are smaller; fever, diarrhoea, recurrent infections, conjunctivitis, arthralgia, lymphadenopathy
Cutaneous asthaenia	Fragile skin that tears easily, very 'stretchy'	Animals often die of acutely aortic rupture
Familial dermatomyositis	Alopecia, pustules, papules, erosions, crusts, on ear tips, face, tail, paws	Muscle atrophy, reproductive problems, megaesophagus, stunted growth, difficulty eating and swallowing
Collagen disorder of the footpads of German Shepherd Dog	Softer than normal footpads, central ulcers in footpads	Dogs develop renal amyloidosis by 2 – 3 years of life
Telogen defluxion/anagen defluxion	Generalised non-inflammatory hair-loss over the entire body; hairs easily epilate	May be a sequela to any major illness, especially fevers and infections. Commonly occurs in small dogs post partum, especially if a dystocia was present
Mast cell tumour	Variable clinical presentation, may be singular or multiple	Gastric ulcers, coagulopathies

FIG. 12.9 Miscellaneous causes of cutaneous and systemic signs.

III Problem-Oriented Approach to Skin Diseases of Cats

13

Pruritus

IAN MASON

In contrast to pruritus in dogs, pruritus in cats can be difficult to recognise as it is often characterised by a range of clinical signs other than overt scratching, licking and biting of the skin. Symmetrical alopecia, miliary dermatitis or eosinophilic skin diseases are usually associated with feline pruritus; these are discussed in *Chapters 14, 15* and *19*. It is not uncommon for two or three of these syndromes to be present in the same cat, either simultaneously or at different stages of the disease.

In many instances, owners are not aware that their cat is pruritic and present it to the veterinarian with what they consider to be spontaneous hair-loss, cutaneous plaques or tiny crusts within the skin (Figs 13.1 and 13.2). However, there are also instances where clients are quite aware that the skin lesions are due to self-trauma. Cats can be somewhat secretive animals and may induce skin trauma out of sight of the owners. In other instances, particularly in cases of self-induced alopecia, the animal simply grooms the coat too vigorously. Many clients do not realise that this is not normal grooming behaviour. One of the challenges to the clinician is to persuade owners that alopecia and skin plaques can be self-induced and not spontaneous problems.

It has been suggested that up to 90% of pruritic cats have flea allergic dermatitis. Irrespective of any other diagnostic criteria, flea allergy should always be considered first.

Figures 13.6 and 13.7 illustrate a suggested diagnostic approach to feline pruritus.

Feline Skin Diseases Primarily Associated with Pruritus

Hypersensitivity

Flea allergic dermatitis

Description. Flea allergic dermatitis (FAD) is probably the most common cause of skin disease in cats. FAD not only leads to pruritus but is also responsible for most cases of feline alopecia, miliary dermatitis and eosinophilic skin disease. The species of flea most frequently associated with feline skin disease is *Ctenocephalides felis*. However, in Europe, hedgehog fleas (*Archeopsylla erinacei*) and rabbit fleas (*Spillopsyllus cuniculi*) may be isolated, the latter predominantly affecting the head

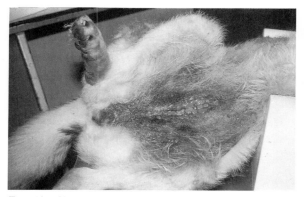

FIG. 13.1 Ventral abdomen of a cat with severe pruritus associated with eosinophilic plaques. Slide courtesy of Richard Harvey.

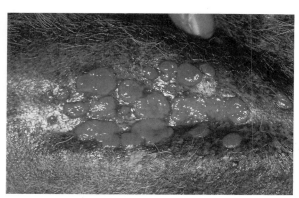

FIG. 13.2 Closer view of Fig. 13.1. Slide courtesy of Richard Harvey.

DIFFERENTIAL DIAGNOSIS OF FELINE PRURITUS	
Hypersensitivity	Flea-bite hypersensitivity Food intolerance/hypersensitivity Atopic dermatitis Insect (mosquito) hypersensitivity
Ectoparasites	*Cheyletiella* spp. infestation (esp. *C. blakei*) Otodectic mange Pediculosis (*Felicola subrostratus*) *Notoedres cati* infestation *Trombicula autumnalis* infestation *Lynxacarus radovsky* infestation Demodicosis
Infectious causes	Bacterial folliculitis Dermatophytosis Poxvirus
Other causes	Contact dermatitis Essential fatty acid deficiency Hypereosinophilia

FIG. 13.3 Differential diagnosis of feline pruritus.

and pinnae. Pruritus results from a hypersensitivity reaction following binding of haptens in flea saliva with dermal collagen.

Clinical signs. FAD can affect virtually any adult cat. Pruritus is moderate to severe. Occasionally owners may be unaware that the cat is pruritic, especially if no self-induced trauma other than hair-loss is present. FAD may be seasonal (many cases start in late summer/early autumn) and some animals in cold geographical locations may recover spontaneously during winter. In many parts of the world, flea allergy is a year-round problem. Affected individuals may also be infested with the tapeworm *Dipylidium caninum*, as the flea is the intermediate host of this parasite.

Clinical signs are variable; self-trauma, severe excoriation, crusting and hair-loss may be seen, especially over the rear half of the dorsum. Flea allergy can also lead to miliary dermatitis,

eosinophilic disease and symmetrical alopecia; the clinical features of these disorders are described in the relevant chapters. Lesions may affect solely the head and neck.

Diagnosis. The presence of fleas, or flea excrement within material brushed from the coat, plus compatible clinical signs are highly suggestive that flea allergy is involved. However, in cats the absence of such direct evidence of flea infestation should not deter the clinician from suspecting FAD. Pruritic cats are frequent and proficient groomers, so that evidence of flea infestation may be rapidly removed from the skin and coat. A response to intradermal injection of flea extract indicates that flea allergy is present but false-negative reactions are common. Probably the best means of establishing the diagnosis is to eradicate fleas thoroughly without making any other management changes or giving any therapy; if pruritus ceases, then FAD was likely to be involved.

Treatment. Flea control is covered in detail in *Chapter 30*.

Prognosis. The prognosis is excellent provided that good flea control remains in force. Under certain climatic conditions this may be impossible and short-term recurrence is seen during the most humid and hot parts of the year.

Food hypersensitivity/intolerance

Description. Dietary intolerance is more common in cats than in dogs. The immunological and pathological mechanisms are unknown and it has been

APPROACH TO FELINE PRURITUS: HISTORY	
Factor	**Differential diagnosis**
Breed Long-haired (Persian, Himalayan, Chinchilla)	Dermatophytosis

Age of onset
    Less than 6 months
    9 months to adulthood
	Dermatophytosis
	Hypersensitivity

Environment/management	Outdoor cats are exposed to more fleas, insects and contact irritants
Seasonality	Fleas; atopy; tromboculidiasis
Gastrointestinal disease	Food allergy
Contagion/zoonosis	Fleas; cheyletiellosis; dermatophytosis

FIG. 13.4 Approach to feline pruritus: History.

APPROACH TO FELINE PRURITUS: PHYSICAL EXAMINATION	
Physical finding	**Differential diagnosis**
Distribution of lesions Head and neck	Atopy; food allergy; ear mites; *Notoedres* infestation; chronic ear disease; aural polyp
Caudal thigh and tail-head area	Flea allergy
Planum nasale and dorsum of the muzzle	Mosquito-bite hypersensitivity; pemphigus foliaceus
Lymphadenopathy	Hypersensitivity (occasional finding)

FIG. 13.5 Approach to feline pruritus: Physical examination.

suggested that there may be more than one mechanism by which reactions to foods may affect the skin and lead to pruritus (Fig 13.8). These putative mechanisms range from true hypersensitivity to toxic, idiosyncratic or pharmacological reactions. Concurrent atopy or FAD have been reported in cases of feline food allergy.

Clinical signs. Any cat can be affected; there is no apparent age, breed or sex predisposition. Pruritus is non-seasonal and most affected cats have been fed the offending food for months or years. Pruritus is said to be poorly responsive to glucocorticoids in cases of feline food intolerance. Food allergy may lead to the other manifestations of inflammatory skin disease discussed elsewhere (symmetrical alopecia (Fig. 13.8), eosinophilic skin disease and miliary dermatitis). However, intense self-trauma, crusting and excoriation may be seen. In the author's experience this can affect any part of the body, although there is some evidence to suggest that the head and neck are most commonly involved.

Diagnosis. Diagnosis is based on the feeding of a hypoallergenic diet for at least 6 weeks. The diet must be based on a source of protein to which the cat has been regularly exposed previously. The diagnosis of food intolerance is discussed in detail in *Chapter 3*.

It is highly likely that *in vitro* testing for food allergy in the cat is as unreliable as it is in dogs.

Treatment. A diet based on foods to which the cat has been shown to be tolerant should be fed. This should be balanced. In many instances, a suitable commercial diet will suffice. Occasionally a home-cooked maintenance diet will be needed.

Prognosis. The prognosis is excellent provided that other hypersensitivities do not develop.

Atopic dermatitis

Description. Atopy is not well documented in cats although it has recently been recognised in this

DIAGNOSTIC PLAN FOR FELINE PRURITUS

1. Rule out flea allergy. Flea allergic dermatitis or flea-bite dermatitis is the most common cause of feline pruritus. A rigorous flea eradication regimen as described in *Chapter 30* should be implemented early in the investigation of pruritic cats — **even if there is no visible evidence of flea infestation**
2. Rule out other ectoparasites

Focused diagnostic tests: Microscopy of skin scrapings; adhesive tape specimens; hair plucks and coat brushings; or trial therapy with antiparasitic agents

3. Screen for dermatophytosis

Focused diagnostic tests: Wood's lamp examination; microscopy of plucked hair shafts; dermatophyte culture

4. *If no ectoparasites or dermatophytes are detected and there is not a response to flea eradication* investigate the role of allergic disease

Focused diagnostic tests: Food: restriction diet; Atopy: Intradermal test, *in vitro* test (RAST/ELISA); Ectoparasites (including fleas): Haematology — an eosinophilia suggests that parasites are involved

5. If no diagnosis:

Focused diagnostic tests: Skin biopsy may produce evidence in support of a diagnosis of bacterial folliculitis, feline poxvirus, dermatophytosis or hypereosinophilia. Blood samples: Clinical haematology and biochemistry, assay of anti-nuclear antibody titre, serology for FeLV and FIV etc., as indicated

FIG. 13.6 Diagnostic plan for feline pruritus.

species. The precise immunology and pathogenesis remain obscure.

Clinical signs. In dogs, foot chewing and face rubbing are regarded as hall-marks of atopic disease. In cats, foot chewing is not a feature although facial pruritus and self-trauma are seen in some cases. Atopic cats usually present with generalised pruritus and resultant self-trauma although the other manifestations of feline inflammatory disease (symmetrical alopecia, eosinophilic disease or miliary dermatitis) may also be present.

Diagnosis. Diagnosis is based on elimination of other allergic diseases, infectious dermatoses and ectoparasite infestation. Definitive diagnosis depends on intradermal skin testing (*Chapter 3*) but this test is more difficult to perform and interpret in cats than in dogs. *In vitro* testing is not yet available for cats.

Treatment. The management of pruritus is discussed in detail in *Chapter 31* and involves attempts to limit exposure to allergens, reduction of flare factors (such as flea exposure) and modification of immune response through the use of medicaments such as antihistamines and (for a few cats) glucocorticoids. Cats are fairly resistant to the development of clinical side-effects when low-dose alternate day prednisone, prednisolone or methylprednisolone therapy is used.

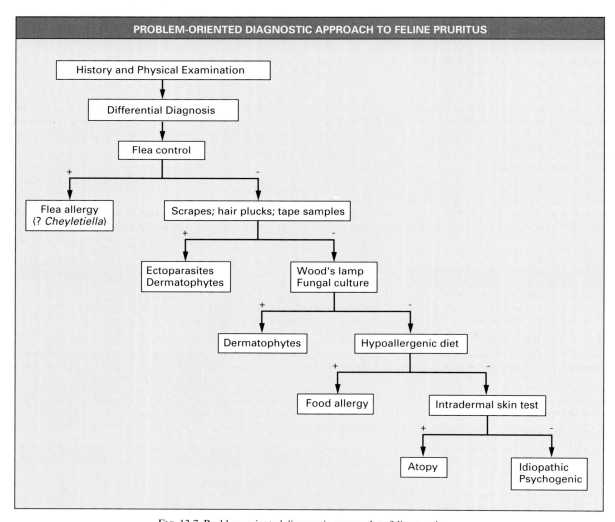

FIG. 13.7 Problem-oriented diagnostic approach to feline pruritus.

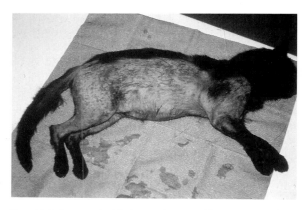

Fig. 13.8 Symmetrical hair-loss due to self-trauma associated with pruritic dermatosis in a cat due to dietary intolerance. Slide courtesy of Richard Harvey.

Anecdotal reports indicate that cats are more likely than dogs to have a beneficial response to hyposensitisation therapy: as many as 80% of cases show improvement within 4–6 months of the onset of therapy.

Prognosis. Atopic dermatitis is incurable and affected cats require lifelong medical management (*Chapter 31*). Many cats respond well to simple therapy such as antihistamines and reduction of flare factors. Similarly, hyposensitisation appears to work well although it may be difficult to formulate a hyposensitisation vaccine in many instances due to the technical difficulties involved in performing intradermal skin tests in this species.

Insect hypersensitivity

Description. Animal skin reactions to insects are discussed in detail in *Chapter 5*. In cats the insects involved most frequently are fleas (see above). It is probable that house dust mites (*Dermatophagoides* spp.) may be involved in feline atopy. Other examples of insect-induced skin disease include wasp and bee stings and mosquito-bites.

Clinical signs. Reactions vary depending on the insect involved and the degree of sensitisation of the host to the allergen or toxin. **Bee or wasp stings** lead to severe, painful, swollen lesions that are sudden in onset. They are not uncommon in cats which are fascinated by and attempt to play with these insects. Lesions are more frequent in the summer. Theoretically anaphylaxis is possible in sensitised animals.

Fly- and mosquito-bites may be local and papular in non-sensitised animals. Pruritus may be present; it may be seasonal and in sensitised animals may be severe and associated with urticaria.

Typically, insect reactions involve areas with short or sparse hair such as the dorsum of the muzzle, pinnae, ventral abdomen and distal extremities.

Mosquito-bites in cats may lead to a visually distinctive facial dermatitis termed **feline mosquito-bite hypersensitivity** (see Plate 21). The incidence of this disorder varies with geographical region. Warm areas with high humidity have more mosquitos and therefore more cases. The disorder is presumed to be a hypersensitivity and predominantly affects the face, especially the dorsum of the muzzle and planum nasale. It is possible that other biting insects may lead to a similar syndrome. The lesions are erythematous eruptions with papules, crusting, swelling and alopecia. In severe cases erosion, ulceration and exudation are present. Chronic cases may have firm nodules. Pruritus varies but is usually moderate. The disease is seasonal, confined to regions of the world where mosquitos are a problem and appears to have no age, breed or sex predispositions.

Diagnosis. History may give important clues that an insect-induced disorder is present. The diagnosis for a cat with a swollen face following a summer afternoon chasing wasps should be easily made. Clinical signs are usually helpful. Wasp and bee stings are quite characteristic and mosquito-bite hypersensitivity is a very distinctive disease clinically. Diagnosis is based on circumstantial evidence and elimination of other disorders from the differential diagnosis. Biopsy and histopathology revealing an eosinophilic perivascular dermatitis with or without collagenolysis and flame figures is supportive evidence that the lesion is insect-induced. Histology results should be interpreted with caution: the comment may be that the lesion is 'consistent with the eosinophilic granuloma complex'. This underscores the advice given in *Chapter 19* that the eosinophilic diseases are simply a reaction pattern and that the true underlying cause should always be investigated.

Treatment. Management varies with the insect involved and the animal's response. Exposure should be prevented by the use of insect repellents and the confinement of cats during the period of risk. Topical and systemic antihistamine and gluco-corticoid therapy may be required for severe cases.

Prognosis. The prognosis is usually favourable, although anaphylaxis is potentially life-endangering.

Endoparasite hypersensitivity

Description. It has been suggested that endoparasites may induce hypersensitivity reactions that affect the skin and lead to pruritus. The authors have seen pruritic cats with endoparasite burdens but many of these have also had flea-allergic dermatitis. It should be remembered that the flea is the intermediate host of the tapeworm *Dipylidium caninum*.

Clinical signs. Clinical signs are generalised or localised pruritus with associated hair-loss, self-trauma and other associated conditions such as eosinophilic skin disease or miliary dermatitis. There may be evidence of adult roundworms or tapeworm segments in faeces.

Diagnosis. Evidence of nematodes, tapeworm segments or parasite eggs on faecal examination may be suggestive of this diagnosis but such findings may be entirely coincidental. Resolution of pruritus following treatment with an appropriate anthelmintic is diagnostic.

Treatment. Systemic anthelmintic therapy is indicated.

Prognosis. The prognosis is excellent provided that reinfestation does not occur.

Ectoparasites

Cheyletiellosis

Description. Cats may become infested with surface parasites of the genus *Cheyletiella*. The usual feline parasite is *C. blakei*, although the rabbit species *C. parasitivorax* may also be involved in cats which hunt. The disease is a zoonosis; human lesions are multiple papules which may have a necrotic centre. This disease is also discussed in *Chapter 15*.

Clinical signs. The clinical signs vary and some affected cats may exhibit only mild signs such as diffuse scaling of the skin surface. At the other end of the spectrum is severe pruritus leading to self-trauma, hair-loss and the manifestations of feline inflammatory skin disease (discussed previously).

Diagnosis. This disorder is underdiagnosed in cats. The pruritic cat is particularly adept at removing evidence of ectoparasites from the skin surface and coat and so microscopy of skin scrapings, hair plucks and adhesive tape specimens may be unrewarding. Of these techniques, the examination of hairs combed from the coat or plucked is likely to be the most rewarding as the eggs of the parasites are attached to the hairs and may be retained in the coat for longer than are the other stages of the parasite's life-cycle. A speculative diagnosis of cheyletiellosis may be made retrospectively following strict topical and environmental antiparasitic therapy. However, it is possible that undiagnosed cases of cheyletiellosis which respond to antiparasitic therapy are ascribed to flea-bite hypersensitivity. It is salutary to note that cheyletiellosis is diagnosed more commonly in flea-free locations.

Treatment. Treatment depends on the use of topical ectoparasiticidal agents and environmental control. Environmental treatment is similar to that described for fleas in *Chapter 30*. Rigorous vacuuming of the carpets will remove shed hair and scale which may contain parasites. An environmental spray containing dichlorvos and fenthion or pyrethroids should be used throughout the dwelling. Animal treatment should include all dogs and cats in the household even if they exhibit no signs of disease; some virtually asymptomatic animals may be carriers. In the UK only one product is licensed for the treatment of this disease: selenium sulphide 1% shampoo. Clearly, there may be practical difficulties in bathing cats and it may be necessary to seek unlicensed alternatives such as carbamates (e.g. carbaryl) and lime sulphur dips. Ivermectin is used extensively in cats in North America and appears to be quite safe. Topical flea preparations may have some effect on *Cheyletiella* spp. but should not be relied upon.

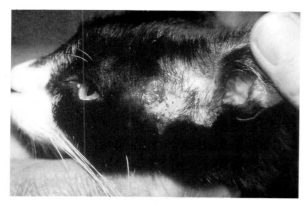

FIG. 13.9 Pruritic facial dermatosis with erythematous crusts associated with *Otodectes cynotis* infection. Slide courtesy of Richard Harvey.

Prognosis. Provided that the cat does not become reinfested, the prognosis is excellent.

Otodectic mange

Description. *Otodectes cynotis* is a common feline parasite and the most common cause of otitis externa in this species (Fig. 13.9, *Chapter 27*). Occasionally ectopic infestation occurs, leading to pruritus.

Clinical signs. Affected cats exhibit otitis externa associated with thick, crumbly brown to black wax along with pruritus. Pruritus predominantly affects the head, although other sites may be involved. Anecdotal reports indicate that the tip of the tail may be affected and it has been suggested that this is because cats sleep with the tip of the tail resting on the side of the head. Pruritus may be associated with erythema, papules, crusting and excoriation as well as all of the other signs and syndromes discussed elsewhere in this chapter.

Diagnosis. Diagnosis is established by finding the parasite on microscopy of scrapings from the skin surface.

Treatment. Otoacariasis should be managed as described in *Chapter 27*. Treatment with a topical acaricidal agent specifically formulated for ears should be administered to all dogs and cats within the household for at least 3 weeks. Management of the aberrant infestation is more difficult. In the UK, the only products licensed for the treatment of ear mites are ear drops. Hence, other licensed products have to be used 'off-label'. Suggested products include ivermectin, lime sulphur, pyrethroids (these should be used cautiously in cats), selenium sulphide and carbamates (e.g. carbaryl).

Prognosis. The prognosis is excellent.

Pediculosis

Description. This is a relatively uncommon cause of pruritus in cats. The parasite is a biting louse *Felicola subrostratus* which may be found around body orifices and long-haired regions. The disease is often associated with poor management (overcrowding and dirty housing) and is usually seen in 'rescued' kittens.

Clinical signs. Variable amounts of pruritus may result from lice infestation. Papules, crusts and excoriations may be present; miliary dermatitis is commonly seen in association with pediculosis in cats. In severe, longstanding infestations, anaemia and debility may be seen.

Diagnosis. The diagnosis is usually straightforward and based on the identification of parasites on the skin and eggs cemented to the hairs.

Treatment. Lice are quite sensitive to most insecticides and so topical therapy with flea sprays or powders is likely to be curative. Therapy should continue for 3–4 weeks. Lice do not survive for long in the environment and so reinfestation is unlikely to be a problem, although it is advisable to treat the environment with an insecticidal agent as a precaution. Lice are host-specific and so only the affected cat and other cats within the household need to be treated.

Prognosis. The prognosis is excellent.

Notoedric mange

Description. *Notoedres cati* is a sarcoptid mite and closely related to *Sarcoptes scabiei*. Infestation with *Notoedres cati*, or notoedric mange, is a syndrome which finds its way into every textbook and on to almost every list of differential diagnoses. However, it is relatively uncommon throughout the world and virtually non-existent in the UK. It is popularly known as **feline scabies** although the use of this term may be misleading as it implies that *Sarcoptes scabiei* is involved. *S. scabiei* var. *canis* has been shown to be an extremely rare cause of skin disease in cats and it may be preferable to reserve the term feline scabies for disease caused by *S. scabiei*, while using the term notoedric mange to describe *Notoedres* infestation.

Clinical signs. Clinically, notoedric mange is very similar to canine scabies (*Chapter 5*). It is a transient zoonosis and may also affect foxes, dogs and rabbits. It is highly contagious between cats by direct contact.

Typically the disease involves the margins of the pinnae, the face, eyelids and neck. However, as with otoacariasis, the feet and perineum may become affected. Presumably this is because the cat sleeps curled up. Intense pruritus and resultant self-trauma and hair-loss are seen along with papules and thickened, wrinkled skin. A tightly adherent yellow-to-grey crust may be present. There is usually a peripheral lymphadenopathy.

Diagnosis. The severe pruritus, distribution of lesions and, if appropriate, contagion to in-contact cats is suggestive of notoedric mange. Diagnosis is confirmed following microscopy of skin scrapings, which will reveal large numbers of sarcoptid mites. *Notoedres cati* can easily be confused with *Sarcoptes scabiei*. It may be worth consulting an expert in mite identification if doubt exists as to the identity of any mite isolated from cat skin.

Treatment. There are no licensed products in the UK for the treatment of feline notoedric mange. Ivermectin has been used safely in the USA. To the author's knowledge, ivermectin is not licensed anywhere in the world for use in cats. Other suggested medicaments include amitraz, although this can be lethal to cats and therefore cannot be recommended. Lime sulphur is available in the USA and is effective against this parasite.

Prognosis. The prognosis is excellent.

Trombiculidiasis

Description. *Trombicula autumnalis* infestation is discussed in detail in *Chapter 5*. In cats, trombiculi-

diasis is very similar to the disease seen in dogs although the mites may also be found on the pinnae as well as the feet. Diagnosis is based on identifying the orange-red parasites on the skin. Treatment is difficult as this is an outdoor, environmental parasite which infests cats that freely roam during late summer. Reinfestation is therefore quite common.

In the UK, only one product is licensed for use in cats: 1% selenium sulphide shampoo. However, it is likely that unlicensed products such as lime sulphur, carbaryl and ivermectin are also effective. Disease only occurs during late summer; during this period reinfestation can be minimised by the use of flea collars and sprays.

Fur mites

Description. *Lynxacarus radovsky* is a small feline fur mite with a very limited geographical distribution: it is predominantly reported in Australia, Hawaii and Florida. Morphologically this mite is extremely similar to the rabbit fur mite *Listrophorus gibbus*.

Fur mites appear to be well-adapted parasites and seldom lead to clinical signs, although slight pruritus has been reported in cats and there is one report of quite significant pruritic skin disease due to *Listrophorus gibbus* in rabbits in the UK. In cats there is usually mild scaling and dullness of the coat; this appearance has been termed 'salt and pepper'. Diagnosis is based on identification of the mites on microscopy of coat brushings, plucked hairs, skin scrapings or adhesive tape specimens. Treatment with insecticidal sprays of lime sulphur dips is said to be curative.

Infectious Causes

Bacterial folliculitis

Description. Bacterial folliculitis is not commonly reported in cats, but this may partly be because pyoderma is difficult to recognise grossly in this species. Little is known of the aetiology and pathogenesis of bacterial folliculitis in cats. Extrapolation from work in other species, such as dogs and humans, suggests that many cases of bacterial skin disease are secondary to another disorder. If this is also true for feline bacterial folliculitis, then investigation and identification of such underlying causes is needed.

Clinical signs. Little information is available regarding the clinical manifestations of bacterial folliculitis in cats. It has been suggested that pruritus with miliary dermatitis is the most typical presentation although there may be some associated hairloss. Most reported cases have had a papular crusted dermatitis with follicular papules and occasionally pustules. Careful examination and investigation is needed to distinguish this disorder from pemphigus foliaceus, in which the pustules are usually interfollicular, and from the other causes of miliary dermatitis (*Chapter 15*).

Diagnosis. Diagnosis is based on elimination of other causes and on histopathology; a neutrophilic folliculitis in the absence of dermatophytes or ectoparasites is suggestive of a bacterial aetiology. Coagulase-positive staphylococci, *Staphylococcus aureus*, *S. intermedius* and *S. hyicus*, appear to be the micro-organisms most commonly involved.

Treatment. Clinical management is based on topical chlorhexidine baths and systemic antibiotic therapy as described for canine pyoderma (*Chapter 32*). The author prefers to use cephalexin at 25 mg/kg b.i.d.

Prognosis. The prognosis is variable. Although an initial response to antibacterial therapy is likely, recurrence may be seen if the underlying factors leading to infection are not identified and addressed.

Dermatophytosis. This disorder is described in detail in *Chapter 15*.

Feline poxvirus infection

Description. Cat pox has only been reported in the British Isles. The disease is usually self-limiting within 1–2 months. However, it may become chronic in immunosuppressed animals, such as those treated inappropriately with glucocorticoids, or infected with FIV or FeLV. Cat pox is zoonotic to immunosuppressed people.

Clinical signs. Feline poxvirus infection may present as an extremely pruritic lesion, although typically the lesions are crusted, ulcerated, alopecic macules, papules or, most typically, nodules. The lesions usually affect the limbs and may resemble eosinophilic plaques or linear granulomata. They may arise at the site of a previous bite or injury, so giving credence to the hypothesis that this is a sylvatic disease with an unidentified wildlife reservoir.

Diagnosis. Diagnosis is by histopathology; poxvirus infection may be readily differentiated from eosinophilic skin disease as the reaction patterns are quite distinct and intracytoplasmic viral inclusion bodies are present in keratinocytes in cat pox lesions.

Treatment. Supportive therapy with topical and systemic antimicrobial agents to prevent secondary bacterial infection is required. **Glucocorticoids are strongly contraindicated.** The use of such drugs may lead to fatal complications.

Prognosis. The prognosis is excellent in uncomplicated cases where glucocorticoids have not been used.

Other Causes

Contact dermatitis

Contact hypersensitivity has not been documented convincingly in the cat. Reactions to environmental substances are more likely to be due to irritant dermatitis than to true allergic disease. The approach to diagnosis of contact dermatitis and the differentiation of contact hypersensitivity and contact irritant dermatitis are discussed in detail in *Chapter 5*.

Essential fatty acid deficiency

Description. It has been shown that both linoleic and arachidonic acid are essential for the cat. This requirement is readily met by most commercial diets fed to cats and so essential fatty acid (EFA) deficiency is unlikely to be encountered in practice. Experimentally induced (EFA) deficiency in growing cats leads to a dry, brittle coat with profuse scale formation.

EFAs are used extensively in the management of allergic and pruritic skin diseases in cats but these animals are not EFA deficient and this benefit is a pharmacological rather than a nutritional effect (*Chapter 31*).

Hypereosinophilia

Description. Hypereosinophilia is a rare syndrome of cats which even less commonly affects the skin, leading to pruritus. The disease is characterised by an idiopathic, presumably immune-mediated persistent blood and tissue eosinophilia. Tissue eosinophilia affects the bone marrow, lymph nodes, liver, spleen and gastrointestinal tract, leading to multisystemic disease.

Clinical signs. In extremely rare cases, the skin is involved leading to severe pruritus, maculopapular erythema and resultant self-trauma. **This disorder should not be confused with the eosinophilic skin diseases discussed in *Chapter 19*.**

Diagnosis. Diagnosis is based on histopathology, which reveals a predominantly eosinophilic dermatitis, and haematology, which shows a moderate to marked eosinophilia (up to 25×10^9/l).

Treatment. There is no effective therapy for this disorder. Treatment with prednisolone at immunosuppressive doses has invariably been unsuccessful.

Prognosis. The prognosis is poor. The disease is not responsive to glucocorticoids and the severity of pruritus usually leads the client to request euthanasia on welfare grounds.

14

Alopecia

IAN MASON

Alopecia is defined as the absence of hair from normally hairy areas. It may be manifested as thinning of the coat or as areas of skin completely devoid of hair, and it may be focal, multi-focal or bilaterally symmetrical.

Congenital alopecia is failure of hair production, e.g. congenital lack of hair or hair follicles. **Acquired alopecia** includes shedding or loss of an existing coat from, for example, endocrine disease or damage to the hair follicle, or as a result of excessive grooming, scratching and biting leading to loss of hair (e.g. pruritus or psychogenic factors).

Feline alopecia is commonly seen in veterinary practice and often incorrectly ascribed to a sex-hormone abnormality resulting from spaying or castration. This erroneous impression is reinforced by the often excellent response seen following the use of hormonal supplements such as testosterone, megoestrol acetate and liothyronine (T3). In fact, acquired feline alopecia is almost always self-induced as a result of pruritus. **The authors do not believe in the existence of feline endocrine alopecia.**

DIFFERENTIAL DIAGNOSIS OF FELINE ALOPECIA	

Alopecia due to failure of hair production	Congenital or genetic alopecias
	  Alopecia universalis (Sphinx Cat)
	  Hypotrichosis
	  Pili torti

Alopecia due to loss of existing hair	Follicular atrophy of degeneration
	Endocrinopathies
	  Hyperadrenocorticism
	  Hyperthyroidism
	  Diabetes mellitus
	Telogen defluxion
	Toxic causes (including drugs and vaccines)
	Nutritional causes (poor diet/malabsorption)
	Alopecia mucinosa
	Alopecia areata
	Folliculitis
	  Dermatophytosis (*Chapter 15*)
	  Bacterial disease (*Chapter 13*)
	  Demodicosis (*Chapter 15*)

Alopecia due to self-trauma	Self-trauma due to pruritus (Fig. 13.3) Psychogenic factors

FIG. 14.1 Differential diagnosis of feline alopecia.

The most common cause of feline alopecia is removal of normal hair as a result of self-trauma due to pruritus. It is always safer to assume that the alopecic cat is a pruritic cat until proved wrong, than to embark on potentially hazardous and empirical hormonal therapy.

The most important step in the investigation of an alopecic cat is to confirm or refute the thesis that the hair has simply dropped out. Figures 14.4 and 14.5 illustrate a suggested approach to feline alopecia.

Feline Skin Diseases Primarily Associated with Pruritus

This section will not discuss hair-loss due to pruritus as such disorders are in *Chapter 13*.

Alopecia Due to Failure of Hair Production

Congenital or genetic alopecia

Description. Genetic factors may lead to feline alopecia although this is quite uncommon. The underlying mechanism may be one of involution (atrophy) of hair follicles or dysplasia (failure of growth and development). Often these diseases arise as a result of misguided breeding programmes.

Clinical signs. The alopecia may be generalised or regional. Clincial signs range from the marked pre-auricular alopecia of some Siamese Cats to alopecia universalis. **Feline alopecia universalis** is a rare congenital disorder which cat breeders have specifically created by their breeding programmes. Affected animals are called Sphinx or Canadian hairless cats and are born without any primary hairs and only a few secondary hairs and whiskers. Sebaceous glands open directly on to the skin surface, which is extremely oily with accumulations of lipid especially

Fig. 14.2 Approach to feline alopecia: History.

APPROACH TO FELINE ALOPECIA: HISTORY	
Factor	**Differential diagnosis**

Breed
  Siamese, Abyssinian and Burmese
  Devon and Cornish Rex
	Psychogenic alopecia
	Congenital hypotrichosis

Age of onset
  Birth to a few weeks
  Less than 6 weeks
	Congenital or genetic
	Dermatophytosis

Recent/concurrent physical or emotional 'stress'	Telogen defluxion; psychogenic alopecia
Intercurrent disease	Metabolic, nutritional or endocrine-induced alopecia
Pruritus	See *Chapter 13*

Previous medication
  Injections (vaccines, wormers)
  Glucocorticoids
	Focal, local alopecia
	Hyperadrenocorticism

Hair in faeces or vomit	Indicates that hair-loss is self-induced

Fig. 14.3 Approach to feline alopecia: Physical examination.

APPROACH TO FELINE ALOPECIA: PHYSICAL EXAMINATION	
Physical finding	**Differential diagnosis**
Short broken hairs	Hair-loss is self-induced
Complete absence of hairs	Hair-loss is not self-induced
Fragile skin	Hyperadrenocorticism; Ehlers–Danlos syndrome
Evidence of self-trauma	See *Chapter 13*

in the nail folds. Affected cats are reluctant to groom this secretion from the skin surface and need frequent bathing. The morality of selectively breeding for such cats is questionable.

Another genetically determined alopecia for which cat owners specifically breed is that exhibited by the Devon and Cornish Rex breeds. In some cats, the alopecia is exaggerated and affected individuals are born with a very thin hair coat which is partly lost within the first few months of life. Rex kittens also have a somewhat wrinkled skin.

Diagnosis. The diagnosis is clinical although in some instances histopathology may be required for conformation. Follicles and skin glands may be absent or dysplastic.

Treatment. There is no treatment although Sphinx cats will require regular bathing with anti-seborrhoeic shampoo and removal of lipid from the nail folds. Alopecic cats may suffer from actinic (sunlight-induced) dermatitis which may develop into squamous cell carcinomata. Owners should be warned not to allow their cats to be exposed to sunlight in summer, using sun-blocks or confinement.

Prognosis. These disorders are seldom life-endangering and in most instances are merely cosmetic. They are incurable.

Pili torti

This is a rare disorder, so far reported only in the UK. Secondary hair shafts are rotated along their long axes leading to diffuse hair-loss by 10 days of age with rapidly developing generalised alopecia, pedal dermatitis and paronychia. All affected kittens reported in the literature have died or been destroyed on humane grounds. The author has seen one affected litter; the product of a brother–sister mating. Diagnosis is made on the basis of history and physical examination. Microscopy of plucked secondary hairs is diagnostic. There is no treatment.

Alopecia Due to Loss of Existing Hair: Follicular Atrophy or Degeneration

Feline symmetrical alopecia (FSA)

Description. This disorder was formerly known as feline endocrine alopecia (FEA). It is a controversial

1. Determine whether the hair-loss is congenital, spontaneous or self-induced. It is imperative that this distinction is made on the very first occasion that the animal is seen and that the client is convinced of the mechanism of hair-loss. History may be valuable (Fig. 14.2)

Focused diagnostic tests: *Trichogram* (or microscopy of plucked hairs): Fractured hairs with normal tips indicate that hair-loss is self-induced; normal tapered tips with a predominance of telogen hairs indicate that hair-loss is not self-induced (*Chapter 3*). Elizabethan collar: Used for up to 2 months, will confirm that the hair-loss is self-induced but this is slower than simply examining the hairs microscopically; it is also less humane

If hair-loss is self-induced, then pruritus is present (see *Chapter 13*) or the disorder is psychogenic, (see later).
If the animal was born without hair then the disorder is genetic or congenital. Histopathology may identify the underlying cause.
If hair-loss is acquired but not self-induced:
2. Rule out demodicosis and dermatophytosis

Focused diagnostic tests: Microscopy of skin scraping, hair plucks and adhesive tape specimens; Wood's lamp examination; fungal culture

3. Rule out bacterial folliculitis

Focused diagnostic tests: Histopathology and bacteriology; response to antibiotic therapy

If no diagnosis, then haematology, histopathology and trial therapies are needed to distinguish between endocrinopathies, telogen defluxion, toxic, acquired hair follicle dysplasia and nutritional disease

FIG. 14.4 Diagnostic plan for feline alopecia.

disorder and most dermatologists, including the authors, are convinced that it does not exist. As our understanding of skin disease advances, so misconceptions regarding the pathogenesis of certain diseases become exposed. In general veterinary practice, 'FEA' is a common clinical diagnosis. However, no endocrine abnormality has ever been convincingly demonstrated in affected cats. It is likely that cases of feline alopecia previously ascribed to an endocrine aetiology were in fact due to self-trauma (as discussed earlier). It has therefore been suggested that the disorder be renamed feline symmetrical alopecia or FSA. FSA is simply a cutaneous reaction pattern and is usually the result of pruritus. The authors have never seen a cat with idiopathic FSA.

Clinical signs. Acquired symmetrical alopecia of the perineum, ventrum, inguinal region, the forelegs from elbow to carpus and the medial aspect of the hindlimbs are the usual presentations of FSA. The condition is seen in entire or neutered animals of any age or breed.

Diagnosis. Cases of FSA should be investigated following the recommendations given in Figs 14.4 and 14.5. Almost all cases are due to allergic or psychosomatic disorders which lead to self-induced hair-loss. In order to confirm this, and to convince the sceptical owner, hair plucks should be examined microscopically for evidence of self-trauma. In

some cases, histopathology is needed to demonstrate that anagen hairs are present so ruling out an endocrine aetiology. The use of an Elizabethan collar is often of value. One particularly useful test is to count circulating eosinophils, as an eosinophilia is usually associated with ectoparasitism, especially flea allergic dermatitis. Cases with eosinophilia should be carefully evaluated for hypersensitivity, particularly FAD.

Treatment. Cats regrow their hair once the underlying cause of their hair-loss has been identified and treated.

Prognosis. The prognosis is good where the cause is due to hypersensitivity or ectoparasitism. Psychogenic alopecia is more difficult to treat.

Hyperadrenocorticism

Description. Hyperadrenocorticism is rare in cats although there are several published series of cases of this disorder. In general, the non-dermatological manifestations of the disease have been reported with little emphasis on the dermatological signs. Both adrenal and pituitary dependent forms of the disease have been recorded.

Clinical signs. Dermatological signs are similar to those reported in other species and include easy bruising of the skin, which may be thin with

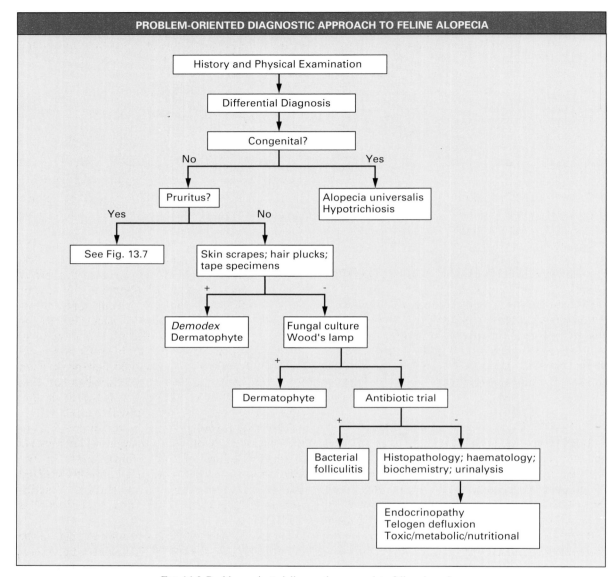

PROBLEM-ORIENTED DIAGNOSTIC APPROACH TO FELINE ALOPECIA

FIG. 14.5 Problem-oriented diagnostic approach to feline alopecia.

prominent vasculature, comedone formation and hyperpigmentation. Bilaterally symmetrical alopecia affecting the trunk and flanks has been reported. The most striking feature of this disease in the cat is that 48% of cases reported in a recent survey had extremely fragile skin, which tore easily on routine handling; this may be confused with cutaneous asthenia (*Chapter 18*). Some iatrogenic cases of feline hyperadrenocorticism have been reported to have medial curling of the pinnae,

although it is probable that this does not occur in the naturally-occurring disease.

Systemic signs include polyuria, polydipsia, concomitant diabetes mellitus, polyphagia and abdominal distension.

Diagnosis. ACTH stimulation and dexamethasone suppression tests have been described for use in cats (*Chapter 3*) but their reliability is unknown.

Treatment. There is no effective treatment. Management with o,p'-DDD (Lysodren or mitotane) has been reported to be of little benefit; this drug is toxic in cats. Ketoconazole (12 mg/kg orally twice daily) has been reported to be of value in some pituitary dependent cases.

Prognosis. The prognosis is poor with short survival times even in cats treated with ketoconazole.

Thyroid disease

Only one case of naturally occurring acquired hypothyroidism has been reported in the cat. It has been shown that radioactive iodine-induced experimental ablation of the feline thyroid does not lead to bilaterally symmetrical alopecia except of the pinnae. This suggests that an intact thyroid gland is not essential for the maintenance of the hair coat of cats.

Occasionally congenital hypothyroidism occurs in kittens. Affected animals do have a generally thin coat but respond well to thyroid supplementation.

Feline hyperthyroidism can affect the skin but does not induce alopecia. Hyperthyroidism is discussed more fully in *Chapter 15*.

Diabetes mellitus

Symmetrical alopecia affecting the groin, perineum, lateral abdomen and hind limbs has been reported in cats with diabetes mellitus. However, there is a high incidence of diabetes in cats with hyperadrenocorticism and it may be this which leads to alopecia. All cats with symmetric alopecia and diabetes mellitus should be evaluated for the presence of hyperadrenocorticism.

Telogen defluxion

Telogen defluxion (which is also termed telogen defluvium or telogen effluvium) is characterised by shortening of the anagen stage of the hair cycle so that many hairs enter telogen simultaneously, with resultant shedding of the hair coat. Telogen defluxion is induced by physical or psychological stresses such as gestation, lactation, surgery, pyrexia and internal disease. The hair-loss is widespread but only temporary. Diagnosis is based on history and physical examination along with elimination of the other disorders listed in Fig. 14.1. Histopathology reveals that all of the hair follicles are in telogen. Although this condition may cause great concern to owners, no therapy is indicated nor effective and the prognosis is excellent with full recovery in a few months.

Toxic, metabolic and nutritional factors

Alopecia due to toxic, metabolic or nutritional factors is surprisingly uncommon in cats. Hair growth requires up to 30% of total nutritional protein requirements and the hair-forming follicular matrix and basal cells are highly active structures and therefore very sensitive to toxic or metabolic insult.

Diseases leading to protein deficiency may be associated with diffuse hair-loss and brittle, dry, easily fractured hairs. These changes particularly affect the trunk. Chronic hepatic or renal disease or malabsorption syndromes (especially protein-losing enteropathies) may lead to such changes. A protein-deficient diet may also lead to alopecia in this way. A thorough diagnostic investigation, especially a full medical history, should lead the clinician to suspect the underlying cause of the hair-loss and investigate and treat accordingly. If the underlying cause can be corrected, the hair will regrow.

The hair-forming tissues are susceptible to the effects of cytotoxic and immuno-suppressive drugs (including glucocorticoids) used in the management of neoplastic and immune-mediated diseases. Such medicaments can lead to generalised alopecia but this is reversible once therapy is discontinued.

Dietary deficiencies are uncommon in cats in the developed world as most are fed balanced commercial diets. Occasionally, unusual diets are fed to cats by owners — usually those who are vegetarians, and who are unaware that cats are obligate carnivores. Alopecia due to nutritional hypovitaminosis A has been reported in cats.

Alopecia mucinosa and alopecia areata

Alopecia mucinosa and areata are extremely rare in the cat.

Alopecia mucinosa appears to be a precursor of epitheliotropic lymphoma (mycosis fungoides) and the prognosis is therefore extremely poor. It has been described in only two cats, in which alopecia associated with fine scaling was confined to the head, ears and neck. Diagnosis is based on histopathology, which reveals a mucinous degeneration of the epidermis and hair follicle outer root sheath. The aetiology and pathogenesis of this syndrome are unknown.

Alopecia areata is characterised by focal or multi-focal areas of alopecia, which are often symmetrical. The underlying skin appears normal. There are no age, breed or sex predilections. Diagnosis is based on histopathology, which reveals a lymphoplasmocytic perifolliculitis and folliculitis. This cellular infiltrate is so folliculocentric that the appearance has been likened to a 'swarm of bees'. Topical and systemic glucocorticoids have been used in this disorder but there is little evidence that they are of any benefit. Some cases recover spontaneously.

Partial pre-auricular alopecia

Occasionally owners may report that their cat is losing hair from between the ear and the eye. This is a physiological phenomenon and no treatment is warranted or indicated. Owners should simply be reassured that this is not pathological.

Alopecia Due to Self-Trauma

Pruritus

Pruritus is a common cause of self-induced hair-loss and is discussed in detail in *Chapter 13*.

Psychogenic factors

Psychogenic alopecia is self-induced as a response to anxiety or, less commonly, boredom. Breeds such as Siamese and Burmese are most commonly affected. Anxiety may be caused by the arrival of a new pet or baby into the cat's established household or a change of environment such as kennelling or moving home. In some cases, the self-trauma is partly the result of psychogenic factors and partly due to a pre-existing pruritic disease. Hence, the psychological stress lowers the itch threshold for an animal which has an asymptomatic pruritic disorder.

Diagnosis is based on history and physical examination. Demonstration that the hair-loss is self-induced may be necessary if the owner is sceptical. Trichograms and the use of Elizabethan collars in order to effect this have been discussed previously. It is imperative that a rigorous investigation of any potential pruritic disease is made, as pruritus is a far more common cause of self-induced hair-loss in cats than is psychogenic alopecia.

Treatment with mood-modifying drugs such as oral diazepam (1–2 mg per cat b.i.d.) may be effective. Occasionally oral clomipramine or phenobarbitone (8–15 mg per cat per day) may be required but there is no published information regarding the toxicity of the latter two drugs in cats. None of the three drugs mentioned are licensed for use in this species. This topic is discussed in further detail in *Chapter 34*. The author recommends that the initiating psychological factor be identified and corrected if possible. Medical treatment should be regarded as the last resort.

15

Scaling and Crusting

KAREN MORIELLO

Scaling and crusting or exfoliative dermatoses have a number of causes including infectious agents, parasitic agents, immune-mediated events and neoplasia (Fig. 15.1). Scaling and crusting lesions are particularly difficult to evaluate and a thorough and methodical diagnostic approach is mandatory. It is important to note that primary seborrhoea is rare in the cat compared with the dog. All cats presented for the problem of scaling should be screened for dermatophytosis via fungal culture.

Selected Feline Skin Diseases Associated with Scaling and Crusting

'Stud tail' or tail seborrhoea

Description. 'Stud tail' is the layperson's term for tail seborrhoea (it was first described in intact male cats). This condition can be seen in intact or surgically neutered male or female cats. The dorsal region, particularly the proximal portion, of a cat's tail is rich in sebaceous glands. These glands can become overactive, producing an abundant amount of oil that causes matting of the fur in this area. Tail seborrhoea is more common in long-haired cats. This may be a breed predisposition or may reflect the cat's inability to groom off excessive amounts of oil.

Clinical signs. Tail seborrhoea is easily recognised. The hair on the dorsal surface of the tail is matted and oily. In some cats, a secondary bacterial infection may be present.

Diagnosis. Definitive diagnosis is made most often by clinical appearance. It is important to examine the underlying skin closely for evidence of a bacterial infection, i.e. pustules, exudation, crusts. If this area is examined with a Wood's lamp, the oil on the coat will produce a blue-green false fluorescence. A dermatophyte culture is indicated in these cats.

Treatment. If the hair is heavily matted, the hair coat on the tail may need to be shaved. The area should be washed daily or every other day with a benzoyl peroxide shampoo; tar-based shampoos are best avoided in cats because they can be severely irritating. The shampoo must be thoroughly rinsed from the hair to prevent the cat from licking and ingesting small amounts of shampoo. These shampoos are not toxic to cats but many owners report that cats will salivate and vomit if they groom these areas excessively.

Prognosis. The prognosis is excellent; this is not a life-threatening disease. Most cats require life-long therapy. If there is no response to antiseborrhoeic shampoos, the area should be biopsied.

DIFFERENTIAL DIAGNOSIS OF EXFOLIATIVE DERMATOSES IN CATS	
Infectious	Dermatophytosis Bacterial pyoderma
Parasitic	Lice Cheyletiellosis Fleas Fur mites *Notoedres, Sarcoptes, Otodectes*
Immune-mediated	Drug eruption Pemphigus foliaceus/erythematosus Systemic lupus erythematosus Feline atopy Feline food allergy
Keratinisation defects	Tail-gland seborrhoea Chin acne Primary seborrhoea
Miscellaneous causes	Cutaneous neoplasia Actinic dermatitis Low humidity Nutritional disorders Sebaceous adenitis

FIG. 15.1 Differential diagnosis of exfoliative dermatoses in cats.

FIG. 15.2 Approach to exfoliative skin diseases: History.

APPROACH TO EXFOLIATIVE SKIN DISEASES: HISTORY	
Factor	**Differential diagnosis**
Breed Brachiocephalic breeds	Primary facial seborrhoea; tail seborrhoea

Age of onset
  More than 10 years
  Less than 1–2 years
	Neoplasia more common
	Dermatophytosis more common

Pruritus	Cutaneous parasites; dermatophytosis; allergic skin disease

FIG. 15.3 Approach to exfoliative skin diseases: Physical examination.

APPROACH TO EXFOLIATIVE SKIN DISEASES: PHYSICAL EXAMINATION	
Physical finding	**Differential diagnosis**
Pruritus	Parasitic skin diseases; allergies
Symmetrical lesions on face, trunk, footpads	Immune-mediated diseases
Dorsal truncal distribution	Fleas; *Cheyletiella* mites
Focal distribution	Tail seborrhoea; chin acne
Alopecia	Dermatophytosis

Feline chin acne or comedone syndrome

Description. This is a relatively common condition of cats involving the chin and lateral commissures of the mouth, with affected cats having comedones in these areas. The face and chin of cats is rich in sebaceous glands.

There are many causes of this condition. Some clinicians believe that it is caused by poor grooming on the cat's part but this belief is not widely held. The sudden development of comedones on a cat's chin should raise the suspicion of feline demodicosis, dermatophytosis, *Malassezia* infection or bacterial furunculosis as possible causes. Gradual development of comedones in a young cat may be due to the infectious agents listed above; however, a keratinisation disorder should also be considered. This is particularly true if the cat has facial fold seborrhoea or tail seborrhoea. Geriatric cats may develop comedones on their chins but this is usually of little clinical significance. Almost all of these cats are as fastidious groomers in their old age as they were as young cats, which suggests that comedones may occur as part of the skin's ageing process in cats.

Clinical signs. Feline comedone syndrome can vary from mild to severe. In mild cases, a few widely scattered comedones may be visible on the chin or around the commissures of the mouth. These rarely cause the cat any discomfort. This presentation is most commonly seen in older cats. In more moderate to severe cases, there may be an acute onset of thick, black discharge on the chin. The affected area may be painful, swollen and exudative. In the most severe form of feline comedone syndrome, the chin is grossly swollen because of the development of furunculosis. Ruptured furuncles discharge a combination of black sebaceous material mixed with blood-tinged purulent exudate. Sometimes oxidised keratin debris will be mistaken for flea dirt. The cat's chin is very painful and the cat resents any manipulation of the area.

Diagnosis. Diagnosis is easily made via clinical signs but diagnostic tests are necessary to determine the underlying cause. A skin scraping for *Demodex* mites should be performed on all cases, especially in older cats. The development of demodicosis in older cats may accompany the onset of feline diabetes mellitus. Impression smears and scrape preparations of the black debris should be performed to look for the presence of *Malassezia* and inflammatory cells. Dermatophytosis should be considered in young cats, show cats and indoor–outdoor cats that suffer an acute episode of moderate to marked severity. A skin biopsy should be considered in severe cases that do not respond to appropriate therapy.

Treatment. Mild cases do not require any therapy if an underlying cause is not identified. Most cats prefer to be left alone and resent any scrubbing of the area. Moderate to severe cases usually benefit

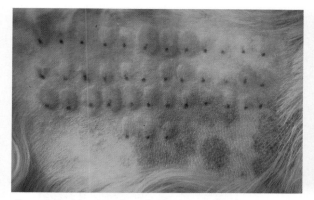

PLATE 1 Positive intradermal allergy test showing numerous strong reactions to inhalant allergens

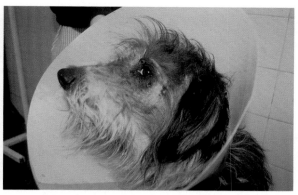

PLATE 2 Sarcoptic mange. Head of affected dog showing alopecia, erythema and self-induced excoriation of the skin. The Elizabethan collar is to prevent further self-trauma.

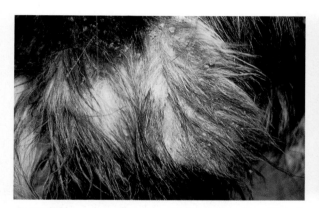

PLATE 3 Close view of a pinna of affected dog from Plate 2 showing crusting, alopecia and erythema.

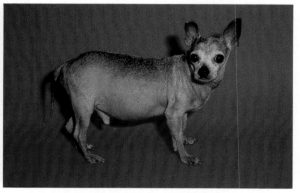

PLATE 4 Canine hyperadrenocorticism. Note pendulous abdomen.

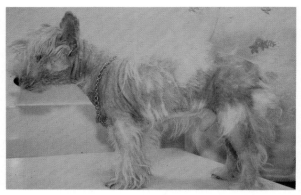

PLATE 5 Epidermal dysplasia in a West Highland White Terrier. Severe erythema, alopecia and epidermal hyperplasia are present.

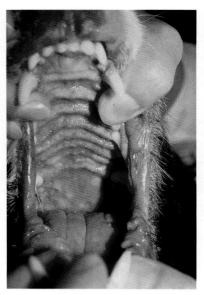

PLATE 6 Ulcerative stomatitis.

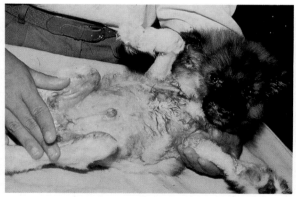

PLATE 7 Cutaneous candidiasis in a young dog receiving immunosuppressive drugs for presumptive graft vs host disease.

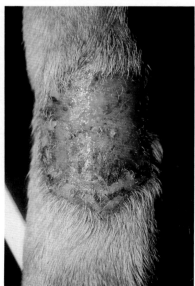

PLATE 8 Ulceration of the anterior aspect of the carpus of a German Shepherd Dog with bullous pemphigoid.

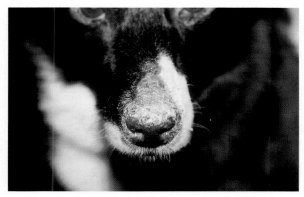

PLATE 9 Dorsum of muzzle of a dog with pemphigus foliaceus crusting and ulceration with depigmentation of the rhinarium.

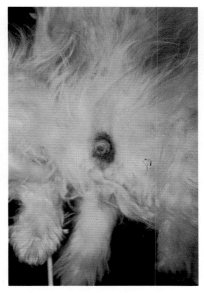

PLATE 10 Intertrigo of the vulvar fold.

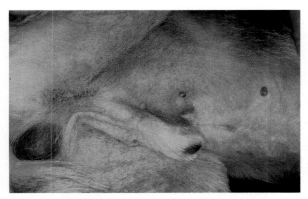

PLATE 11 Superficial folliculitis affecting ventral abdomen of a German Shepherd Dog showing papules, alopecia, hyperpigmentation and erythema.

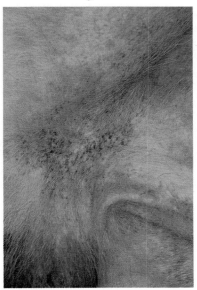

PLATE 12 Close view of Plate 11 to show detail.

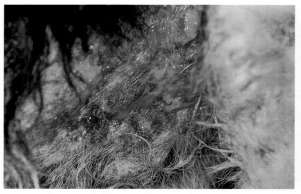

PLATE 13 Deep pyoderma of the flank of a German Shepherd Dog. Severe lesions are present with ulceration, hyperpigmentation and exudation.

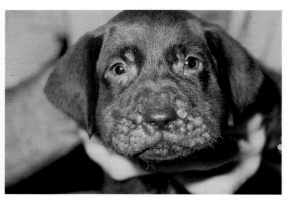

PLATE 14 Juvenile cellulitis.

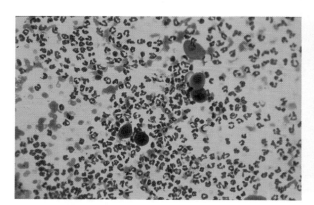

PLATE 15 Impression smear of exudate found in pemphigus foliaceus. Note the large blue cells—acantholytic cells.

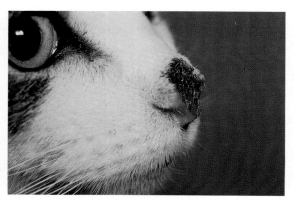

PLATE 16 Feline nasal squamous cell carcinoma.

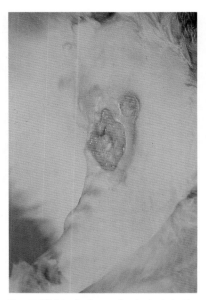

PLATE 17 Atypical mycobacteriosis in the cat affecting posterior aspect of the hock. Note the large ulcer and the dermal nodules.

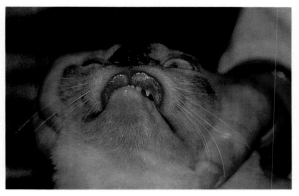

PLATE 18 Feline indolent ulcer.

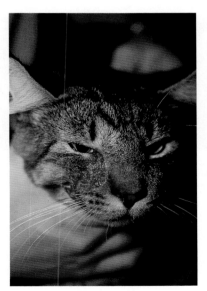

PLATE 19 Feline eosinophilic plaque.

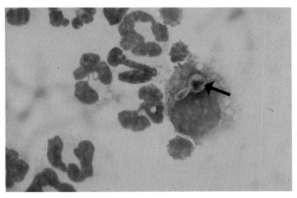

PLATE 20 Microscopic appearance of *Sporothrix schenkii* organisms.

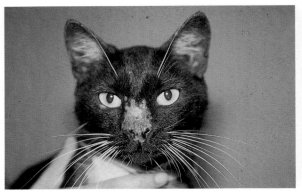

PLATE 21 Feline insect hypersensitivity.

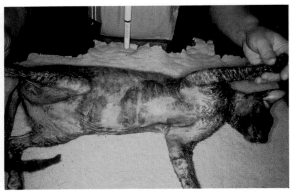

PLATE 22 Cat with generalised ulcerative skin disease. This cat was atopic.

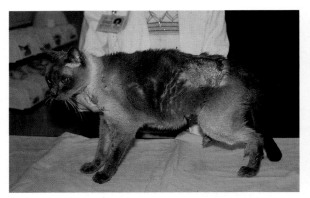

PLATE 23 Cat with feline hyperadrenocorticism.

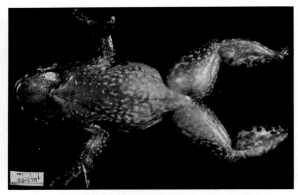

PLATE 24 Septicaemia in a frog: 'red leg disease'. Slide courtesy of the University of California, School of Veterinary Medicine, Zoological Medicine Department.

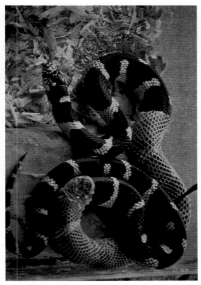

PLATE 25 Normal ecdysis in a snake.
Slide courtesy of Dr Dale DeNardo,
University of California, Berkeley.

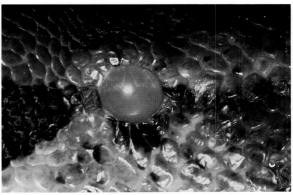

PLATE 26 Normal spectacular clouding as part of the
normal ecdysis in a snake. Slide courtesy of Dr Chris Murphy,
School of Veterinary Medicine, University of Wisconsin.

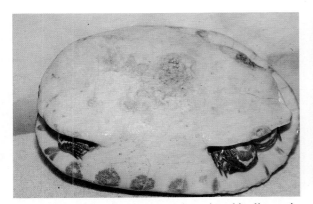

PLATE 27 Septicaemic cutaneous ulcerative skin disease in
a turtle.

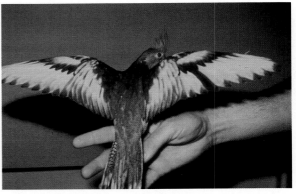

PLATE 28 Achromatosis in cockatiel with experimental choline
deficiency. Slide courtesy of Dr Thomas Rhodybush, Placerville.

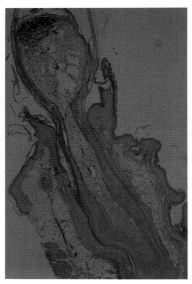

PLATE 29 Histological section of a feather follicle from a bird with PBFD. Slide courtesy of Dr Julie Langenberg, International Crane Foundation, Wisconsin.

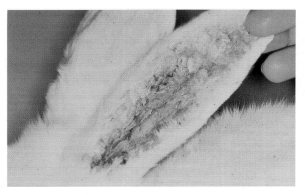

PLATE 30 Ear mite infestation in a rabbit. Slide courtesy of the University of California-Davis, Department of Zoological Medicine teaching file.

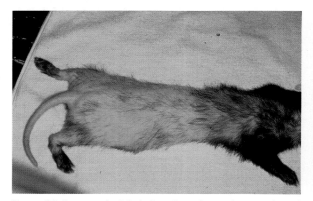

PLATE 31 Symmetrical hair-loss in a ferret due to adrenal gland disease.

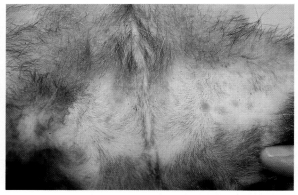

PLATE 32 Benign mast cell tumours in a ferret.

from therapy. If an underlying cause is identified, specific therapy for that disease along with topical therapy should result in resolution of the chin seborrhoea. (The reader is referred to other sections in the book for information on specific therapies.)

DIAGNOSTIC PLAN FOR EXFOLIATIVE SKIN LESIONS IN CATS

When presented with a cat with the problem of scaling and crusting it is helpful to determine the distribution of the lesions. There are several exfoliative skin diseases of cats that have a specific regional distribution of lesions. In general, the most important and useful in-house diagnostic tests are skin scrapings, dermatophyte cultures and flea combings for parasites

1. When presented with a cat with the problem of exfoliative dermatitis, it is important to determine whether or not the cat is pruritic. If pruritus is a significant component of the history or physical examination, the diagnostic plan for pruritus should be pursued (*Chapter 13*)

2. *If pruritus is not a significant component of the history,* determine if there is a recent drug history. If the cat is currently receiving any recent or chronic drug therapy, consider a cutaneous drug eruption. Cutaneous drug eruptions in cats are commonly seen on the head, face and ears. If possible, all drugs should be discontinued for a period of 3–7 days and the patient reassessed prior to beginning an in-depth diagnostic evaluation

3. *If pruritus and a recent drug history are not components of the patient's history or physical examination,* determine the most representative pattern for the exfoliation (localised or generalised/symmetrical)

Localised Exfoliation and/or Oily Seborrhoea

1. *If the area of oily seborrhoea is on the dorsal tail,* consider tail seborrhoea. *If the area is on the chin or commissures of the mouth,* consider feline chin acne or feline comedones

> **Focused diagnostic tests**: Skin scrapings for *Demodex* mites should be performed. Impression smears or scrape preparations from the area of seborrhoea should be performed and examined for *Malassezia* and bacteria. A fungal culture should be considered, as dermatophytes can also cause these lesions

2. *If the skin scrapings and cytology specimens are negative for micro-organisms,* consider the diagnosis of chin acne or tail seborrhoea. A response to therapy trial should be considered

3. *If there is a good response to therapy,* it should be continued indefinitely. *If there is no response to therapy,* a skin biopsy should be performed to confirm or deny the presence of a primary disorder or keratinisation. Dermatophytosis should be considered

> **Focused diagnostic tests**: A skin biopsy and a dermatophyte culture (if not already done) should be performed

Facial Crusting

1. *If the exfoliation is limited to the face and ears,* consider dermatophytosis and parasitic infestations (*Otodectes, Notoedres*). *If exudation is present,* consider pemphigus and eosinophilic skin diseases

> **Focused diagnostic tests**: Numerous skin scrapings should be performed to look for parasites. A dermatophyte culture should also be taken. Cytological examination of exudate for inflammatory cells and acantholytic cells should also be done. This is especially important if the medial pinnae are involved

2. *If skin scrapings, dermatophyte culture and cytological examination of exudate are negative or non-diagnostic,* a skin biopsy should be performed

> **Focused diagnostic tests**: A skin biopsy should be obtained to look for evidence of cutaneous neoplasia, pemphigus, actinic dermatitis or eosinophilic infiltrates in the skin. If eosinophils are found in the skin, allergic skin disease (atopy, food allergy or flea allergy) should be suspected

Generalised or Symmetrical Exfoliation and Oily Seborrhoea

1. *If the exfoliation or seborrhoea is symmetrical on the face or trunk or generalised in distribution,* consider parasitic agents and dermatophytosis

> **Focused diagnostic tests**: Numerous skin scrapings for mites and flea-combing for lice, fleas and *Cheyletiella* mites should be performed. These mites are difficult to find and hair/scale debris may need to be digested and then examined

2. *If no parasites are found,* a response to antiparasite therapy should be evaluated. It may be very difficult to identify cutaneous ectoparasites on cats due to their fastidious grooming behaviour

> **Focused diagnostic tests**: A 3–4 week course of flea control should be initiated and the cat re-examined. Many cats with cutaneous parasites are not reported by their owners to be very pruritic; pruritus should not be used as the sole criterion for choosing this test

3. *If there is no response to flea control therapy and the cat is still very scaly,* a trial course of ivermectin should be considered. Ivermectin therapy will eliminate the suspicion of cheyletiellosis; not all cases of *Cheyletiella* infection resolve with flea control

> **Focused diagnostic tests**: Oral or subcutaneous ivermectin (200 μg/kg) every 2–3 weeks for three treatments is recommended. Alternatively, lime sulphur dip (22 g/l (4 oz/gal) of warm water) used every 5 days for six to eight therapies will be equally as effective

Continued

DIAGNOSTIC PLAN FOR EXFOLIATIVE SKIN LESIONS IN CATS

4. *If there is no response to antiparasite therapy,* consider the possibility of an autoimmune skin disease, cutaneous neoplasia, dietary deficiency or chronic exposure to low humidity

> **Focused diagnostic tests:** Numerous skin biopsies are recommended from multiple areas to look for compatible histological findings of an autoimmune skin disease (e.g. pemphigus), cutaneous neoplasia or a disorder of keratinisation. If systemic lupus erythematosus is strongly suspected, then an ANA test should be submitted. If eosinophils are found on skin biopsies in notable numbers, allergic skin disease should be considered

5. *If the skin biopsies are non-diagnostic,* consider systemic diseases such as feline immunodeficiency virus, FeLV and diabetes mellitus

> **Focused diagnostic tests:** Blood should be submitted for haematology, serum biochemistry panel and FIV and FeLV testings

6. *If these tests are normal,* then it may be reasonable to consider the possibility that the cat is atopic or food-allergic. Generally, these diseases are pruritic; however, some cats are not markedly pruritic and owners do not report significant pruritus

> **Focused diagnostic tests:** A food trial and/or intradermal skin testing should be performed (*Chapter 3*)

FIG. 15.4 Diagnostic plan for exfoliative skin lesions in cats.

In all cases of feline chin seborrhoea–furunculosis, it is important to impress upon the owner that the lesions should not be squeezed or pinched. Squeezing these lesions is painful for the cat and may cause more inflammation. If the cat will tolerate it, warm compresses on the chin three to four times per day are soothing. Gentle scrubs with benzoyl peroxide shampoo are very useful but may be irritating to some cats. Topical benzoyl peroxide gel or vitamin A cream daily may be beneficial in some cats but can be irritating to others. If frank furunculosis is present oral antibiotics are necessary. Cephalexin (20 mg/kg t.i.d.), ampicillin–clavulanic acid (2 mg/kg t.i.d.), or lincomycin (10 mg/kg b.i.d.) are effective. The length of therapy is variable depending upon the severity of the lesions. In general, deep pyodermas should be treated for 4–6 weeks. If *Malassezia* is found, ketoconazole or itraconazole (10 mg/kg once a day) for 30 days is recommended. Anecdotally, isotretinoin (1 mg/kg daily) has been reported to benefit some cats with severe cystic comedone syndrome.

Prognosis. The prognosis is good; this is not a life-threatening disease. Mild cases may resolve without therapy. Severe cases may not resolve completely or the cats may have relapses throughout their lives.

Facial seborrhoea of Persian cats

Description. Facial seborrhoea of Persian cats is an inherited disorder of keratinisation. The condition is chronic and there is no cure; treatment is lifelong.

Clinical signs. Cats with facial seborrhoea often have excessively flat faces. In this condition, thick black debris will mat the hair coat and will accumulate around the nose, mouth, eyes and folds (Fig. 17.2). The cats are otherwise healthy, except for this cosmetic defect.

Diagnosis. A tentative clinical diagnosis may be made via clinical appearance. Skin scrapings for *Demodex* mites and impression smears for bacteria and *Malassezia* should be performed. Skin biopsies are not very useful in making a definitive diagnosis but may be beneficial in helping to rule out feline demodicosis and/or *Malassezia* infection.

Treatment. Treatment is lifelong and affected cats require face washing two to three times per week with an antiseborrhoeic shampoo. Benzoyl peroxide, tar or tar-and-sulphur combinations are all acceptable choices. It may be necessary to rotate various shampoos as some cats may find one shampoo too irritating or no longer respond to the active ingredient. Washing a Persian cat's face is no easy task and they hate it.

Prognosis. The prognosis is excellent; this is not a life-threatening disease. Unfortunately, the condition is lifelong and requires constant care. It is important to stress this to the cat's owner. Affected cats should not be bred.

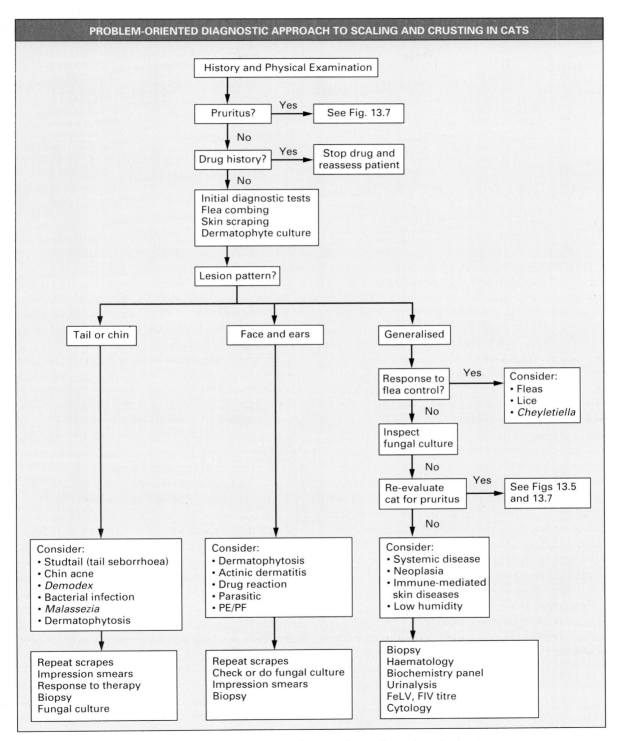

PROBLEM-ORIENTED DIAGNOSTIC APPROACH TO SCALING AND CRUSTING IN CATS

History and Physical Examination

Pruritus? — Yes → See Fig. 13.7

No

Drug history? — Yes → Stop drug and reassess patient

No

Initial diagnostic tests
Flea combing
Skin scraping
Dermatophyte culture

Lesion pattern?

Tail or chin | **Face and ears** | **Generalised**

Response to flea control? — Yes → Consider:
• Fleas
• Lice
• *Cheyletiella*

No

Inspect fungal culture

No

Re-evaluate cat for pruritus — Yes → See Figs 13.5 and 13.7

No

Consider:
• Studtail (tail seborrhoea)
• Chin acne
• *Demodex*
• Bacterial infection
• *Malassezia*
• Dermatophytosis

Consider:
• Dermatophytosis
• Actinic dermatitis
• Drug reaction
• Parasitic
• PE/PF

Consider:
• Systemic disease
• Neoplasia
• Immune-mediated skin diseases
• Low humidity

Repeat scrapes
Impression smears
Response to therapy
Biopsy
Fungal culture

Repeat scrapes
Check or do fungal culture
Impression smears
Biopsy

Biopsy
Haematology
Biochemistry panel
Urinalysis
FeLV, FIV titre
Cytology

FIG. 15.5 Problem-oriented diagnostic approach to scaling and crusting in cats.

Actinic dermatitis and squamous cell carcinoma

Description. Actinic dermatitis is a solar-induced pre-neoplastic condition that is seen in light-coloured cats. It may affect the preauricular area, ears, face and eyelids. Squamous cell carcinomas in cats are the sequelae to actinic dermatitis and may occur in any of these areas. The lesions may be very symmetrical.

Clinical signs. Actinic dermatitis is seen in light-coloured cats (e.g. white cats, lilac point Siamese cats) that are sunbathers. The affected areas are erythematous and scaly and may have ulcerations and erosions. The affected skin may be thickened. These areas are frequently pruritic. Severe ulceration is suggestive of squamous cell carcinoma.

Diagnosis. Definitive diagnosis is made by skin biopsy for either condition. Several different skin biopsies from various stages of the lesions should be submitted; diagnostic lesions may be found in only one portion of a biopsy. If lesions are present only on ear margins, a full-thickness resection should be performed. Actinic dermatitis is characterised by epidermal hyperplasia with marked dysplasia. Squamous cell carcinomas are easily recognised by the dermatopathologist because of the characteristic neoplastic changes. Trabeculae of squamous cells from the epidermis are seen extending into the dermis with the development of 'keratin pearls'.

Treatment. The treatment of choice for actinic dermatitis is to limit sun exposure of the cat. Since this is (realistically) very difficult to accomplish, benign neglect is often the owner's choice. The development of actinic dermatitis into a squamous cell carcinoma is a slow process. The owners may attempt to apply sun-screen (SPF 20 or greater) to the cat's face but most cats rapidly groom off the creams. If the owners are willing, they can purchase plastic sun-screens to fit their windows; these are designed to block the UV light. It is important to have the screens installed in every window where the cat can sunbathe and to make sure that the screens are secured so that the cat cannot sneak behind them. The treatment of choice in private practice for squamous cell carcinoma is surgical excision.

Prognosis. The prognosis is guarded for both actinic dermatitis and squamous cell carcinoma. Most older cats that develop actinic dermatitis usually develop squamous cell carcinomas late in life and die of other causes. Young cats that develop either condition are at greater risk for a shortened lifespan, especially if the skin lesions are in areas that are not surgically resectable.

Cutaneous drug eruption

Description. Cutaneous drug eruptions may occur from any systemic drug administered to the cat or any topical agent applied to the cat's skin.

Clinical signs. The clinical signs are extremely variable and may include any combination of erythema, scaling, ulceration, hair-loss and pruritus. The onset may be slow or rapid. The most common site for cutaneous drug eruptions is the skin in the preauricular area and ears. In some cats the condition is clinically and histologically indistinguishable from pemphigus foliaceus.

Drug eruptions in cats are relatively rare and can mimic almost any known skin disease. Lesions may develop slowly or acutely and can occur weeks after the drug has been administered. Facial crusting with or without ulceration is a common presenting complaint. The two most common drugs in the author's practice associated with exfoliative drug eruptions are sulphonamides and methimazole.

Diagnosis. Definitive diagnosis can be very difficult and is usually made by exclusion of other more common causes, resolution of clinical signs with cessation of drug therapy, and skin biopsy. Cats at risk are those receiving systemic drugs, or receiving topical ointments to their skin, particularly the ears. Skin scrapings and fungal cultures should be taken, to rule out infectious causes. All drugs should be stopped and the cat re-examined 5–7 days later. If the reaction is severe or if there is risk in stopping a systemic drug, then a skin biopsy should be taken. The inflammatory pattern seen in a cutaneous drug eruption is extremely variable and the pathologist should be given a very thorough history. One of the most common drugs to cause facial crusting in cats, in the author's experience is methimazole.

Treatment. The treatment of choice is discontinuation of the drug. Symptomatic therapy may be necessary; however, the use of glucocorticoids is controversial.

Prognosis. The prognosis is variable, depending upon the severity of the drug eruption. In most cases, the lesions resolve in a few days to weeks.

Parasitic mite infestations causing facial crusting

Description. Infestations of *Notoedres cati*, *Sarcoptes* (rare), *Cheyletiella* spp. and *Otodectes* mites may cause facial crusting. These conditions are usually pruritic.

Clinical signs. Parasitic infestations may appear similar to each other. The cat usually demonstrates facial pruritus with excoriations on the head, face and neck. Depending upon the severity of the infestation, crusting may be mild to marked. Erythema, ulceration and secondary bacterial infections are common. *Notoedres cati* causes intense pruritus and scaling. Mites may also be found in the nailbeds. Ear mite infestations are usually less severe. Feline *Sarcoptes* infestations are relatively rare and may have some geographical variation in appearance. Feline cheyletiellosis is usually associated with generalised infestations; scaling and exfoliation on the dorsal surface of the cat's body is common.

Diagnosis. Definitive diagnosis is made by skin scraping and identification of the mite infestations. Mites are almost always found in *Notoedres cati* infestations but may not be found in feline scabies or in ear mite infestations because the pathophysiology of these diseases involves a Type 1 hypersensitivity response. In these cases, a presumptive diagnosis can often be made via response to therapy.

Treatment. These mite infestations are extremely susceptible to lime sulphur sponge-on dips (antifungal/antiparasitic), systemic ivermectin and pyrethrin sponge-on dips. Pyrethrin sprays have variable efficacy and should not be used when a response to therapy is being used as a diagnostic test. It is difficult to spray cats thoroughly without causing toxicity and severely annoying the cat.

Prognosis. Excellent.

Parasitic skin infestations causing generalised scaling

Description. Fleas, lice, *Cheyletiella* spp. and *Lynxacarus* spp. mite infestations can all cause diffuse scaling and crusting.

Clinical signs. Parasitic infestations can present with diffuse scaling and crusting of the hair coat and miliary dermatitis. The scaling may be due to the parasite (e.g. *Cheyletiella*) or to the response of the epidermis to the presence of the parasite. Pruritus is usually present but it may be absent in some cases of cheyletiellosis. The degree of scaling in these parasitic infestations varies from mild to severe. Hairloss is more common in flea infestations than in other parasitic skin infestations in cats. Lesions induced by fleas on cats may have a lumbosacral, neck or generalised distribution. *Cheyletiella* mite infestations classically have a dorsal distribution of lesions but commonly are generalised. In *Cheyletiella* mite infestations and lice infestations, the scale is a combination of parasites and egg sacs, which appear as white specks attached to hairs. Lice eggs or nits are much larger than the egg sacs of *Cheyletiella* mites. *Lynxacarus* mite infestations are similar in appearance to *Cheyletiella* infestations.

Diagnosis. Definitive diagnosis of all of these infestations is made by finding and identifying the parasites. Flea-combing and careful examination of the debris with a magnifying lens or dissecting microscope is the most cost- and time-effective diagnostic tool. Fleas and lice can be seen without magnification. *Cheyletiella* and other mites can be difficult to find in cats because of their fastidious grooming. Skin scrapings and adhesive tape preparations may be less reliable than flea-combing for locating these mites. In some cases, response to either flea control or antiparasiticidal therapy may be the diagnostic tool of choice.

Treatment. Specific therapy for these parasites is outlined in *Chapter 30*. *Cheyletiella* mites, lice and *Lynxacarus* are susceptible to ivermectin and to lime sulphur, in addition to most topical insecticides used to kill fleas. All in-contact animals must be treated.

Prognosis. The prognosis is excellent as these are not life-threatening diseases. Reinfestation from the environment is of concern with both fleas and *Cheyletiella* mites. The environment should be thoroughly cleaned and treated with a spray designed for environmental flea control. The owners should be warned about the zoonotic implications of fleas and *Cheyletiella* mites.

Dermatophytosis

Description. Feline dermatophytosis is most commonly caused by *Microsporum canis*. This

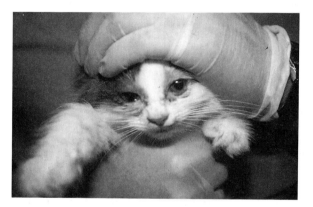

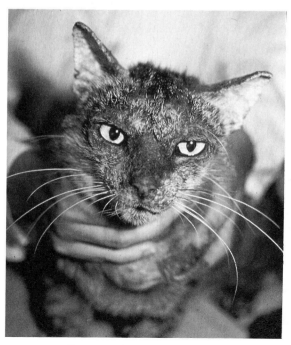

Fig. 15.6 Feline dermatophytosis.

organism invades growing hairs and the epithelium, causing hair-loss, and is the most common infectious cause of scaling. It is not part of the normal fungal flora of healthy pet cats. Strays, or kittens and cats from catteries and animal shelters with chronic dermatophytosis, pose the greatest public health risk. Young and debilitated cats are more prone to infection.

Clinical signs. Feline dermatophytosis is highly variable in clinical presentation. It is the author's opinion that fungal cultures should be performed for all cats with skin disease, particularly young cats, to determine whether dermatophytosis is a cause of skin disease. Clinically, cats present with varying degrees of hair-loss, scaling, and pruritus. Lesions in young cats tend to be more inflammatory. Early lesions usually begin on the face, ears and muzzle. Lesions are rapidly spread to other parts of the body via grooming and fomite exposure (infected bedding, brushes etc.). Early lesions may be difficult to see. As the lesions develop, hair-loss, scaling and erythema are common. Gross lesions of dermatophytosis may be focal, multi-focal or generalised. Pruritus is variable and the author has seen lesions of dermatophytosis that are clinically identical to eosinophilic plaques caused by flea infestations. Feline dermatophytosis can mimic miliary dermatitis, flea allergy dermatitis, symmetrical alopecia, pemphigus foliaceus (Fig. 15.7), hyperaesthesia and self-mutilation syndrome, and chronic conjunctivitis.

Diagnosis. Definitive diagnosis requires documenting the presence of the organism. This is done most time- and cost-effectively in practice via fungal culture. The details of making a diagnosis are discussed in *Chapter 3*.

Treatment. Treatment is discussed in detail in *Chapter 32*.

Prognosis. The prognosis for feline dermatophytosis is excellent because this disease is not life-threatening. There is, however, preliminary experimental evidence that inbred cats may have an inherited cell-mediated defect making them more susceptible to dermatophytosis and more difficult to cure.

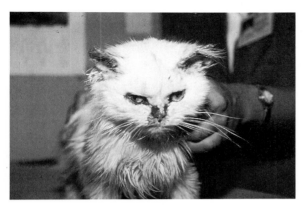

FIG. 15.7 Cat with pemphigus foliaceus.

Allergic skin diseases

Description. Cats with flea-allergy dermatitis, atopy or food allergy can develop exfoliative skin disease.

Clinical signs. Feline flea-allergy dermatitis, atopy and food allergy are described in detail under pruritic causes of feline skin disease (*Chapter 13*). The pruritus associated with these diseases may cause hair-loss, scaling and mild miliary dermatitis. Additionally, seborrhoea may be the only sign of feline atopy or food allergy in a small number of cases.

Diagnosis. See *Chapters 3* and *13*.

Treatment. See *Chapters 13* and *31*.

Prognosis. Allergic skin diseases are not life-threatening and the prognosis is excellent. The prognosis for control of the pruritus is much more variable, depending upon the cause and the ability to control the cat's pruritus.

Autoimmune skin diseases

Description. In general, autoimmune skin diseases are uncommon in cats. The diseases most likely to be encountered are feline **pemphigus foliaceus**, **pemphigus erythematosus**, **drug eruptions** and possibly **lupus erythematosus**. Feline pemphigus foliaceus and erythematosus are the most common of the autoimmune skin diseases. Pemphigus is caused by the development of autoantibodies

against the intercellular cement substance. When these autoantibodies bind to the intercellular cement, there is a loss of cell cohesion and the development of vesicles and pustules. The inflammatory mediators that are released are strongly chemotactic for neutrophils, which quickly migrate into the vesicles. The neutrophil-packed vesicles appear clinically as pustules; they rupture easily and are the source of the crusting.

Drug eruptions can be caused by a Type 1, 2, 3 or 4 hypersensitivity reaction. They can mimic auto-immune skin diseases and need to be differentiated from them. Lupus erythematosus is caused by a Type 3 reaction or immune complex reaction; it is extremely rare in cats and usually presents as a multisystemic disease.

Clinical signs. Clinically, pemphigus foliaceus and pemphigus erythematosus are very similar. The only difference is that the distribution of pemphigus erythematosus is limited to the head. Pemphigus foliaceus is more generalised and involves the head, neck, face, ears, paws and trunk (Fig. 15.7). Pustules will form in any area of the skin, but are most visible in the thinly haired areas. Pemphigus is characterised by symmetrical crusting. Nasal, periocular and inner pinnae crusting is very typical. Some cats will present with crusting on only the face and feet. The nailbeds may exude a black to green exudate or be thickly crusted. Intact pustules are most likely to be seen in the inner pinnae and around the mammae. Affected cats are often depressed and anorectic and have a marked lymphadenopathy. Pruritus is variable. In rare cases, cats will have lesions on the ears only for months before the disease becomes more generalised. These cats are often presented with the complaint of recurrent otitis externa.

Lupus erythematosus is a rare disease in cats. It is usually a multisystemic disease and the most common dermatological signs are marked exfoliation and mucocutaneous ulceration.

Diagnosis. Definitive diagnosis of an autoimmune skin disease in cats requires a skin biopsy. Biopsy selection is critical and many skin samples should be collected and submitted for routine histopathology. It is very important to remember **not** to scrub or wipe the skin biopsy sites: the crucial pathological changes are very superficial and are easily damaged. Cats may need to be hospitalized to get primary lesions. A very detailed history should be provided for the pathologist and, if possible, photographs of the patient should be included. Because pemphigus foliaceus can mimic dermatophytosis, a fungal culture should be performed on suspect patients. Ancillary diagnostic tests including impression smears of the exudate for acantholytic cells and bacterial culture and sensitivities should be undertaken to rule out these diseases (Plate 15).

Drug eruptions and lupus erythematosus are more difficult and costly to diagnose. If a drug eruption or lupus erythematosus is suspected, obtain a complete blood count, urinalysis, serum chemistry profile and antinuclear antibody test.

Treatment. Treatment of autoimmune skin diseases is outlined in *Chapter 31*. In general, drug eruptions in cats are treated by discontinuing the offending drug and administering any supportive therapy that is indicated. The use of glucocorticoids is highly controversial and of questionable value.

Prognosis. The prognosis for autoimmune skin diseases in cats varies from guarded to excellent depending upon the severity of the skin signs, the cat's response to therapy and the cat's tolerance for the immunosuppressive drugs used to control the signs. In most cases of pemphigus, the prognosis for a good quality of life is very good to excellent. The prognosis for lupus erythematosus is more difficult to predict. The prognosis for a drug eruption is also variable depending upon how severely affected the cat is and how quickly it recovers.

Temperature and humidity as causes of scaling

Description. The quality of an animal's hair coat is determined by a number of factors including nutrition, general health, grooming and the ambient temperature and humidity. Excessively warm temperatures and low humidity will dry the hair coat of cats housed indoors. Cats are notorious for sunbathing and for sleeping in front of forced-air heating vents: their universal heat-seeking behaviours will exacerbate the problem.

Clinical signs. Cats with this condition will have excessive scaling in their hair coat and may be mildly pruritic. Owners will often complain that the cat conducts excessive static electricity. This problem is usually one of house cats and is seasonal; it occurs during the winter months.

Diagnosis. A definitive diagnosis is made via the history and clinical signs and by eliminating cutaneous parasites from the differential diagnosis. Skin scrapings and flea-combings should be performed to look for *Cheyletiella* mites and fleas. A dermatophyte culture is indicated to rule out dermatophytosis.

Treatment. The most obvious treatment is to prevent the cat from sunbathing and from sleeping in front of or near heating vents but this presents practical difficulties. The owners should be instructed to increase the humidity in the home via a humidifier. If they do not have a humidifier, then containers of water can be placed near heating ducts to mimic the effects of a central humidifier. The owners can use a moisturiser on the cat's hair coat to decrease scaling and minimise the excessive conduction of static electricity. Most cats do not mind conducting static electricity as long as they do not get 'sparked' on the nose. Oil-free moisturisers work well and are very acceptable to both patient and owner.

Prognosis. The prognosis is excellent.

Systemic diseases

Description. Any systemic illness which affects a cat's health for a significant period can cause a change in the hair coat. The skin uses up to 30% of the cat's dietary protein intake each day to build and repair the epidermis and hair. Any disease that affects the cat's liver, kidneys or gastrointestinal tract will decrease available nutrients for the skin. Cats with hyperthyroidism commonly have excessively oily and scaly hair coats. Cats receiving inadequate nutrition, particularly those on 'fad owner diets' (e.g. vegetarian diets) are at risk. Pregnant and nursing queens will often have a very poor hair coat. In addition, cats infected with feline leukemia virus or feline immunodeficiency virus may have poor hair coats.

Clinical signs. The dermatological changes that are most common in cats with systemic illness include an oily and matted coat, excessive shedding and scaling. In most cases (but not always) the owners will report that the cat is grooming itself less than usual.

Diagnosis. Definitive diagnosis of 'poor grooming' in cats is relatively easy. The affected cat almost always shows clinical signs of illness. Attention should be directed at identifying the underlying systemic cause. Young cats with poor hair coats should be thoroughly examined for evidence of intestinal parasites, poor nutrition or FeLV/FIV. Older cats are much more likely to have liver, kidney or thyroid disease.

Treatment. Refer to a textbook of internal medicine for treatment of non-dermatological diseases.

Prognosis. The prognosis varies from poor to excellent depending upon the cause of the underlying skin disease.

Cutaneous neoplasia

Description. The most common cutaneous neoplasia in cats associated with excessive scaling is cutaneous lymphoma or cutaneous epitheliotropic lymphoma. In this neoplasia, there is an abnormal accumulation of T lymphocytes in the epidermis.

Clinical signs. The most common clinical signs are erythema, scaling and nodules in the skin. The lesions may be localised, but are most commonly generalised. Lymphadenopathy is common. The cat may be febrile, depressed or anorectic or it may be completely normal.

Diagnosis. Definitive diagnosis is made via skin biopsy. In addition, radiographs of the abdomen and chest and a bone marrow aspirate should be performed to determine the extent of the disease.

Treatment. To date, there is no satisfactory treatment for this disease in cats. Consult with a local veterinary oncologist for the most current treatment recommendations.

Prognosis. The prognosis for this disease is guarded.

16

Pustular Dermatoses

IAN MASON

Pustular dermatoses are seldom encountered in feline practice. Only few pustular disorders have been reported in this species and all of them are uncommon or rare (Fig. 16.1).

Pustules are spaces within the epidermis or immediately beneath it which are filled with inflammatory cells. They may develop from papules as a result of exocytosis of inflammatory cells into the epidermis. Pustule formation requires breakdown of adhesion between epidermal cells. Oedema and influx of inflammatory cells may lead to physical separation of the epidermis. Alternatively, intercellular bonds may be broken down by epidermolytic toxins from bacteria or by autoimmune mechanisms as in the pemphigus group of diseases. Pustules may contain micro-organisms such as bacteria or they may be sterile.

Feline pustular diseases are quite distinct clinically and diagnosis is usually based on microscopic examination of stained smears from lesions, bacterial and fungal culture and histopathology of biopsy material. History is of limited value in the diagnosis of these diseases (Fig. 16.2). This is partly because most of them are so rare that there are insufficient data on such risk factors as age, sex or breed incidence to enable clinicians to raise or lower the index of suspicion of a particular diagnosis on the basis of such criteria.

Skin Diseases Associated with Pustules

These disorders are discussed in detail elsewhere in the text, as shown in Fig. 16.1.

DIFFERENTIAL DIAGNOSIS OF FELINE PUSTULAR DERMATOSES	
Immune-mediated disease	Pemphigus group 　Pemphigus foliaceus (see *Chapter 15*) 　Pemphigus erythematosus (see *Chapter 15*) 　Pemphigus vulgaris (see *Chapter 17*) 　Lupus erythematosus (see *Chapters 15* and *17*) 　Drug eruption (see *Chapter 15*)
Bacterial disease	Chin acne (see *Chapter 15*) Bacterial folliculitis (see *Chapter 15*)
Contact allergy and irritant dermatitis	(see *Chapters 5* and *13*)

FIG. 16.1 Differential diagnosis of feline pustular dermatoses.

APPROACH TO FELINE PUSTULAR DERMATOSES: HISTORY	
Factor	**Differential diagnosis**
Contact with irritant, acidic or caustic substances	Contact irritant dermatitis

FIG. 16.2 Approach to feline pustular dermatoses: History.

APPROACH TO FELINE PUSTULAR DERMATOSES: PHYSICAL EXAMINATION	
Physical finding	**Differential diagnosis**
Pads affected	Allergic or irritant contact dermatitis
Paronychia	Pemphigus foliaceus
Lesions confined to face	Chin acne; pemphigus erythematosus
Fever;x systemic disease	Pemphigus foliaceus; systemic lupus erythematosus

FIG. 16.3 Approach to feline pustular dermatoses: Physical examination.

FIG. 16.4 Diagnostic plan for feline pustular dermatoses.

DIAGNOSTIC PLAN FOR FELINE PUSTULAR DERMATOSES

Focused diagnostic tests:

1. Microscopy of smears from pustules. Allows assessment of role of bacteria and other micro-organisms and may reveal immune cells and acantholytic cells (pemphigus)

2. Evaluate response to antimicrobial therapy. Resolution of lesions indicates that bacterial folliculitis is present

3. Histopathology of intact pustules may lead to a definitive diagnosis. Special stains may be indicated

17

Ulcerative Skin Lesions

KAREN MORIELLO

The terms **ulcer** and **erosion** refer to defects in the skin caused by inflammation, self-trauma or auto-immune or infectious processes. Clinically, ulcers and erosions are very similar. An ulcer is defined as a defect or loss of epidermis that extends to or beneath the basement membrane. An erosion only involves the loss of the most superficial layers of the skin. In this chapter, the term **ulcerative** will encompass both erosive and true ulcerative skin diseases (Figs 17.1 and 17.2, Plate 16).

Ulcerative skin diseases may be very subtle or dramatic in clinical appearance (Plate 16). Obvious ulcers are usually noticed by clients. Ulcerative diseases of the mucous membranes, especially the mouth, are often foul-smelling. When presented with a cat with ulcerative skin lesions, it is important to determine rapidly if the cause is self-traumatic, infectious, neoplastic, metabolic or auto-immune/immunological.

This chapter discusses, the diseases in which ulceration is a part of the pathogenesis and therefore, nearly always a clinical feature.

Selected Skin Diseases of Cats Characterised by Ulceration

Feline indolent ulcer

Description. Feline indolent ulcer is also referred to as a rodent ulcer or eosinophilic ulcer. The pathogenesis of this lesion is unknown, but an underlying allergic aetiology is suspected because it occurs very commonly in cats with food allergy, atopy, or flea allergy. Although an infectious aetiology has not been demonstrated, some lesions may be the result of a bacterial infection because they resolve with antibiotic therapy.

Clinical signs. Feline indolent ulcers occur most commonly on the upper lips (Plate 18). Lesions may be unilateral or bilateral. Clinically, they appear as a

DIFFERENTIAL DIAGNOSIS OF ULCERATIVE SKIN LESIONS IN CATS	
Focal areas	Feline indolent ulcer
	Feline eosinophilic plaque
	Sporotrichosis
	Feline idiopathic ulcerative dermatosis
	Spider-bites
Face and nasal lesions	Sporotrichosis and cryptococcoses
	Neoplasia (squamous cell carcinoma and lymphoma)
	Insect-bite hypersensitivity
	Drug eruptions
	Pemphigus complex
	Thermal injuries
Mucocutaneous	Uraemia
	Pemphigus vulgaris
	Systemic lupus erythematosus
	Drug eruptions
	Respiratory viruses (Herpes virus, calicivirus)
	Bacterial infections
Generalised	Miliary dermatitis
	Drug reaction
	Toxic epidermal necrolysis/erythema multiforme
	Infectious agents
	Cutaneous neoplasia
	Thermal injury

FIG. 17.1 Differential diagnosis of ulcerative skin lesions in cats.

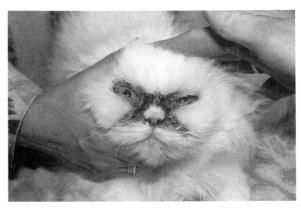

FIG. 17.2 Facial seborrhoea affecting a Persian cat. Close apposition of skin in facial folds leads to increased humidity, accumulation of skin secretions, maceration of the epidermis and secondary bacterial infection. Slide courtesy of Richard Harvey.

FIG. 17.3 Approach to cats with ulcerative skin disease: History.

APPROACH TO CATS WITH ULCERATIVE SKIN DISEASE: HISTORY	
Factor	**Differential diagnosis**
Age of onset 　　Less than 1 year 　　More than 5 years	Indolent ulcers Neoplasia
Pruritus before onset of lesion	Eosinophilic plaques due to allergy
History of 'sunbathing'	Solar damage; squamous cell carcinoma
History of drug exposure	Drug reaction; toxic epidermal necrolysis; 　　erythema multiforme; candidiasis
Signs of systemic illness	Systemic lupus erythematosus; uraemia/renal 　　failure
History of slow onset	Neoplasia; systemic fungal infection; 　　autoimmune skin diseases
History of abrupt/acute onset	Drug reactions, toxic epidermal necrolysis

FIG. 17.4 Approach to cats with ulcerative skin lesions: Physical examination.

APPROACH TO CATS WITH ULCERATIVE SKIN LESIONS: PHYSICAL EXAMINATION	
Physical finding	**Differential diagnosis**
Lesions in white or sun-exposed areas	Actinic dermatitis; squamous cell carcinoma
Destructive nasal lesions and/or nasal 　　discharge	Cryptococcus; squamous cell carcinoma
Focal ulcerative lesion on lips/gums 　　(symmetrical or asymmetrical)	Indolent ulcer
Focal ulcerative/exudative lesion dermatitis	Eosinophilic plaque; idiopathic ulcerative
Ulceration associated with sloughing of skin	TEN; thermal burn; SLE; cellulitis
Mucocutaneous ulceration	Uraemia, SLE; drug reaction

focal area of ulceration — the area appears to be 'melting away'. The margins may be slightly raised and the depressed crater may have a yellow hue. The ulcer may become large and may be very disfiguring to the cat. Indolent ulcers are most common in young cats but may occur in cats of any age. The sudden development of this lesion in an older cat is of concern because of the possibility of it mimicking a neoplastic process.

Diagnosis. Diagnosis is made most often via clinical signs. It is prudent to perform impression smears on these lesions to look for neoplastic cells. Lesions in cats that do not respond to conventional therapy should be biopsied.

Treatment. Because many of these lesions are single occurrences and owners are greatly distressed by the appearance of the lesion, the author treats all lesions first and pursues specialised diagnostic tests if the lesion recurs. These lesions are treated most commonly with glucocorticoids; injectable glucocorticoids are most popular and most effective, e.g. 20 mg/cat SC of methylprednisolone acetate every 2 weeks until the lesion is healed. It is unnecessary to perform intralesional injections, in the author's opinion, although some dermatologists feel this is very beneficial. Intralesional injections are painful and difficult to perform. Exudative acute lesions may respond to oral antibiotic therapy: trimethoprim potentiated sulphonamides 30 mg/kg *per os* twice daily. (See *Chapter 19* for more information.)

Prognosis. The prognosis is generally good. Most lesions will resolve within several months with appropriate therapy. Lesions that are recurrent or non-responsive to therapy require a skin biopsy to rule out other causes. Cats with recurrent indolent ulcers often have an underlying allergic disease and should be evaluated for food allergy, flea allergy and atopy. These lesions can be very difficult to resolve in some cats. Recurrent lesions are often associated with underlying allergic skin disease.

Feline eosinophilic plaque

Description. Feline eosinophilic plaque is a term used to describe a clinical lesion commonly seen in cats. Eosinophilic plaques are usually a clinical sign of an underlying allergic skin disease. They are also doscussed in *Chapter 19*.

Clinical signs. Eosinophilic plaques are focal areas of intense pruritus (Plate 19). The cat self-traumatises the pruritic area and hair-loss, exudation

---

DIAGNOSTIC PLAN FOR ULCERATIVE SKIN LESIONS

1. At the initial visit, determine if the cat has been traumatised or exposed to a caustic agent, or may have suffered a thermal injury

2. At the initial visit, consider the possibility of a systemic drug reaction. Cats most commonly develop drug reactions on their face but generalised drug reactions characterised by ulceration and sloughing of the skin do occur

> **Focused diagnostic tests**: Impression smears should be carried out to determine if infectious agents are present. If the specimen is very cellular, it should be examined closely for the presence of eosinophils, plasma cells and mast cells. These cells are very suggestive of an eosinophilic plaque or ulcer and an underlying allergic aetiology. Eosinophilic plaques or ulcers can develop quite suddenly and if the patient is receiving a systemic drug it could be difficult to differentiate the two, based on history and physical examination alone. If there is a recent drug history, discontinue any systemic or topical drugs for 3 – 7 days and re-examine the patient

3. If the lesion has developed acutely, determine if the cat is pruritic. If the cat is pruritic, there is a high probability that the lesion is an eosinophilic plaque. If pruritus is a strong component of the history, see *Chapter 13*

Focal Area of Ulceration

1. If there is a focal area of ulceration, consider the possibility of a feline indolent ulcer, feline eosinophilic plaque, sporotrichosis, spider-bite or feline idiopathic ulcerative dermatitis. Feline indolent ulcers classically occur on the lips and may be unilateral or bilateral. These lesions are most often diagnosed via clinical signs; however, squamous cell carcinomas can mimic these lesions. Eosinophilic plaques occur acutely and feline idiopathic ulcerative dermatitis is a relapsing chronic condition. Sporotrichosis can develop acutely; however, most cats present with non-healing wounds

> **Focused diagnostic tests**: Skin scrapings can be performed but *Notoedres cati* is the only parasite that is likely to be found to account for a focal area of ulceration. Flea-combing may reveal fleas as a potential cause of pruritus. The most important diagnostic test is an impression smear, which should be carefully examined for the presence of bacteria and fungal organisms, inflammatory cells, eosinophils and mast cells and neoplastic cells. Unfortunately, ulcerative neoplastic lesions are difficult to diagnose via impression smears because inflammatory cells are often predominant

2. If the skin scraping is negative, the next step will depend upon the results of the impression smear. If the impression smear is diagnostic (e.g. allergic aetiology), treat appropriately. If the impression smear is non-diagnostic, a skin biopsy is indicated

> **Focused diagnostic tests**: Perform a skin biopsy using a long elliptical excision. Histological examination of an ulcer is rarely diagnostic and skin biopsy punches sample too small an area for an accurate diagnosis. Diagnostic histological changes and infectious agents are often found at the margins. If the lesion is exudative, impression smears for Gram stain and acid-fast stains should be sent to the diagnostic laboratory or performed in-house. Depending upon the results of the biopsy and bacterial stains, wedge biopsies for culture may need to be submitted

Ulcerations of the Face and Nose

1. If lesions are limited to the nose, consider the possibility of neoplasia and infectious diseases, especially if a nasal discharge or sinusitis is present

> **Focused diagnostic tests**: The most cost-effective diagnostic approach is to perform impression smears and skin biopsies. Impression smears should be examined for the presence of infectious agents, especially *Cryptococcus*. Skin biopsies from several representative areas should be examined

2. If lesions include the nose and face, with or without the ears, consider the possibility of pemphigus, drug eruptions, neoplasia and insect hypersensitivity. Facial miliary dermatitis and eosinophilic plaques are also a consideration

> **Focused diagnostic tests**: Impression smears should be examined for infectious agents, inflammatory cells (eosinophils and neutrophils) and neoplastic cells. If the impression smears are non-diagnostic or do not strongly suggest a cause, a skin biopsy should be obtained

Mucocutaneous Ulcerations

1. A careful examination of the mucocutaneous junctions should be performed. If ulcerations are limited to the oral mucosa, consider gingivitis, stomatitis, uraemia/renal failure. The patient should be carefully examined to determine if signs of systemic illness are present

> **Focused diagnostic tests**: Serum urea nitrogen and creatinine concentrations should be determined to confirm the presence of uraemia and secondary ulceration

2. If the cat is not uraemic or if uraemia is not suspected, consider the possibility of an anaerobic infection, aerobic infection, viral infection, drug reaction, caustic agent/toxin, mucocutaneous candidiasis, pemphigus vulgaris or systemic lupus erythematosus. If an upper respiratory infection or conjunctivitis is present, infectious viral agents are highly likely. The latter are most common in young cats and/or cats with no history of vaccination and a strong history of exposure, i.e. stray cats

Continued

DIAGNOSTIC PLAN FOR ULCERATIVE SKIN LESIONS

Focused diagnostic tests: Because of the wide range of aetiological causes and the potential life-threatening nature of some of these diseases, skin biopsies are indicated at first presentation. Impression smears should be obtained for cytological examination and Gram stain. If large numbers of bacteria and degenerate neutrophils are present, anaerobic and aerobic bacterial cultures should be obtained. Conjunctival swabs may show inclusion bodies, which helps to diagnose infectious viral agents. General skin biopsies should be obtained. The cat should be carefully examined for the presence of vesicles or bullae. These lesions require biopsy via an elliptical excision under a short-acting anaesthetic agent. If these lesions are not visible, then a very wide elliptical excision including the ulcer and several millimetres of margin should be submitted for routine histopathology. If the patient is showing signs of systemic illness or if the mucocutaneous ulceration is severe and widespread, request haematology, serum biochemistry panel, urinalysis and antinuclear antibody test to determine if systemic lupus erythematosus is present. If the initial biopsies are non-diagnostic, the patient should be hospitalised and examined every few hours for the development of vesicles/bullae. These lesions are very transient and should be collected when seen

Generalised or Multifocal Areas of Ulceration

1. If there is generalised ulceration or multifocal areas of ulceration, consider pruritic skin diseases and the possibility of severe life-threatening skin disease. It is important at this point to determine, again, whether or not the cat is pruritic. Many cats with intense pruritus will cause severe self-trauma, with dramatic ulceration of the skin. Severe ulceration can also occur with thermal burns, drug reactions, TEN and EM, neoplasia and some cutaneous infectious agents

Focused diagnostic tests: Because of the severity of the lesions and the potential life-threatening nature, a rapid diagnosis must be established. Impression smears and *numerous* skin biopsies from a variety of skin sites should be obtained. If the impression smears show suspect infectious agents or sepsis, bacterial and fungal cultures should be obtained. Haematology, urinalysis, serum biochemistry panel and antinuclear antibody tests should be submitted if systemic lupus erythematosus is suspected

FIG. 17.5 Diagnostic plan for ulcerative skin lesions.

---

and ulceration are the result. The area is often thickened, exudative, crusted, ulcerated and erythematous. Miliary dermatitis is common in cats with eosinophilic plaques. Lesions may occur anywhere on the body but the face and neck are common areas.

Diagnosis. In most cases, a diagnosis is made via clinical signs. Impression smears will show an inflammation. Because these lesions are often secondarily infected, neutrophils and bacteria may be more readily seen on cytological inspection of an impression smear than eosinophils and mast cells. Skin biopsy is usually 'diagnostic' but it is important to remember that this is a clinical entity associated with an allergy: a diagnosis of 'eosinophilic plaque' is not an end-point. The vast majority of eosinophilic plaques are associated with flea allergy dermatitis. Recurrent eosinophilic plaques are suggestive of food allergy or atopy.

Treatment. Treatment of an eosinophilic plaque is a two-stage therapy. The first stage is to relieve the discomfort of the lesion. Management of these lesions is very similar to that of 'hot spots' or areas of pyotraumatic dermatitis in dogs. Cats with these lesions are intensely pruritic and will respond to the traditional therapy of glucocorticoids, e.g. 20 mg methylprednisone SC every 2 to 3 weeks until the lesion resolves. Alternatively, the author has found

that cats with markedly exudative lesions show a much better response to oral antibiotics for 2 to 3 weeks and an Elizabethan collar. The area should be gently cleansed with a chlorhexidine scrub and a mild antibiotic ointment applied to the area (e.g. mupirocin cream). The second stage of therapy is to determine the underlying cause of the eosinophilic plaque. Fleas and flea allergy dermatitis are the most common causes. Recurrent plaques are often the result of atopy and food allergy.

Prognosis. The prognosis for these lesions is excellent, provided that initial relief from the pruritus is supplied and the underlying cause is identified. Some early cases of feline idiopathic ulcerative dermatitis may begin as eosinophilic plaques (see below).

Feline idiopathic ulcerative dermatitis

Description. Feline idiopathic ulcerative dermatitis is a rare skin disease of cats. It occurs most commonly between the scapulae. The aetiology is unknown; however, it has been proposed that it is caused by a hypersensitivity to a subcutaneous injection of a vaccine or other medication. This syndrome has been seen in cats with no history of an injection at the site of the lesion and it is likely that the syndrome has multiple causes.

Clinical signs. Clinically, a focal ulcer develops at the site of the lesion (which is almost always between the shoulder blades). Owners report that the cat will mutilate this area, if allowed. The area may have a thick crust and the surrounding hair is often matted with debris. The site may feel thickened upon palpation. The area is usually painful to the cat and even mild sensations such as pin-pricking may evoke a strong negative response from the cat.

Diagnosis. Definitive diagnosis may be difficult. It is important to rule out the possibility that the lesion may be an eosinophilic plaque. Histological examination of a skin biopsy specimen may be the most useful aid. Dense infiltrates of eosinophils and mast cells are not present in lesions of ulcerative dermatitis but are very common in lesions of eosinophilic plaques. There is usually minimal inflammation in the dermis and some fibrosis may be seen.

Treatment. To date, there is no one effective therapy for these lesions. Intralesional glucocorticoids, antibiotics, buspirone, diazepam and wide surgical excision are all options, but have been unrewarding clinically in the author's experience. Most cases require some type of restraint device to keep the cat from traumatising itself.

Prognosis. The prognosis is guarded for a cure.

Sporotrichosis

Description. Sporotrichosis is an cutaneous fungal disease of cats that is caused by the dimorphic fungus, *Sporothrix schenkii* (Plate 20). In the skin, this organism is present in the yeast form. It is an opportunistic pathogen that invades the skin via a traumatic wound. The organism is common in garden soil and in sphagnum moss. The latter is commonly used by florists in ornamental plant designs. The author knows of two house-cats that developed sporotrichosis after the introduction of a potted plant containing this moss. The owner reported that the cats frequently dug in the potted plants and may have been exposed to the organism in this manner.

Clinical signs. Sporotrichosis most commonly occurs as an ulcerated non-healing wound in cats. The lesions may be acute or chronic. They often resemble eosinophilic plaques and will spread quite readily to the other areas of the body. Some cats will develop cutaneous nodules that ulcerate.

Diagnosis. This disease is readily diagnosed via an impression smear. However, it is advisable to submit several unstained air-dried slides to a diagnostic laboratory for confirmation. The organism is very pleomorphic and can appear as round to cigar-shaped intracellular organisms. It can also be diagnosed via skin biopsy and culture. Sporotrichosis is a reasonable differential diagnosis in indoor–outdoor cats with non-healing wounds.

Treatment. This disease is of serious zoonotic concern and infected cats should be hospitalised until the ulcerative lesions have healed and are no longer exudative and moist. Anyone handling the cat should wear long rubber gloves — preferably large-animal obstetric sleeves. This organism will readily penetrate open wounds in humans and create very painful and debilitating lesions. The treatment of choice is itraconazole (10 mg/kg once or twice daily). Therapy should be continued for at least 30 days. Itraconazole is well tolerated by cats, although some can become anorexic and depressed. Topical wound management is not necessary but, if desired, warm soaks of the lesions with gauze sponges soaked in 20% NaI are best. Systemic NaI is also an effective treatment but it is poorly tolerated by cats and is less effective than itraconazole.

Prognosis. The prognosis for cure is excellent. The major concern with treatment of this disease is the zoonotic implications.

Spider-bites and venomous insect-bites

Description. The inquisitive nature of cats makes them prime candidates for spider, centipede and millipede bites. In addition, wasps and other flying insects may also sting cats, usually in self-defence. In most cases, these bites are not life-threatening and often go unnoticed.

Clinical signs. Most cats are bitten on the face or paws. The initial bite may be swollen or slightly painful to the cat. Oedema and swelling may also be seen. If the bite occurs on the foot, lameness may be apparent. The bite may heal without being noticed by the owner. If the insect has injected a venom, an area of local ulceration or abscessation may develop. In rare cases, severe cellulitis and sloughing of the skin may occur.

Diagnosis. Unless the bite is observed, it is almost impossible to make a definitive diagnosis. A presumptive diagnosis may be made from the history, clinical signs and biopsy. Histologically, severe necrosis of the dermis with oedema, haemorrhage and vasculopathy are typical of toxic reactions. Inflammatory cells are common, but eosinophils are not typically very common.

Treatment. Lesions should be treated symptomatically. This may involve no therapy at all, antibiotic therapy or warm soaks.

Prognosis. The prognosis is good unless the bite severely damages facial tissue, interfering with eating and breathing.

Insect hypersensitivity

Description. Recently, flying and biting insects have been recognised as a cause of facial dermatitis in cats. This syndrome is most commonly recognised in cats that go outdoors, especially in the evening when mosquitoes and midges are present. The pathogenesis is believed to be due to a hypersensitivity reaction to the bite of flying insects. This disease is seasonal, occurring most commonly when these insects are prevalent.

Clinical signs. Cats with insect hypersensitivity have relatively symmetrical lesions on the face, ear tips, nose or footpads; the thinly haired areas are most commonly affected (Plate 21). The skin is pruritic and the cat traumatises itself. The ears, nose and face ulcerate and the lesions mimic autoimmune skin diseases. Cutaneous ulceration of the footpads is common. This clinical syndrome was described as a manifestation of the eosinophilic granuloma complex before the cause was recognised.

Diagnosis. Definitive diagnosis requires a skin biopsy. Histologically, skin biopsy specimens are very similar to what is described for inflammatory eosinophilic skin diseases of cats: perivascular accumulations of eosinophils and mast cells and collagen necrosis. In many cases, a presumptive clinical diagnosis can be made via history, clinical signs, season of exposure and response to treatment. Lesions will resolve if the cat is housed indoors for several weeks, however many owners will request more aggressive therapy. This disease will respond to oral or systemic anti-inflammatory doses of glucocorticoids.

Treatment. Housing the cat indoors is the best permanent treatment and the best preventive measure. This disease is very responsive to oral or systemic glucocorticoids. Injectable methylprednisolone (20 mg/cat every 2 weeks until the lesions resolve) is very effective. If owners cannot or will not house their cat indoors, the cat should be sprayed with a flea spray that contains a repellent before being allowed outdoors. Alternatively, the cat could be housed indoors during the early evening and morning hours when it is most likely to be bitten. Unfortunately, due to the nature of cats, they tend to frequent areas in gardens and fields that will expose them to biting insects all day.

Prognosis. The prognosis is excellent as this is not a life-threatening disease.

Drug eruptions (also see TEN and EM)

Description. Cutaneous drug eruptions can be caused by immunological (Type 1–4 hypersensitivities) and non-immunological mechanisms. Drug eruptions are unpredictable and can occur with the administration of even very small amounts of topical, oral, or parenteral drugs.

Clinical signs. There are many clinical presentations of drug eruptions in cats, including urticaria, maculopapular eruptions, erythroderma, exfoliation, vesicular-bullous eruptions, lichenoid eruptions, erythema multiforme and toxic epidermal necrolysis. The most common site for cats to exhibit cutaneous drug reactions is on the face, particularly in the preauricular area. In cats, the most life-threatening are erythema multiforme (EM) and toxic epidermal necrolysis (TEN). These reactions are acute and often involve the mucous membranes. Early signs include a rash, fever, malaise, and vesicles in the mucous membranes. As the inflammatory process continues the skin may develop full-thickness sloughs and ulceration. This may occur anywhere on the body.

Diagnosis. Definitive diagnosis can be difficult. The most compelling clinical findings are the sudden development of lesions, the history of exposure to a systemic drug, and the absence of other reasonable differential diagnoses. In some drug reactions, skin biopsy may be diagnostic, e.g. EM and TEN. A skin biopsy is recommended in all cases.

Treatment. The cornerstone of treatment is early recognition of the possibility of a drug reaction and the withdrawal of the offending agent. The lesions should be managed as open wounds. Silver sulphadiazine cream is an effective antibacterial agent that can be used to keep wounds moist. In severe reactions where there is marked sloughing of the skin,

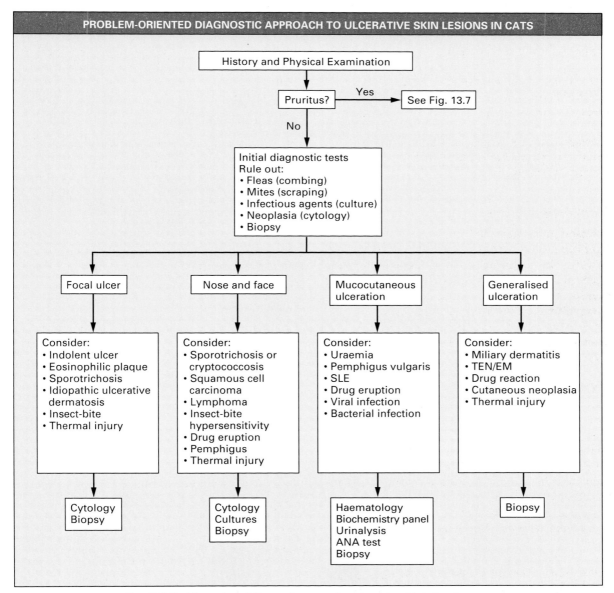

FIG. 17.6 Problem-oriented diagnostic approach to ulcerative skin lesions in cats.

systemic antibiotics may be useful and necessary. Fluids, electrolytes and parenteral nutrition may be necessary in some cats. To date, the use of systemic glucocorticoids is highly controversial. The use of glucocorticoids is only clearly indicated in patients that are rapidly deteriorating and are in shock.

Prognosis. The prognosis is guarded in all cases of cutaneous drug reactions.

Mucocutaneous ulceration secondary to uraemia

Description. Cats with renal failure, diabetes mellitus or feline hyperadrenocorticism can present mucocutaneous ulceration because of uraemia. Cats with severe life-threatening autoimmune skin diseases also may develop prerenal azotaemia.

Clinical signs. Refer to an internal medicine textbook for a detailed description of feline diabetes mellitus and hyperadrenocorticism. Cats with systemic illnesses causing stomatitis or ulceration usually have fetid breath and oral ulcerations. Signs of systemic illness (anorexia, depression, dehydration etc.) are usually obvious. In some serious autoimmune skin diseases, e.g. systemic lupus erythematosus and drug eruptions, prerenal azotaemia can develop. It can be difficult to distinguish these diseases based upon clinical signs alone.

Diagnosis. Minimally, serum creatinine and blood urea nitrogen concentration tests should be determined in cases where uraemia is suspected. More appropriately, cats presented with mucocutaneous ulceration should be carefully evaluated with a complete serum chemistry panel, complete blood count, urinalysis and antinuclear antibody test.

Treatment. Refer to an internal medicine textbook.

Prognosis. Variable depending upon severity, response to treatment and underlying cause.

Viral causes of mucocutaneous ulceration

Description. Feline Herpes virus, calicivirus, rhinotracheitis, feline immunodeficiency virus and leukaemia virus can cause mucocutaneous ulcerations in cats.

Clinical signs. Mucocutaneous ulcerations caused by feline Herpes, rhinotracheitis and calicivirus are usually accompanied by signs of conjunctivitis and upper respiratory infection. Cats infected with either FeLV or FIV may have stomatitis and gingivitis along with numerous other clinical signs.

Diagnosis. Reliable serological tests are available for FIV and FeLV infections. Most cases of feline Herpes, calicivirus or rhinotracheitis virus can be diagnosed tentatively on the basis of history and clinical signs. Virus isolation is possible but it is neither practical nor cost effective in a clinical practice situation. Cats with these latter infections are usually young or strays with no history of vaccination.

Treatment. There is no specific treatment. Supportive care should be administered as needed.

Prognosis. Ulcerations heal very quickly on the mucous membranes of animals. Cats that can be supported adequately usually do well. Cats with FeLV or FIV infections have an uncertain prognosis due to the nature of these infections.

Pemphigus vulgaris

Description. Pemphigus vulgaris is a very rare autoimmune skin disease of cats. In this disease, autoantibodies bind to desmosomes and cause intercellular damage. This results in the formation of intraepidermal vesicles, bullae and pustules. In pemphigus vulgaris, this reaction tends to be localised to the mucocutaneous junctions.

Clinical signs. This disease results in large fragile vesicles and bullae that rupture creating erosions and ulcers. These ulcers may occur at any mucocutaneous junction — mouth, genitals, eyelids and nose. It is possible that lesions may extend into the oesophagus and the lips may also be involved. Because of the pain from the ulcers, affected cats are often anoretic and depressed. This disease may be clinically indistinguishable from systemic lupus erythematosus and epitheliotropic lymphoma.

Diagnosis. Definitive diagnosis requires an excisional skin biopsy of an intact vesicle or bulla. These lesions are very fragile and should be obtained immediately when they are seen. A short-acting anaesthetic agent should be administered to the cat to facilitate obtaining the specimen. Histologically, pemphigus vulgaris is characterised by a suprabasilar cleft leading to the formation of a bulla. These clefts may extend into hair follicles if samples are taken from junctional areas of hair and non-haired skin. The classic 'row of tombstones' or rounded basal cells at the base of the cleft may be visible. Many specimens will have secondary inflammation present. Additionally, a complete blood count, serum chemistry panel, urinalysis and antinuclear antibody (ANA) test should be performed to help differentiate this disease from systemic lupus erythematosus.

Treatment. Treatment of pemphigus vulgaris is described in *Chapter 31*.

Prognosis. The prognosis is variable. There have been so few cases of feline pemphigus vulgaris reported that it is difficult to comment accurately on the outcome of the disease. Management, especially in the early stages, is time-consuming and costly if extensive nursing care is needed.

Systemic lupus erythematosus

Description. Systemic lupus erythematosus (SLE) is a rare autoimmune skin disease caused by the deposition of antigen–antibody complexes in the tissues. It is a multisystemic disease with a wide variety of clinical presentations.

Clinical signs. This disease is rare in the cat but Siamese cats may be predisposed. Mucocutaneous ulceration with or without cutaneous erythema, scaling, crusting, depigmentation and alopecia may be seen. Ulcers may be seen on the footpads, as well as on the oral mucosa and skin. The face, ears and legs are most commonly affected. In addition to skin signs, other organs may be involved causing lameness, anaemia, kidney failure, liver failure, weakness or anorexia.

Diagnosis. Definitive diagnosis is made by ruling out other causes of the skin disease. A skin biopsy, ANA test, complete blood count, urinalysis and serum chemistry panel should be performed on suspect cases. Additional diagnostic tests, e.g. radiographs and joint aspirates, may be necessary in some cases. The histological findings in systemic lupus erythematosus are variable. In some cases, the skin biopsy specimens are non-diagnostic. Classically, there is a lichenoid band of inflammation at the basement membrane. Basal cell vacuolation and vesiculation may be present in some cases.

Treatment. Treatment of SLE can be complicated and difficult; referral to a specialty care clinic may be indicated for initial management (*Chapter 31*).

Prognosis. The prognosis is guarded. This disease is not curable and although most cases can be medically managed to provide a reasonable quality of life for the cat, relapses are common.

Skin Diseases Causing Generalised Ulceration

Cats presenting with generalised ulcerations are extremely rare in clinical practice. One common clinical syndrome that can be mistaken for generalised ulceration is **miliary dermatitis**. Many clients will describe miliary dermatitis as widespread multifocal ulcerations of the skin, and in some cases it may appear that this is the case. Miliary dermatitis is easily recognised clinically and is discussed in *Chapter 19*.

Generalised ulceration *not* caused by miliary dermatitis of the skin of cats is a life-threatening condition (Plate 22). The potential causes include drug eruptions, TEN/EM, burns, neoplasia and infectious agents. It is critical to establish a diagnosis as quickly as possible and stabilise the patient. Skin biopsies, impression smears, a complete blood count, ANA test, urinalysis and a serum chemistry profile panel should be obtained immediately upon presentation. The skin biopsy, impression smears and ANA test should narrow the differential diagnosis list. The other fluid analysis tests will help to determine what type of supportive care is necessary.

Hydration and electrolytes in patients with widespread ulceration need to be monitored. If the cat is eating and drinking, intravenous fluids are not necessary. The protein and fluid losses from the wounds are remarkably great and these cats should be fed a very high-protein and calorie-dense diet. Wounds can be managed in a wide variety of ways but at initial presentation open wound management techniques are preferred, until the patient is stable and the cause is determined. Initially, the wound should be cleansed with sterile saline. When flushing wounds, care should be taken to avoid creating pockets of dead space that will collect fluid and harbour bacterial growth. The wound should be kept moist and covered. This may be difficult in some cats. Silver sulphadiazine cream is an excellent antibacterial cream used in burn patients but unfortunately it will clump on the skin and collect debris if used without an occlusive bandage. Sterile non-stick gauze pads and appropriate wrapping can be used over the cream. If this is not possible, pre-packaged, sterile, gel-impregnated bandage dressings may be used. These are expensive and they may adhere to the edges of the wound and be difficult to remove. An inexpensive alternative is sterile gauze sponges impregnated with petroleum jelly or simply sterile petroleum jelly to protect the wound until a decision on wound closure can be made. Refer to surgical texts for more information on wound management.

18

Nodules, Non-Healing Wounds and Common Skin Tumours

KAREN MORIELLO

A **nodule** describes any mass that is present in the skin or subcutaneous tissue. A **non-healing wound** is any wound that does not heal within the expected period of time after appropriate conventional therapy (medical or surgical).

Nodules, tumours and non-healing wounds in cats are less common than other skin diseases, e.g. eosinophilic lesions but they are usually more serious in nature. Nodules and non-healing wounds can be caused by infectious or parasitic agents,

DIFFERENTIAL DIAGNOSIS OF NODULAR AND NON-HEALING WOUNDS IN CATS	
Bacterial	Cutaneous bacterial granuloma Actinomycosis and nocardiosis Staphylococcal furunculosis (chin acne) Cat-bite abscess Opportunistic mycobacterial infections Feline leprosy
Fungal	Kerion Mycetoma and pseudomycetoma Phaeohyphomycosis Cryptococcosis Blastomycosis Histoplasmosis Coccidioidomycosis Sporotrichosis Miscellaneous opportunistic algae and fungi
Hypersensitivity reactions	Arthropod-bite granulomas Eosinophilic granulomas and lesions
Parasites	Arthropod-bite granulomas Cuterebra larvae
Immune-mediated	Sterile nodular panniculitis Sterile nodular granuloma and pyogranuloma Plasma cell pododermatitis
Neoplasia	Round cell tumours Epithelial tumours Spindle cell tumours Feline pox
Miscellaneous	Foreign bodies Cutaneous xanthoma Fragile skin syndrome

FIG. 18.1 Differential diagnosis of nodular and non-healing wounds in cats.

foreign bodies, or neoplasia. Appropriate therapy requires a definitive diagnosis, which is impossible to make by simple clinical examination alone. The diagnostic approach and aetiologies for nodules and non-healing wounds are similar. The most useful and cost-effective diagnostic tests are cytological examination of tissue imprints, skin biopsies and cultures.

Selected Skin Diseases Characterised by Nodular and/or Non-Healing Wounds

Eosinophilic granulomas and plaques

Eosinophilic granulomas and plaques are discussed in detail in *Chapters 17* and *19*. Eosinophilic plaques usually have an underlying allergic aetiology and are usually more ulcerative than nodular; however, they can present as non-healing 'wounds'. Eosinophilic granulomas are true granulomas via histological criteria. These lesions probably have an underlying allergic aetiology and are often present in association with an eosinophilic plaque or ulcer.

Mosquito-bite hypersensitivity

This disease can look like a non-healing wound on the nose/face (see *Chapter 17* and Plate 21 for details).

Arthropod-bite granuloma

Description. Nodular lesions at the site of a bite or sting of various arthropods are relatively common. The most common arthropod to cause these reactions are **ticks**. The reaction is believed to be due to a Type 4 hypersensitivity reaction to the bite.

Clinical signs. These lesions are not commonly reported by clients because they are not easily

FIG. 18.2 Approach to nodules and non-healing wounds: History.

APPROACH TO NODULES AND NON-HEALING WOUNDS: HISTORY	
Factor	**Differential diagnosis**
Breed	Certain types of tumours (see *Appendix*) Pseudomycetomas — long-haired cats
Age of onset More than 5 years	Tumours
History of trauma	Foreign body; opportunistic fungal or bacterial organism
Travel to areas with endemic diseases	Deep fungal; leishmaniasis
Outside cat	Trauma; foreign body; tick-bites; cat-bites
Systemic signs of illness	Systemic fungal; opportunistic fungal; bacterial; algae; neoplasia
History of diabetes mellitus and/or megestrol acetate	Cutaneous xanthoma

FIG. 18.3 Approach to nodules and non-healing wounds: Physical examination.

APPROACH TO NODULES AND NON-HEALING WOUNDS: PHYSICAL EXAMINATION	
Physical finding	**Differential diagnosis**
Fever; signs of systemic illness	Systemic mycoses; opportunistic infectious agents; systemic neoplasia
Ocular disease	Lymphosarcoma; systemic mycoses
Solitary lesion	Foreign body; abscess; cutaneous neoplasia; arthropod-bite granuloma

Multiple lesions, with or without exudation	Deep pyoderma; systemic mycoses;
	  opportunistic infectious agent panniculitis;
	  actinomycoses; nocardiosis; sporotrichosis;
	  fungal mycetoma or pseudomycetoma;
	  feline leprosy; cutaneous xanthoma

Acute lesions with inflammation	Fungal kerion; foreign body; abscess neoplasia

Slowly developing lesion with minimal
  inflammation
	Fungal mycetomas; opportunistic infectious
	  agents; foreign bodies; neoplasia; atypical
	  mycobacterial infections

Lesions on footpads	Plasma cell pododermatitis; eosinophilic granuloma

FIG. 18.4 Characteristics of nodules and non-healing wounds in cats.

CHARACTERISTICS OF NODULES AND NON-HEALING WOUNDS IN CATS	
Mixed inflammatory infiltrate with increased eosinophils	Eosinophilic granulomas and diagnosis Arthropod-bite granuloma Mosquito-bite hypersensitivity Spider-bites Plasma cell pododermatitis
Mixed inflammatory infiltrates with neutrophils predominating	Foreign body reaction Cutaneous xanthoma Fungal kerion Opportunistic fungi and algae infection Systemic fungal infections Actinomycoses and nocardiosis Opportunistic mycobacterial infection Cutaneous leishmaniasis Panniculitis Feline leprosy Feline pox
Neutrophilic infiltrate	Staphylococcal infection Streptococcal infection Cat-bite abscess

DIAGNOSTIC PLAN FOR NODULES AND NON-HEALING WOUNDS

When presented with a cat with the problem of nodular lesions or non-healing wounds, the most important task is to determine if the aetiology is infectious or neoplastic. Because many of the diseases that cause nodular or non-healing lesions are potentially life-threatening, efforts should be directed at rapidly answering that question. The most useful in-house diagnostic screening tool is cytological examination of the nodule or wound

1. Perform a fine needle aspirate, impression smear of exudate, tissue imprint or scraping of the margin of the lesion. Collect at least three or four specimens. The slides should be stained with a quick stain and examined under increasing magnification

2. Determine the predominant cell population of the specimen. Infectious and inflammatory skin diseases are characterised by the presence of obvious numbers of inflammatory cells (neutrophils, macrophages, eosinophils, other cells). Neoplastic skin diseases are characterised by very cellular specimens with homogeneous cell types

Specimen Contains Predominantly Inflammatory Cells

Estimate the approximate percentage of neutrophils and mixed inflammatory cells in the specimen (macrophages, neutrophils, plasma cells, lymphocytes, other cells)

1. If the specimen contains 80–90% neutrophils, the most likely causes are infectious diseases. The presence of large numbers of degenerate neutrophils strongly suggests a bacterial aetiology. The most common cause of a neutrophilic exudate in the cat is an abscess. Depending upon the patient's clinical history and physical examination, no further diagnostic testing may be needed at this point. If the presentation is atypical or the lesion is recurrent, continue as described

> **Focused diagnostic tests:** Obtain additional cytological specimens, if necessary, for Gram stain and special staining and search for an organism. If no infectious agent is found or suspected, submit an aerobic bacterial culture. If lesions are rapidly progressing, the patient is debilitated, or clinical impression warrants it, submit a biopsy at the initial examination. In general, however, biopsies are not usually necessary at initial examination unless cultures and cytological examination do not identify a pathogen

2. If the specimen contains a mixed inflammatory cell population consisting of neutrophils, macrophages and other cells, determine whether or not eosinophils are prominent in the specimen

3. If eosinophil numbers are increased in the specimen, the most likely causes are hypersensitivity and/or parasitic skin disease

> **Focused diagnostic tests:** Skin scrapings should be performed to rule out demodicosis and nematode infestations. Skin biopsy is required for a definitive diagnosis

4. If eosinophil numbers are not increased and neutrophils are prominent with macrophages, consider bacterial, fungal, parasitic and non-infectious inflammatory causes

> **Focused diagnostic tests:** The most cost-effective approach at this point is to submit several representative cytological specimens with a skin biopsy to an appropriate reference laboratory. Ideally, cultures for aerobic and anaerobic bacteria and deep fungal organisms should be submitted at the time the biopsy is collected. If there are cost constraints, it is acceptable to wait for the pathology report before submitting cultures provided that the cat is not systemically ill or rapidly deteriorating. If a definitive diagnosis is not made or if the histological report indicates a pyogranulomatous pattern of inflammation, tissue should be submitted for aerobic, anaerobic and fungal culture. It is critical to remember to ask the pathologist to perform special stains at the initial processing or else there may be a delay in making a definitive diagnosis. In most reference laboratories, special stains are not routinely performed unless requested

Specimen not Containing an Inflammatory Cell Population

1. If the specimen is acellular without a marked predominance of tissue cells, re-aspirate the specimen and/or perform a skin biopsy. Neoplasia or an infectious disease process cannot be ruled out

2. If the specimen is very cellular and contains a homogeneous tissue cell population, strongly consider neoplasia. Small to medium-sized individual cells with discrete borders are suggestive of round cell tumours. Large round, oval or caudate cells in sheets or clumps are suggestive of epithelial tumours. Small to medium cells with spindle shapes and tails of cytoplasm are suggestive of spindle cell tumours

> **Focused diagnostic test:** Unless confident with the cytological diagnosis, e.g. mast cell tumour or lymphoma, perform a skin biopsy for a definitive diagnosis

FIG. 18.5 Diagnostic plan for nodules and non-healing wounds.

found in the skin. The initial lesion usually begins with swelling and erythema at the site of the bite. A firm nodule forms in the skin at the site. The most common site in the cat is the head and shoulder region and probably represents areas where it is difficult for cats to remove ticks.

Diagnosis. Definitive diagnosis requires a skin biopsy but a clinical diagnosis alone may suffice if the history is strongly supportive of a known arthropod-bite at the site.

Treatment. In general, lesions will spontaneously regress and no treatment is required. If necessary, oral prednisolone (0.5–2.2 mg/kg/day for 7 to 10 days) is curative.

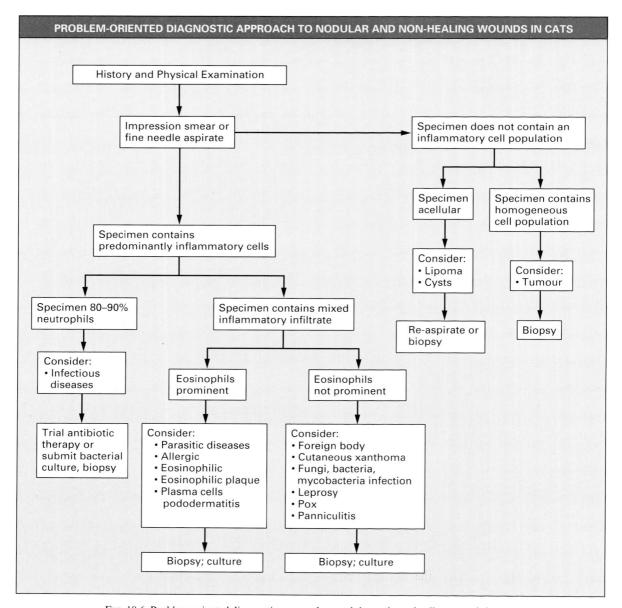

FIG. 18.6 Problem-oriented diagnostic approach to nodular and non-healing wounds in cats.

Prognosis. The prognosis is excellent.

Spider-bites

Description. Spider-bites are rarely documented in veterinary medicine. Geographical location will dictate which species of spider are venomous. Although cats frequent woodpiles, basements and vacated buildings, they are rarely presented for spider-bites.

Clinical signs. Clinical signs may vary from non-detectable to nodular lesions, to widespread tissue necrosis. The face and forelegs are most commonly affected. Erythema and swelling are present at the site of most bites. Marked swelling, vesicles and skin necrosis can occur within 6–12 hours of the bite depending upon the species. Systemic reactions to spider-bites may include salivation, nausea and diarrhoea, ataxia and convulsions. These signs may occur within 6–48 hours of the bite.

Diagnosis. Definitive diagnosis is difficult unless there is a strong supporting history of a known bite in the affected area. Histological findings are non-specific and may be compatible with severe vasculitis, severe bacterial infection, severe foreign body reaction, arthropod-bite granuloma and other infectious diseases.

Treatment. Treatment includes supportive care and appropriate wound management.

Prognosis. This depends upon the clinical signs exhibited by the patient. However, if life-threatening signs are not observed the prognosis is good.

Plasma cell pododermatitis

Description. Plasma cell pododermatitis is a relatively rare skin disease of cats. It is thought to have an immune-mediated or allergic aetiology but the exact pathogenesis is unknown.

Clinical signs. This disease affects multiple footpads. The larger footpads are more commonly affected by a uniform swelling. The footpads often have a silvery, cross-hatched appearance to them from the swelling. In general, the cat is not lame. In severe cases, the footpads may ulcerate and drain a haemorrhagic fluid. Affected individuals should be carefully examined for the possible coexistence of plasma cell stomatitis or renal disease.

Diagnosis. Definitive diagnosis is made via skin biopsy. A deep wedge biopsy from an affected footpad should be submitted; do not submit punch biopsies because they are rarely deep enough to be diagnostic. Histologically, the normal dermis and adipose tissue of the footpad are infiltrated with plasma cells. Neutrophils may be present if there has been ulceration and secondary inflammation.

Treatment. Treatment is not always necessary because many cats are asymptomatic and the disease may spontaneously regress. If the cat is lame or treatment is deemed necessary, a series of therapies may be required before the lesions go into remission. Initial therapy with 4.4 mg/kg s.i.d. of prednisolone is recommended. Lesions may not resolve for several weeks. Once the lesions have resolved, the dose

of prednisolone can be gradually tapered. If there is no response to prednisolone, chrysotherapy is an alternative. See *Chapter 31*.

Foreign body reactions

Description. Foreign body reactions are caused by the penetration of a variety of foreign material but most commonly organic and plant matter, cactus spines, porcupine quills, fibreglass, gravel and grass awns. Additionally, a foreign body reaction can occur at the site of retained suture material, ruptured hair follicles (keratin is very inflammatory in the skin) and malicious acts, for example rubber bands placed on extremities or air gun pellets. Air gun pellets will often take hair with them into the subcutaneous tissue.

Clinical signs. The very early stages of foreign body penetration are rarely observed by either the veterinarian or owner. Mild erythema, a small wound and exudation may be present. As the foreign matter penetrates into tissue via muscular movement, a host reaction develops. A nodule, draining tract or non-healing wound at the entry site develops. Secondary bacterial infections are common and furunculosis may develop, especially with interdigital foreign body reactions. Secondary infections with *Staphylococcus*, *Nocardia* and *Actinomyces* spp. are common.

Diagnosis. Definitive diagnosis requires finding evidence of the foreign material. This may be via exploration of tracts and removal of the material or via skin biopsy. It is critical to inform the pathologist that a foreign body reaction is suspected so that the specimen is examined with special stains and polarised light. The latter helps to identify keratin and fibreglass particles. In some cases, radiographs and fistulograms may be needed to locate the foreign body.

Treatment. Effective treatment requires a thorough search for all of the penetrating material and its removal. Because of the risk of secondary infections, the exudate should be cultured and appropriate antibiotic therapy instituted. Foreign body reactions due to keratin are difficult to treat because keratin is so inflammatory in tissue and impossible to remove surgically. Chronic recurrent deep pyoderma on the chin is a common sequela to ruptured hair follicles in cats.

Prognosis. The prognosis is excellent for patients in which a solitary foreign body is found and removed, provided that no secondary bacterial infections are present. The prognosis for cats with chin furunculosis due to foreign body reactions from keratin or dirt is guarded. Occasionally, cats with chronic chin furunculosis have atopy or a fungal mycetoma.

Cutaneous xanthoma

Description. Cutaneous xanthomas are granulomatous reactions caused by the deposition of cholesterol and triglycerides in tissue macrophages. This occurs when there are abnormally elevated levels of plasma cholesterol and triglycerides. In cats, this has been observed in individuals with spontaneous diabetes mellitus or diabetes mellitus secondary to megestrol acetate, and hereditary hyperchylomicronaemia and also in individuals with no detectable underlying cause, i.e. idiopathic.

Clinical signs. Xanthomas may be single or multiple and appear as white to yellow plaques and/or nodules in the skin. Some masses ulcerate and will drain an inspissated, caseous, necrotic material. The most common sites are the footpads, face, trunk and bony prominences.

Diagnosis. Definitive diagnosis requires a skin biopsy. Histologically, macrophages with foamy cytoplasm are visible in large sheets. Cholesterol clefts and small numbers of neutrophils may be present. Special stains show lipid in the macrophages.

Treatment. There is no specific treatment for the xanthomas. Therapy should be directed at identifying and treating the underlying metabolic abnormality.

Prognosis. The prognosis is good if the underlying metabolic disease is treatable and controllable. The cutaneous xanthomas will spontaneously resolve in several months.

Fungal kerion

Description. A fungal kerion is an acute inflammatory lesion caused by a dermatophyte. The most commonly isolated dermatophyte is *Microsporum gypseum*. Fungal kerions can occur with any of the dermatophytes but they are most common with the geophilic organisms.

Clinical signs. There is no age, breed or sex predilection; however, cats that spend a great deal of time outdoors are at increased risk. Fungal kerions are also more common in warm climates. The typical lesion usually occurs on the nose or extremity and is alopecic, exudative and erythematous. Lesions are usually solitary but they may be multiple, especially on the feet, and they may be painful or pruritic.

Diagnosis. Definitive diagnosis requires a biopsy. Fungal cultures are usually negative because of the intense inflammation at the lesion site. Most lesions are markedly improved, if not totally resolved, by the time the histopathology report is received.

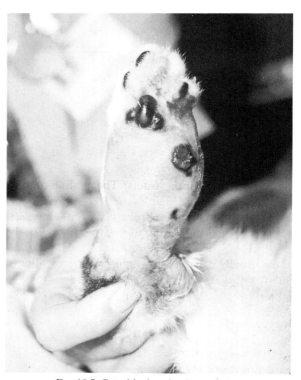

FIG. 18.7 Cat with phaeohyphomycosis.

Treatment. Lesions are self-curing and require no treatment. Some cats will benefit from warm compresses and antibacterial scrubs to remove crusting debris. Topical antifungal ointments, creams or gels are not usually necessary.

Opportunistic infections with fungi and algae

Description. There are many miscellaneous cutaneous infections of the skin with opportunistic fungi and algae. The various terms used to subdivide or subclassify these infections include mycetoma and phaeohyphomycosis (Fig. 18.7). **Mycetomas** can be caused by either bacteria or fungi and are characterised by swelling, exudation, draining tracts and the presence of tissue granules (usually microscopic). In cats, mycetomas can also be caused by dermatophytic fungi, *Microsporum canis*, and are commonly referred to as a 'pseudomycetoma'. **Phaeohyphomycosis** and **zygomycosis** are clinically indistinguishable from mycetomas. Phaeohyphomycosis is caused by dematiaceous fungi (pigmented fungi), such as *Alternaria*, *Drechslera* and *Curvularia*. It is relatively rare and is most common in tropical and semi-tropical regions. Almost all of these infections are caused by traumatic inoculation of the organism into the skin or exposure of traumatised skin to contaminated soil or water.

Clinical signs. The clinical signs of infection depend upon whether or not the organism has a tendency only to invade the skin and subcutaneous tissues or to spread systemically. Most of the organisms that cause mycetomas and phaeohyphomycosis produce only cutaneous or subcutaneous infections. Infection is most common on the extremities and usually presents as slowly developing nodules with draining tracts. The nodule/tumour is usually cool and painless to the touch, which helps to differentiate it from bacterial abscesses. Occasionally, small granules may be present in the exudate. Animals with systemic opportunistic infections usually present with signs of systemic illness, such as weight-loss, lethargy, fever, and respiratory signs (coughing, nasal discharge). Concurrent systemic involvement is most common with *Aspergillus*, *Pacilomyces*, *Prototheca* and *Phythium* spp.

Diagnosis. Definitive diagnosis requires a skin biopsy and culture of a wedge of tissue for bacteria and fungi.

Treatment. Definitive identification of the organism is necessary to determine whether or not treatment is possible. In the rare instance of bacterial mycetomas, antibiotic therapy is usually very effective combined with surgical excision. Unfortunately, most of the organisms that cause fungal mycetomas and phaeohyphomycosis are not susceptible to the systemic antifungal agents that are currently available. Effective therapy requires surgical excision, and amputation in many instances. No successful therapy is known for systemic opportunistic fungal, algal, or phythiosis infections. The development of newer antifungal agents may be promising as potential therapies. Dermatophytic mycetomas caused by *M. canis* are best treated with surgical excision and systemic antifungal therapy (*See Chapter 32*).

Prognosis. Prognosis for localised opportunistic infections is poor to guarded. The prognosis for systemic opportunistic infections is grave.

Systemic fungal infections

Description. The systemic mycoses are fungal infections that invade internal organs and then disseminate secondarily to the skin. In rare instances, these organisms may involve only the skin. The systemic mycoses include *Blastomyces dermatitides*, *Coccidioides immitis* and *Histoplasma capsulatum*. Inhalation of spores from contaminated environments is the most common route of infection. *Cryptococcus neoformans*, *Paecilomyces* spp., *Candida albicans* and *Aspergillosis* spp. can also causes systemic mycoses in debilitated hosts. Systemic fungal infections are rare in cats.

Clinical signs. Systemic signs of illness include fever, weight-loss, lethargy, coughing, nasal discharge, diarrhoea, neurological signs and ocular signs. The cutaneous lesions usually present as nodular to ulcerated lesions that may be solitary or multiple. Early lesions may begin as patches of erythema that quickly develop into nodular lesions, which ulcerate. Regional lymphadenopathy is common and often dramatic.

Diagnosis. Definitive diagnosis can often be made via cytological examination of exudate. Organisms of blastomycosis, coccidioidomycosis, histoplasmosis and cryptococcoses are very characteristic in appearance. Skin biopsy may also be definitive. Culture of infected tissue, skin biopsy and serum fungal titres are the best triad of diagnostic tests when an infective agent is not easily identified on cytologic examination of exudate.

Treatment. Systemic antifungal therapy is the treatment of choice for these infections. (Refer to the references for a detailed discussion of treatment options.) Therapy is time-consuming and expensive and a thorough familiarity with antifungal drugs, complications of use and ancillary therapy is necessary and beyond the scope of this book. Referral to a veterinary specialist may be indicated. Prior to the initiation of therapy, a careful and complete physical examination, including an ophthalmological examination, is necessary to determine the full scope of the infection.

Prognosis. The prognosis is guarded.

Actinomycosis and nocardiosis

Description. Infections with *Actinomyces* spp. and *Nocardia* spp. are rare and are usually the result of trauma with penetrating wounds, especially foreign bodies such as quills and grass awns. Cutaneous nocardiosis may develop secondary to pulmonary nocardiosis in debilitated hosts.

Clinical signs. Infections for both of these organisms take weeks to months to develop. Systemic signs of fever, weakness, lethargy, pyothorax, dyspnoea, and neurological signs may be present in nocardiosis. Cutaneous lesions begin as granulomas that may progress to subcutaneous abscesses and cellulitis, with ulcerated nodules and draining tracts. Fine granular material may be present in the exudate. The exudate of nocardiosis is brownish red and has been described as 'tomato soup'.

Diagnosis. Definitive diagnosis can be made via cytological examination of exudate, bacterial culture, and skin biopsy. *Actinomyces* spp. are Gram-positive, non-acid-fast filamentous anaerobic rods. *Nocardia* spp. are Gram-positive, partially acid-fast, branching filamentous aerobes.

Treatment. Effective therapy depends upon locating and removing any penetrating foreign body, if

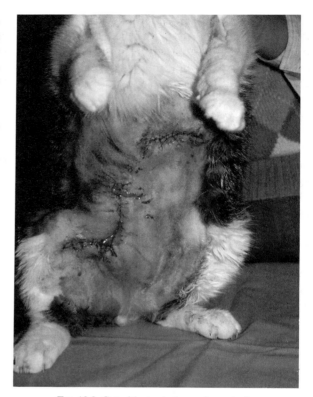

FIG. 18.8 Cat with atypical mycobacteriosis.

one is present. Actinomycosis can be treated with penicillin (100,000 units/kg/day), sulphonamides (10 mg/kg b.i.d.) or trimethoprim-potentiated sulphonamide (30 mg/kg b.i.d.). Nocardiosis is not particularly responsive to penicillin. Effective therapy requires surgical drainage of the lesion and several months of effective antibiotic therapy based upon culture and sensitivity.

Opportunistic mycobacterial infections

Description. Opportunistic mycobacterial infections refer to several species of atypical mycobacteria than can cause cutaneous infections. These organisms are atypical because they are rapid growers on laboratory media when compared with other groups of mycobacterial organisms. The most commonly isolated atypical Mycobacterium are *Mycobacterium fortuitum*, *M. chelonei* and *M. smegmatis* (Fig. 18.8, Plate 17). These organisms are free-living and are found in soil and standing water.

Clinical signs. Many cats with these infections have a history prior treatment for cat-bite abscesses and surgery to remove abscessed or necrotic fat. These organisms are inoculated into the skin via a traumatic injury and subsequent contamination of the wound with soil or water harbouring the organism. The infection takes weeks to months to develop. The hallmark of this infection is a chronic, non-healing, recurrent abscessing wound with draining tracts and fistulas (Fig. 18.8). Lesions may occur anywhere but these organisms have a predilection for the inguinal region. Systemic signs are usually absent.

Diagnosis. Definitive diagnosis is made by finding the acid-fast organisms in smears, culture and/or skin biopsy. These organisms can be extremely difficult to find because large numbers are not usually present in the skin. The most cost-effective approach is to submit several unstained air-dried tissue imprints for acid-fast staining, several large deep wedges of tissue for culture and several large sections of tissue for skin biopsy. It is important to remember that tissue for culture or biopsy should not be collected with a skin biopsy punch, but rather a deep wedge incision using a scalpel blade. The organisms tend to be found in the deep dermis/panniculus and a skin biopsy punch may collect too superficial a sample to be fruitful. The laboratory should be told that these organisms are suspected, to ensure that they are cultured appropriately.

Treatment. Lesions usually regress spontaneously but this may take months to years. Wide surgical excision coupled with antimicrobial therapy is the treatment of choice. Antibiotic therapy should be based upon culture and sensitivity. Some newer antimicrobial agents have been very effective in the treatment of this disease. Clofazimine (8–12 mg/kg *per os* once daily), ciprofloxacin (10–15 mg/kg *per os* b.i.d.) and enrofloxacin (5 mg/kg *per os* b.i.d.) have been reported as effective therapies.

Prognosis. The prognosis is guarded to good depending upon response to therapy.

Cutaneous leishmaniasis

Description. Leishmaniasis is a rare multisystemic disease with cutaneous manifestations. It is caused by the obligate intracellular protozoa, *Leishmania* spp. The organism is transmitted by sandflies of the genera *Lutzomyia* and *Phlebotomus*. The infection begins in the skin and then disseminates to internal organs.

Clinical signs. The most common clinical signs are a non-pruritic exfoliative dermatitis. Nodules and ulcers occur as the disease progresses. Symmetrical lesions on the face characterised by periorbital rings of alopecia and scaling are common. Depigmentation of the planum nasale may occur. Peripheral lymphadenopathy is common. Systemic signs of infection include fever, malaise, weight-loss, muscle atrophy, coagulopathy, polyarthritis and renal failure.

Diagnosis. Definitive diagnosis requires identification of the organism in macrophages. Organisms may be found in fine needle aspirates of peripheral lymph nodes, bone marrow or spleen. The organism may also be cultured in specialised diagnostic laboratories. An indirect fluorescent antibody test is available but it is only diagnostic for *Leishmania donovani*. Positive titres indicate exposure to the organism, not active infection.

Treatment. Several agents are available for the treatment of leishmaniasis; it is recommended that in the US National Center for Disease Control be contacted before initiating therapy to ensure that the most current therapy is used. All of these agents are expensive and potentially toxic, and there is no guarantee that the agent will be eliminated from the body. Sodium stibogluconate (10–50 mg/kg) and meglumine antimonate (100 mg/kg) are the two most commonly used drugs. Both are administered daily by by IV, IM or SC injection. Itraconazole may also be effective against this agent.

Prognosis. The prognosis is poor because relapses are common.

Panniculitis

Description. Panniculitis is inflammation of the subcutaneous fat and this disease is rare in the cat. The most important task a veterinarian has when trying to evaluate a patient with a nodule in the subcutaneous fat is to determine the aetiology:

infectious, neoplastic or sterile (idiopathic). Fat necrosis may occur secondary to and surrounding neoplasias. In cats, vitamin E deficiency or pansteatitis is of special concern when there have been questionable feeding practices.

Clinical signs. Clinically, panniculitis is most common on the dorsal trunk, but lesions may extend to the extremities. Depending upon the clinical syndrome, lesions may be solitary or multiple and firm to fluctuant. Large nodules may rupture a haemorrhagic exudate or a thick, oily discharge. Scarring is common and this may cause the skin to become tightly adhered to the underlying tissue. Hair may or may not regrow in severely affected areas, depending upon the damage to the hair follicles. Systemic signs may include fever, anorexia, depression and lethargy. Cats with pansteatitis are commonly painful and systemically ill.

Diagnosis. Definitive diagnosis of the cause of panniculitis is expensive and time-consuming. The most cost-effective test to perform initially is a skin biopsy, provided that the results of skin biopsy can be obtained within a few days. This will allow you to determine whether or not neoplasia is present. If you suspect a delay or if the cat is showing systemic signs and the nodules are rapidly developing, the nodules should be cultured at the time of first examination. Because the lesions are so deep in the skin, samples for histopathological examination should not be collected with a skin biopsy punch. It is preferable to submit an entire nodule for examination. If the nodule is larger than 0.5 cm, it should be transected in several planes to allow for adequate fixation. If it is not possible to submit an intact nodule, then a deep wedge of tissue should be submitted. It is critical to inform the pathologist that you are interested in ruling out infectious agents. Intact nodules should be submitted for aerobic, anaerobic and deep fungal culture. If neoplasia and infectious agents are ruled out, it is cost-effective to screen the cat for systemic lupus via an ANA test, complete blood count, serum chemistry panel and urinalysis. If these tests are normal or negative, the most likely diagnosis is sterile nodular panniculitis.

Treatment. Treatment depends upon the aetiology. Sterile nodular panniculitis may be treated surgically if there is a solitary lesion or just a few lesions that can be removed surgically. In most cases, however, systemic glucocorticoids are necessary. Prednisolone (2 mg/kg *per os* once daily) is administered until the lesions completely resolve, which is usually in 4–8 weeks. Therapy should be stopped at this point as some cats will remain in remission. Adjunct vitamin E (400 IU *per os* b.i.d.) has been useful as an adjunct or single therapy agent in some cats.

Prognosis. The prognosis for sterile nodular panniculitis is good but there may be permanent scarring of the skin and permanent hair-loss.

Feline leprosy

Description. Feline leprosy is a rare disease caused by an acid-fast bacterium with an unknown mode of transmission. The infectious agent is believed to be transmitted via bites from infected cats or rats but some researchers have speculated that fleas, mosquitoes and ticks may also transmit the disease.

Clinical signs. Lesions are most commonly seen on the head extremities. Lesions usually begin as single or multiple nodules that gradually increase in size. Ulceration of larger nodules is common. The lesions are asymptomatic. Regional lymphadenopathy is common. Young cats that go outside are most commonly affected.

Diagnosis. Definitive diagnosis requires a skin biopsy and a bacterial culture for atypical Mycobacterium. Intact nodules should be submitted or a deep wedge biopsy and culture. If granulomatous inflammation and acid-fast organisms are present, feline leprosy and atypical mycobacteriosis are the most likely differential diagnoses. A diagnosis of feline leprosy can be made if the bacterial culture for atypical mycobacteria is negative.

Treatment. Clofazimine (2–3 mg/kg once daily for 30–60 days) has been reported as effective. Surgical removal is also curative in some cases.

Prognosis. The prognosis is good.

Feline poxvirus infection

Description. This newly emerging skin disease of cats was first identified in the late 1970s. It is now accepted that the causative agent is a species-specific poxvirus. Outbreaks of the disease have been limited to Europe.

Clinical signs. There is no age, sex, or breed predilection for the infection. Lesions usually appear as multiple, well-circumscribed lesions that develop into crusted papules, plaques and nodules. Some authors describe craters and ulcer-like lesions. The face, paws and dorsal lumbar areas are most commonly affected. Individuals may or may not show signs of systemic illness including fever, anorexia, lethargy, pyrexia, vomiting, diarrhoea, conjunctivitis, dyspnoea and jaundice.

Diagnosis. Definitive diagnosis requires a skin biopsy, serological testing and/or virus isolation. In practice, skin biopsies and serology are most cost effective and available. Histologically, ballooning degeneration and eosinophilic intracytoplasmic inclusion bodies are characteristic.

Treatment. Cats will recover spontaneously. Signs of systemic illness should be treated symptomatically. As with all infectious skin diseases, glucocorticoids are contraindicated.

Sterile granuloma and pyogranuloma syndrome

Description. This disease syndrome encompasses a relatively common group of diseases all characterised by granulomatous skin lesions that are sterile. Histologically, the disease is manifested by a marked histiocytic infiltrate of the skin. It is believed that the cause may be immune dysfunction associated with persistent antigenic stimulation. This disease is rare in the cat.

Clinical signs. Lesions may develop in cats of any age. Nodules or plaques ranging in size from 0.5 cm to 2 cm that are firm, well demarcated and partially alopecic are most common. Lesions usually occur first on the muzzle and spread to the trunk and distal extremities. Lesions may wax and wane, are non-pruritic and do not rupture. Systemic signs are usually absent.

Diagnosis. See comments for panniculitis. It is critical to rule out infectious agents and neoplasia

as the cause of the nodules since therapy involves the use of immunosuppressive drugs.

Treatment. The treatment of choice is oral prednisolone (1–2 mg/kg once daily) until lesions completely resolve, usually in 3–4 weeks. Alternate-day therapy should be continued for an additional 2–3 weeks. It may or may not be possible to discontinue therapy because lesions commonly recur. An alternative therapy for this disease is native or PEG-L-asparaginase. This is a chemotherapeutic agent that is administered via intramuscular injection once weekly. Lesions usually resolve within three to four treatments and the disease can be kept in clinical remission using intermittent therapy (once or twice monthly treatments). The dose is 10,000 IU per treatment. This is an excellent alternative therapy for this disease because the drug has few side-effects and is easy to administer. Unfortunately, the drug is expensive.

Cat-bite abscess

Description. This is one of the most common medical problems of cats that go outside or live in multi-cat households.

Clinical signs. Affected cats may or may not be systemically ill depending upon the severity of the abscess. Cats with abscesses that have not spontaneously ruptured will present with fever, depression, anorexia and soreness/pain in the site of the abscess. Frequently, two small puncture wounds and/or scabs from the bite may be found in the area of the abscess. The face, extremities, tail base and inguinal region are commonly affected. Intact male cats are more commonly affected.

Diagnosis. In most cases, a definitive diagnosis is made via history and clinical signs. Cytological examination of the exudate will reveal septic inflammation. Further diagnostics are not necessary unless the abscess does not respond to conventional therapy. These lesions respond rapidly to therapy; lesions not responding to therapy require aggressive diagnosis (e.g. culture biopsies). In those rare instances, additional cytological smears should be examined and bacterial cultures and skin biopsies submitted for analysis.

Treatment. Effective therapy requires that the abscess be incised, flushed with large quantities of sterile water or a dilute antibacterial solution, and then allowed to drain. Owners may elect to apply warm compresses to the lesion but however most cats will prefer to groom the area themselves and remove any exudate. Antibiotic therapy is not necessary in every case but, if used, should be for 5–7 days. Amoxicillin is an excellent and inexpensive choice. Castration will decrease the incidence of fighting.

Prognosis. The prognosis is excellent but many cats become chronic 'victims' and may require confinement to the home.

Fragile Skin

Spontaneous tears in the skin of cats are rare. Fragile skin syndrome may be caused by feline hyperadrenocorticism, cutaneous asthenia or drug eruptions (Plate 23). Feline hyperadrenocorticism is most commonly seen in older cats, although the author has seen one cat with iatrogenic hypercortisolaemia that had fragile skin. Cutaneous asthenia (Ehlros-Danlos syndrome), a hereditary skin disease, is usually clinically evident in younger cats. The hallmark of cutaneous asthenia is very stretchy or extendable skin. As the cat ages, spontaneous ruptures will occur. These cats are often put down at the owner's request or die of aortic rupture. Drug eruptions that cause acute necrosis of the skin or dermal oedema may cause the skin to be fragile.

Tumours

Cytological specimens devoid of inflammatory cells and comprised of cellular homogeneous cell populations are very suggestive of skin tumours, either benign or malignant. A definitive diagnosis is best obtained via a skin biopsy. See the *Appendix* for a summary of pertinent clinical information on tumours in cats.

19

Eosinophilic Skin Diseases

IAN MASON

Feline eosinophilic skin diseases (formerly known as the **eosinophilic granuloma complex**) include three very common conditions which affect the skin and occasionally the oral cavity of cats:

- Eosinophilic or indolent ulcers (see also *Chapter 17*).
- Eosinophilic plaques (*Chapter 17*).
- Eosinophilic collagenolytic ('linear') granulomata.

There is histological evidence that **feline miliary dermatitis** now called **papulocrustous dermatitis** is similar to eosinophilic plaque although the lesions are smaller and crusted. Papulocrustous dermatitis is another cutaneous reaction pattern, rather than a specific disease. It may be associated with pruritus, scaling and crusting and ulceration. Reference to this syndrome will therefore be found in the relevant sections of this book (see Fig. 19.2). The differential diagnosis and management of eosinophilic plaque and miliary dermatitis are almost identical.

The eosinophilic dermatoses are not diagnoses in themselves; they are simply skin reaction patterns (as are canine pyoderma and keratinisation disorders). In most instances the eosinophilic diseases are secondary to an underlying primary disease.

Nomenclature of the Eosinophilic Skin Diseases

The term 'eosinophilic granuloma complex' is no longer used for these diseases as only the eosinophilic collagenolytic granulomata are happily described by this term. Histologically so-called 'eosinophilic' indolent ulcers may be devoid of eosinophils and show no evidence of granuloma formation. Similarly, eosinophilic plaques show no evidence of granuloma formation although tissue eosinophilia is a feature. Despite the widely differing histological appearances of these disorders, it is still convenient for clinicians to consider them as a group as their aetiology, diagnosis and management are so similar. This poses the question of what to call the group. One authority has made the

DIFFERENTIAL DIAGNOSIS OF FELINE EOSINOPHILIC SKIN DISEASES	
Hypersensitivity	Flea-bite hypersensitivity Food intolerance/hypersensitivity Atopic dermatitis Insect (mosquito) hypersensitivity Endoparasite hypersensitivity
Ectoparasites	*Cheyletiella* spp. infestation (esp. *C. blakei*) Otodectic mange Pediculosis (*Felicola subrostratus*) *Notoedres cati* infestation *Trombicula autumnalis* infestation *Lynxacarus radovsky* infestation
Infectious causes	Bacterial
Other causes	Genetic factors

FIG. 19.1 Differential diagnosis of feline eosinophilic skin diseases

CAUSES OF PAPULOCRUSTOUS (MILIARY) DERMATITIS	
Infectious	Dermatophytosis Bacterial folliculitis Viral infections
Parasitic	Fleas Lice *Cheyletiella* *Otodectes* *Trobicula* (chiggers) *Notoedres* and *Sarcoptes* (rare) *Demodex* Cat fur mite Endoparasites
Allergic	Flea-bite hypersensitivity Mosquito and biting fly hypersensitivity Atopy Food allergy Drug reactions
Miscellaneous causes	Nutritional Epitheliotropic lymphoma Immune-mediated skin disease Idiopathic

FIG. 19.2 Causes of miliary dermatitis.

tongue-in-cheek suggestion of 'eosinophilic granuloma confusion'; the authors of this book will use the term '**eosinophilic skin diseases**'.

Aetiology and Pathogenesis

The vast majority of cases of eosinophilic skin disease in cats result from inflammation — typically hypersensitivity reactions, ectoparasitism or both. Genetic factors may be involved in some instances and it has been suggested that bacteria may be involved in some cases.

Inflammatory skin diseases in cats are associated with a cellular infiltrate rich in mast cells and eosinophils. Mast-cell degranulation in tissue leads to the release of a wide range of inflammatory mediators and other substances. Some of these substances are chemotactic for eosinophils. However,

eosinophils are also attracted to parasites, micro-organisms and immune-complexes. Eosinophil granules contain substances with various activities, the net effects of which are to reduce inflammation and to damage parasites. Other eosinophil products damage collagen, leading to collagenolysis.

Numerous primary feline dermatoses are associated with the development of eosinophilic disease (Fig. 19.1). Many of these primary disorders have also been shown to lead to other patterns of feline skin disease such as papulocrustous dermatitis, alopecia and pruritus as well as eosinophilic skin disease. However, it is not possible to predict which pattern a particular cat will develop. Cats may exhibit more than one of these patterns or more than one eosinophilic disease, either simultaneously or at different times. Comparison of Fig. 19.1 with Fig. 13.4 will show many disorders common to

DIAGNOSTIC PLAN FOR FELINE EOSINOPHILIC SKIN DISEASE

History and Clinical Examination

Diagnosis is often evident on clinical signs although other disorders such as ulcers and granulomatous lesions due to micro-organisms, foreign bodies and neoplasia (see *Chapters 17* and *18*) should be considered as possible causes

Focused diagnostic tests: Microscopy of skin scrapings and impression smears. Unstained skin scrapings examined under low power will enable the elimination of ectoparasites from the differential diagnosis. Stained scrapes or impression smears will identify neoplastic cells and possibly infectious micro-organisms. Eosinophilic diseases will usually have numerous eosinophils present but secondary bacterial infection may complicate the picture and neutrophils and bacteria may predominate. **Histopathology** is a definitive means of establishing a diagnosis of eosinophilic skin disease in cats. However, this should not be regarded as a specific diagnosis; the underlying factors listed in Fig. 19.1 should be diligently investigated

Investigate Underlying Causes

The approach to the investigation of inflammatory diseases such as ectoparasitism and hypersensitivity which lead to eosinophilic skin diseases is covered in detail in *Chapter 13*

FIG. 19.3 Diagnostic plan for feline eosinophilic skin disease.

CLINICAL MANIFESTATIONS OF FELINE EOSINOPHILIC DERMATOSES

Disease	Clinical signs	Diagnosis	Comments
Eosinophilic/indolent ulcer (*Chapter 17*)	Ulceration of upper lip	Clinical signs Histopathology	In older cats, must differentiate this from neoplasia
Eosinophilic plaque	Self-trauma; hair-loss; exudation; ulceration; thickened skin. Affects the face, neck, abdomen and medial thighs	Clinical signs Histopathology Cytology	Intense pruritus. Very similar in clinical behaviour to feline papulo-crustous dermatitis
Collagenolytic granuloma	Variable. Classically: Linear raised alopecic, yellow-to-erythematous bands. Especially affects posterior aspect of hind-limbs but can occur elsewhere. Alternatively: Papules, nodules, plaques. Bridge of nose, oral cavity, feet, pinnae. Lesions: Swollen, firm; on chin	Clinical signs Histopathology	

FIG. 19.4 Clinical manifestation of feline eosinophilic dermatoses.

both. Figure 19.3 shows a diagnostic approach to the eosinophilic dermatoses.

Clinical Manifestations of Eosinophilic Skin Disease

Figure 19.4 summarises the clinical and diagnostic features of these disorders. Feline eosinophilic (or indolent) ulcers and feline eosinophilic plaque are discussed in detail in *Chapter 17*.

Eosinophilic collagenolytic (or linear) granulomata

Description. Eosinophilic granulomata primarily affect young cats, with females more commonly being affected. There are no breed predilections. The eosinophilic granuloma is the only one of the three patterns of eosinophilic skin disease that is characterised by true granuloma formation and collagenolysis.

Clinical signs. The lesions can vary considerably in appearance. The 'classic' lesion is the raised linear, yellow-to-erythematous lesion extending along the posterior aspect of the hindlimbs. Some individuals may present with such linear band-like lesions elsewhere on the body. Alternatively, the lesions may be circumscribed papules, nodules or plaques affecting the bridge of the nose (as in mosquito-bite hypersensitivity), oral cavity, feet, pinnae or perianal area. In some instances collagenolytic granulomata may be present as firm, palpable nodules affecting the rostral aspect of the chin.

Diagnosis. In most cases, the diagnosis is clinical, especially where linear granulomata are present. Impression smears are helpful but secondary infection may complicate the results with neutrophils and bacteria being more common than eosinophils. Histopathology will confirm that an eosinophilic collagenolytic granuloma is present; this obligates the clinician to search for the underlying cause.

Treatment. Ideally, these lesions are managed by identification and correction of the underlying cause. The treatment of idiopathic cases is discussed in *Chapter 31*.

Prognosis. The prognosis varies depending on the underlying cause. Cases resulting from food or flea hypersensitivity have an excellent prognosis, whereas idiopathic cases may require long-term symptomatic management.

Diseases Leading to Feline Eosinophilic Skin Disease

Hypersensitivity

Flea-bite hypersensitivity, food intolerance/hypersensitivity, atopic dermatitis and endoparasite allergy are discussed in detail in *Chapter 13*. Eosinophilic skin diseases have been reported following insect-bites. Two particular phenomena are recognised:

- mosquito-bite hypersensitivity affecting the bridge of the nose and leading to eosinophilic collagenolytic granulomata
- flea-bite hypersensitivity, leading to eosinophilic plaque.

Insect hypersensitivity is discussed in more detail in *Chapters 5, 17 and 18*.

Ectoparasitism

These disorders are discussed in detail in *Chapter 13*.

Bacterial Disease

No pathogenic bacteria other than contaminants have been isolated from eosinophilic lesions. However, there have been anecdotal reports in which indolent ulcers and eosinophilic collagenolytic granulomata have responded to systemic antimicrobial therapy. There have been no controlled studies and it is conceivable that the response is not solely due to the effect of the drug on bacteria, but that there may also be an anti-inflammatory effect resulting from the use of such drugs.

Genetic Factors

Although the majority of cases of eosinophilic skin disease in cats are due to hypersensitivity or ectoparasitism, there have been reports that genetic factors may be involved. Studies on a colony of related specific pathogen-free cats, which exhibited all three manifestations of eosinophilic skin disease, showed that atopic dermatitis and food allergy were not involved. The colony was free of fleas and other parasites. Evidence was found which suggested a heritable mode of transmission and it was proposed that these lesions can develop spontaneously in genetically predisposed cats.

One of the authors of this text has seen a number of Turkish Van cats in the UK with linear granulomata. No primary disease has been identified and, in view of the extremely limited gene pool of this breed in this country, it is possible that genetic factors are involved.

Treatment of Idiopathic Cases of Feline Eosinophilic Dermatoses

Traditionally, treatment has been based on the use of oral or systemic glucocorticoids. Recently there has been increasing evidence that some cases are responsive to antibiotics. Therefore, there is an argument for evaluating response to antibiotics before using glucocorticoids. The management of feline eosinophilic diseases is covered in detail in *Chapter 31*.

20

Cutaneous Manifestations of Systemic Disease

KAREN MORIELLO

Many skin diseases are either cutaneous markers of systemic disease or are associated with systemic signs. These diseases are summarised in Figs 20.1–20.9. The reader is referred to the text and bibliography for more detailed information.

CUTANEOUS AND SYSTEMIC SIGNS OF DISEASES CAUSED BY IMMUNE-MEDIATED DISEASES		
Disease	**Cutaneous signs**	**Systemic signs**
Atopy	Chronic pruritus, alopecia, excoriations of face, abdomen and legs	In rare cases, associated with signs consistent with feline asthma
Food hypersensitivity	Pruritus of face, abdomen, legs	Gastrointestinal signs, vomiting, diarrhoea
Pemphigus complex	Symmetrical crusting of face, ears, trunk, footpads, paronychia	Fever, depression, lameness, anorexia
Pemphigus vulgaris	Mucocutaneous ulceration, oral ulceration	Fever, anorexia, depression, pain in mouth
Systemic lupus erythematosus	Mucocutaneous ulcers, scaling, footpad ulcers, ear margin necrosis	Fever, depression, anorexia, thrombocytopenia, polymyositis, pericarditis, myocarditis, neurological signs, lymphadenopathy
Vasculitis	Purpura, haemorrhagic bullae, necrosis of skin, ulcers	Fever, depression, anorexia, pitting oedema, polyarthropathy, myopathy
Toxic epidermal necrolysis	Acute onset of vesicles, bullae and necrosis of skin. Epidermis will slough. Mucocutaneous junctions, footpads and oral mucosa are most commonly affected	Fever, anorexia, lethargy, cutaneous pain, depression
Relapsing polychondritis	Swollen, erythematous ears; curled deformed ears	Fever, lameness, can mimic SLE
Feline hypereosinophilic syndrome	Generalised maculopapular erythema, severe pruritus, marked excoriation	Fever, depression and signs associated with organ specific infiltration of eosinophils

FIG. 20.1 Cutaneous and systemic signs of diseases caused by immune-mediated diseases.

CUTANEOUS AND SYSTEMIC SIGNS OF DISEASES CAUSED BY BACTERIAL ORGANISMS		
Disease	**Cutaneous signs**	**Systemic signs**
Subcutaneous abscesses	Hard to fluctuant subcutaneous swelling, pain, exudation	Fever, depression, anorexia
Cutaneous tuberculosis	Nodules on head, neck, legs; yellow-to-green pus	Anorexia, fever, weight-loss, lymphadenopathy
Nocardiosis	Non-healing wound, red-brown exudate, draining tracts	Fever, depression, dyspnoea pyothorax, weakness, neurological signs

FIG. 20.2 Cutaneous and systemic signs of diseases caused by bacterial organisms.

CUTANEOUS AND SYSTEMIC SIGNS OF DISEASES CAUSED BY VIRUSES		
Disease	**Cutaneous signs**	**Systemic signs**
Feline leukaemia virus	Chronic, recurrent pyodermas, paronychia, poor wound healing, seborrhoea, pruritus, rapid nail growth	Anaemia, lymphosarcoma, generalised debilitation, or asymptomatic carrier
Feline immunodeficiency virus infection	Pustular dermatitis, stomatitis, gingivitis	Recurrent infections, stomatitis, generalised debilitation
Feline poxvirus infection	Crusted papules, plaques, nodules and ulcers on the face, limbs, paws and trunk	Anorexia, lethargy, pyrexia, vomiting, diarrhoea, dyspnoea, conjunctivitis and jaundice
Feline Herpes virus infection	Cutaneous ulcers in the mouth and skin	Conjunctivitis and upper respiratory infection, fever, anorexia
Feline calcivirus infection	Swollen painful feet, ulceration of the footpads, vesicles on tongue, palate and lips	Conjunctivitis and upper respiratory infection, fever, anorexia

FIG. 20.3 Cutaneous and systemic signs of diseases caused by viruses.

CUTANEOUS AND SYSTEMIC SIGNS OF DISEASES CAUSED BY FUNGAL ORGANISMS		
Disease	**Cutaneous signs**	**Systemic signs**
Sporotrichosis	Ulcerated nodules, hair-loss, serosanguinous exudate	Fever, depression, signs associated with organ specific invasion: Bone, respiratory tract, spleen, central nervous system
Systemic mycoses	Non-healing wounds, draining tracts, papules, nodules, serosanguinous exudate	Fever, weight-loss, depression, cough, nasal discharge, uveitis, central nervous system signs
Cryptococcoses	Papules and nodules that ulcerate, erosions on the nose	Fever, depression, central nervous system signs, nasal discharge, uveitis

FIG. 20.4 Cutaneous and systemic signs of diseases caused by fungal organisms.

CUTANEOUS AND SYSTEMIC SIGNS OF DISEASES CAUSED BY PARASITES		
Disease	**Cutaneous signs**	**Systemic signs**
Ticks	Cutaneous nodules at site of bite	Tick-bite paralysis
Demodicosis	Hair-loss, pruritus, scaling	Associated with feline diabetes mellitus, feline hyperadrenocorticism, hyperthyroidism
Fleas	Pruritus, hair-loss, scaling, miliary dermatitis	Anaemia in severe infestations
Notoedres	Crusting, intense head and facial pruritus	Lymphadenopathy

FIG. 20.5 Cutaneous and systemic signs of diseases caused by parasites.

CUTANEOUS AND SYSTEMIC SIGNS OF DISEASES CAUSED BY ENVIRONMENTAL CONDITIONS		
Disease	**Cutaneous signs**	**Systemic signs**
Burns	Superficial: Erythema, oedema, pain Deep: Hard skin, sloughing, necrosis, purulent discharge, odour	If > 25% of body is involved systemic signs may include: Shock, renal failure, anaemia, respiratory infections, sepsis
Snake-bite	Rapid and progressive oedema, pain, local haemorrhage, sloughing of the skin	Shock, increased bleeding thrombosis, sepsis, respiratory compromise, cardiac abnormalities, neurological signs
Thallium toxicosis (rodenticide and cockroach poison)	Ulceration, hyperaemia of mucous membranes, alopecia and erythema and necrosis of skin especially on the ears, axillae, posterior abdomen, genitalia and mucous membranes	Early signs: Vomiting, diarrhoea, depression Later signs: Nephrosis, polyneuritis, necrosis of skeletal muscle and myocardial muscles. Inflammation of liver, tongue, pancreas

FIG. 20.6 Cutaneous and systemic signs of diseases caused by environmental conditions.

CUTANEOUS AND SYSTEMIC SIGNS OF DISEASES CAUSED BY NUTRITIONAL CONDITIONS		
Disease	**Cutaneous signs**	**Systemic signs**
Fatty acid deficiency	Alopecia, erythema, scaling, increased sebum production, pruritus, skin thickening	Associated with intestinal malabsorption, pancreatic disease, chronic liver disease
Vitamin E deficiency	Cutaneous masses in the skin, i.e. steatitis	Pain on gentle palpatation of the abdomen, fever, anorexia, lethargy, excitability
Zinc-responsive dermatitis	Thinning of the hair coat, slow hair growth, marked scaling of the skin, ulceration of the mouth	Slow growth

FIG. 20.7 Cutaneous and systemic signs of diseases caused by nutritional conditions.

CUTANEOUS AND SYSTEMIC SIGNS OF DISEASES CAUSED BY ENDOCRINE DISEASES		
Disease	**Cutaneous signs**	**Systemic signs**
Feline hyperadrenocorticism	Fragile skin that easily tears, hair-loss, bruising	Difficult to diagnose. Often seen in conjunction with feline diabetes mellitus
Feline hyperthyroidism	Oily seborrhoea	Polyuria, polydipsia, weight-loss, tachycardia, cardiomyopathy, hypertension

FIG. 20.8 Cutaneous and systemic signs of diseases caused by endocrine diseases.

MISCELLANEOUS CAUSES OF CUTANEOUS AND SYSTEMIC DISEASES		
Disease	**Cutaneous signs**	**Systemic signs**
Autoimmune haemolytic anaemia, SLE, thrombocytopenia, DIC	Ear margin necrosis	Fever, depression, anaemia, bleeding disorders (see specific disease)
Panniculitis	Single or multiple subcutaneous nodules in the trunk. Lesions may drain a serosanguinous to yellow-brown oily fluid	Fever, pain, depression, arthralgia — depending upon the underlying cause
Xanthomas	Hard yellow pustules and plaques in the skin	Associated with naturally occurring and drug-induced feline diabetes mellitus. Has been associated with hereditary hyperlipoproteinaemia
Chediak–Higashsi syndrome	Seen in Persian Cats with blue-smoke hair and partial oculocutaneous albinism	Bleeding disorders, photophobia
Cutaneous asthenia	Fragile skin that tears easily and is very 'stretchy'	Cats die of sudden aortic rupture

FIG. 20.9 Miscellaneous causes of cutaneous and systemic diseases.

IV Problem-Oriented Approach to Skin Diseases of Non-Domestic Pets

21

Skin Diseases of Pet Fish

JOANNE PAUL-MURPHY and KAREN MORIELLO

The Environment

Skin problems in pet fish, like most health problems of fish, require a knowledge of the aquarium system. The veterinarian should have basic knowledge of water quality, disease control and nutrition. Although the scope of this chapter does not allow a detailed discussion of these topics, we will briefly mention some key points. Most fish diseases are associated with water quality problems, overcrowding, poor disease control and poor nutrition.

Water Quality

Fish derive their oxygen from water and they must ventilate a volume of water 10 to 30 times greater than the volume of air breathed by the average dog or cat to obtain the same amount of respiratory air. Oxygen is utilised by the fish, plants and bacteria in the tank.

Oxygen saturation decreases when temperature decreases or salinity increases. Hypoxic fish 'gill' more rapidly and may be seen 'piping' (gulping air) at the surface. A good rule of thumb is to recommend 1.5 to 2.0 l of air percolated through the water per hour for each litre of water in the aquarium. The rate can be estimated by measuring the time taken to fill a beaker inverted over the air pump.

Most aquariums are closed systems, therefore acidity, salinity and nitrates can increase rapidly. Aquariums need to be routinely cleaned and given partial water changes. For the novice pet fish owner, removing and replacing 20% of the water every 7 to 10 days will decrease particulate material along with routine cleaning of the filter. Clients with multiple tanks and/or large tanks should invest in a commercially available water-testing kit to monitor pH, salinity and ammonia concentrations.

Most clients with pet fish obtain water for their tanks from public water supplies, which often contain chlorinated and fluorinated water. In some regions, the water is also very hard and alkaline. Most water can be dechlorinated by 'ageing' the water for several days prior to adding it to the tank. Water hardness can be reduced by adding distilled or deionised water, or by boiling the hard tapwater and decanting the upper portion of the water for the fish tank. Water travelling in metal pipes can carry enough metal ions to cause a toxicity problem; water for the fish tank should be collected from an outside tap to minimise this problem.

Filtration of the water in an aquarium is a critical part of water quality and involves both mechanical and biological systems. Mechanical filters come in a wide array of sizes and capacities and often contain activated charcoal. The size of the filter should be matched to the size of the tank. Biological filters may take more than 3 weeks before enough time and nutrients have accumulated for bacteria (i.e. *Nitrobacter* spp. and *Nitrosomas* spp.) to colonise the filter system. During this time toxic levels of ammonia and nitrate can accumulate. Biological filters are created by adding food for the bacteria and allowing time for the populations to become established. Before adding fish to the tank, these filters should be allowed to develop for several weeks by adding fish waste to the water, or high protein fish feed, or by adding ammonium chloride at 5 mg/l per day to the tank until the filter is established. The filter is considered 'established' when ammonia and its by-products are undetectable.

Overcrowding

Overcrowding and 'mismatch' of species are common problems in tanks owned by novice hobbyists. The carrying capacity of a tank depends upon the size of fish, frequency of feeding, water temperature, biofilter conditioning, water quality and compatibility of various species. In general, 1 inch of fish per gallon of water is a good rule of thumb. The personalities of fish vary just as much as the personalities of dogs and cats and clients should inquire about this when purchasing fish.

Nutrition

Clients should inquire about the specific nutritional requirements of the species of fish that they are purchasing or they should refer to a fish handbook to obtain information. Problems occur when low quality fish foods are used or fish are not fed at appropriate intervals, i.e. over or underfeeding. If small children are in the house, overfeeding tends to be the most common problem.

Quarantine

Good quarantine procedures can help to prevent introduction of infectious diseases into established aquariums. Quarantine procedures may include dips in fresh water, low salinity and low concentrations of copper treatments to eliminate asymptomatic carriers of common ectoparasites.

History Taking and Physical Examination

To make a diagnosis, the client must bring in the affected fish or a selected group of clinically affected fish (Fig. 21.1). This is most easily accomplished by transporting the fish in strong plastic bags or glass jars with lids. The client should be instructed to transport the fish in water obtained from the tank

DIFFERENTIAL DIAGNOSIS OF SKIN DISEASES OF PET FISH	
Discolorations of the skin	Ichthyophthirius multifiliis ('ich' or 'white spot') Ichthyobodo necatrix ('slime disease') Oodinium spp. ('gold dust disease')
Flashing or pruritus	Flatworms
Nodules	Myxobolus spp. Henneguya spp. Myxisium spp.
Cutaneous haemorrhages	Aeromonas spp. Pseudomonas fluorescens Vibrio anguillarum Streptococcus spp.
Fin rot	Flexibacter columnaris
Cutaneous fungal infections	Saprolegnia and related genera

FIG. 21.1 Differential diagnosis of skin diseases of pet fish.

and only fill the transport container two-thirds full to allow for adequate aeration. Questions to ask the fish owner should focus on the tank (size, filter, length of time owned, filter system, heater and water temperature), the water quality (frequency of water changes, source and type of water, pipes in-house, water tests performed), the fish (type, number, appetite, activity, number affected, skin changes, spots, swimming activity, location in tank) and epidemiological questions (number of fish in tank, how many new fish, plants, snails, or other changes).

The examination should rely heavily on a thorough history and review of the husbandry. The second priority is analysis of the water. After a thorough observation of the fish's behaviour, a very rapid but complete physical examination can be done. Be prepared to take skin scrapings. Skin and gill biopsies are best performed on anaesthetised fish.

Fish with skin diseases present either with signs of systemic illness or more commonly with abnormalities on their skin that are apparent to the client. Signs of systemic illness in a fish include depression, anorexia (best observed in surface-feeding fish), drifting aimlessly through the water, inverted swimming (head-standing), gulping air (piping) or lethargy. 'Flashing' describes a fish turning on its side and making a rapid semicircular swimming motion in order to rub against surfaces in the tank. This is usually a sign of a pruritic fish. Colour changes are either increases or decreases in the intensity of colour. Darkening of colour can be associated with reproductive activity (increases in colour intensity), gastrointestinal signs (usually limited to head) and stress (usually the whole body). Paleness of the skin may be a sign of bacterial or viral infections in fish. An excess of mucus on the skin or fins, pinpoint haemorrhages or white spots are suggestive of parasitic or infectious aetiologies. Frayed fins can be caused by other aggressive fish in the tank or may be due to ectoparasites. Selecting a moribund fish for necropsy may be the most rapid diagnostic tool if infectious skin disease is suspected.

Initially, the fish should be examined in the container to note the behaviour and specific lesions. It is often necessary to obtain specimens from the fish. Fish should be examined with a strong light source and a magnifying loupe. Fish should be handled only with wet latex gloves and restrained on smooth surfaces; they should never be restrained on moistened rough surfaces such as paper towels or cloth towels. This is to prevent damage to the skin and mucous layer. Most skin diseases of fish require either microscopic examination of skin scrapings, microscopic examination of skin biopsies, or sacrifice of the patient and culture and histopathology of the entire fish. The latter is generally unacceptable to most clients with pet fish and is usually only cost-effective for hobbyists or commercial breeders. Examination of dead fish is non-productive — they are often autolysed, the parasites will have abandoned the host and numerous saprophytic organisms will have invaded so confusing the diagnosis.

Sampling Techniques

Skin Scrapings and Impression Smears

Skin scrapings and impression smears can be taken from an unanaesthetised fish, but the procedures need to be done rapidly and safely. If the practitioner is inexperienced, then anaesthesia of small, excitable and expensive fish is recommended. Damaging the skin when obtaining a diagnostic sample can be very detrimental to delicate fish. To sample an awake fish, bring the fish to the surface in a small soft net, press a glass microscope slide to the lesion or gently scrape the lesion with the edge of the microscope slide. It is very important to scrape in the direction of the scale growth. An impression smear may contain mucus, leucocytes and possibly bacteria, protozoans or algae hyphae. Place a drop of tank water on the glass microscope slide and then place a cover-slip on the sample. The microscopic examination must be performed immediately. Low power and low illumination should be used to scan the slide for motion, i.e. parasites. The magnification should be increased to examine small organisms. Vital stains, e.g. new methylene blue or lactophenol cotton blue can be applied after the initial wet mount scan.

Fin Biopsy

Tail or fin biopsies can be easily obtained from an unanaesthetised fish. The fish is spread over your fingertips and a small triangular wedge of fin is cut from between the spines. The small piece of fin should be placed on a glass slide, a drop of tank water placed on top of it, and the preparation had a cover-slip placed on it. It should be examined immediately.

Gill Biopsy

Gill biopsies can be easily obtained from unanesthetised fish but the technique needs to be practised to be done quickly and safely. Inexperienced clinicians may be more comfortable anaesthetising delicate or expensive fish. In small fish, the gill is gently lifted with a finger or iris scissors. The small curved blade of the iris scissors is inserted into the gill so that the edge of a single gill lamella drapes on to the blade. A few tips of the primary lamella are cut and withdrawn with the scissors. The specimen is placed on a glass microscope slide, a drop of tank water is put on top of it and the preparation had a cover-slip placed on it. It should be examined immediately.

Selected Skin Diseases of Pet Fish

'White spot' disease

Description. This disease is very contagious in aquariums. The causative agent is *Ichthyophthirius multifiliis* (or *Cryptokaryon irritans* in saltwater fish), a common parasite with a complicated life cycle that includes stages on the fish and other stages in the environment. It is the trophont feeding stage that causes the white spots of discolouration on a fish's skin that give the disease its name. When the trophont has finished feeding, it matures and drops to the bottom of the tank. There it encysts again and divides to produce a large number of theronts—the active, free-living ciliated stage—which embed themselves in the skin and gills of fish, developing into trophonts.

Clinical signs. The infection is easily transmitted into a 'clean' tank by an infected fish. Signs usually begin within 7–10 days of introduction of new stock. The predominant clinical signs are small white spots on the skin and gills. Heavy infestations may produce listlessness and flashing.

Diagnosis. Definitive diagnosis is made by microscopic examination of the skin or gills. A gentle scraping of one or more of the white spots provides enough material for cytology. Unstained wet mounts and squash preparations are best examined. A drop of tank water should cover the specimen; examination of the cover-slipped specimen under low power with reduced light is recommended. The theronts are round or oval with a crescent-shaped macronucleus. These slow moving organisms vary in size from 30 μm to 1 mm in size and have cilia all around the body.

Treatment. There is no effective treatment against the encysted stage and all treatment is directed at eliminating the free-living or theront stage. First, the water temperature should be increased to 26°C for several days. Theronts are heat sensitive but fish may be stressed by an increase in tank temperature as well. Second, heavy filtration using diatomaceous earth filters should be installed to reduce the numbers of free-living theronts. A complete water change including changing the gravel and debris is recommended but the fish will need to be kept in another 'conditioned' tank while the primary tank is being disinfected or treated. Alternatively, the infected fish can be transferred to a fresh tank daily for 7 days. There is no consistent recommendation for an antiparasiticidal treatment of the tank; some authors recommend environmental treatment alone and others recommend adjunct chemotherapy. Newer recommendations include using praziquantel, 10 mg/l for a 3 hour bath; however, acetic acid (vinegar), 2.0 ml/l for a 30 second dip, or formaldehyde (37%) for up to 1 hour every 3 days for three treatments are also effective. The volume of formaldehyde varies with water quality; 0.4 ml/l for soft water, 0.5 ml/l for hard water and 0.6 ml/l for salt water. Formaldehyde can be very toxic. Copper sulphate is extremely toxic and is not recommended for use in home aquariums unless water quality can be monitored.

Prognosis. The prognosis is fair to good, depending upon the severity of the infestation. Fish that have survived infestation are believed to be immune.

Slime disease

Description. *Ichthyobodo necatrix* is a parasite of freshwater fish and is common in goldfish. Tropical fish kept in water temperatures above 25°C do not have problems with ichthybodiasis. *Ichthyobodo* is a commensal organism and environmental changes or a change in health status can promote its proliferation. Most outbreaks occur in primary fish producer facilities, but occasional infection may be seen in pet fish.

Clinical signs. These parasites feed directly on sloughed skin and gills of the fish. An excessive amount of mucus is produced and a whitish film coats the body. Excess mucus on the gills will lead to respiratory distress and high mortality. Fish may rub themselves on the tank surfaces (flashing) or become listless.

Diagnosis. Definitive diagnosis is made by cytological examination of unstained skin scrapings or gill biopsies. The parasite is small (7 μm), transparent and comma-shaped and moves erratically when unattached to epithelial cells. Microscopic examination should be done quickly because the parasites die rapidly on the slide.

Treatment. See treatment recommendations for **white spot**. Small numbers of fish can be dipped.

Prognosis. The prognosis is guarded.

'Velvet' or 'gold dust' disease

Description. *Oodinium* is an ectoparasite that can infect the skin, fins and gills of freshwater, brackish and saltwater fish. *Amyloodinium ocellatum* is the marine parasite of tropical fish. These parasites are common problems in pet shops and are easily transmitted by inanimate objects between tanks. An asymptomatic carrier fish can introduce the organism into an aquarium.

Clinical signs. This dinoflagellate invades the skin of fish and causes the skin to appear gold, rust or coral in colour. The skin and fins appear to have thin, dusty patches. Common names include 'velvet disease' in marine tropical fishes or 'gold dust disease' in freshwater tropical fish. Early signs include rapid breathing, flashing and petechial haemorrhages of the skin.

Diagnosis. Definitive diagnosis is made by examining microscopic wet mounts of skin and gill biopsies. The organism is non-motile and forms pear-shaped cysts.

Treatment. Effective treatment is difficult because the life cycle involves a resistant encapsulated to-mont stage. Reinfection can occur under stressful situations. The organism may be treated by maintaining a level of 0.1–0.2 mg/l of ionic copper in the water for 14–21 days. Copper test kits should be used to measure the copper concentration in the tank every other day and more copper should be added if indicated. Copper can be very toxic in freshwater systems.

Prognosis. The prognosis is guarded and reinfection is common.

Flatworms

Description. There are many flatworm parasites, including trematodes and cestodes of freshwater and saltwater fishes. These organisms have a pre-dilection for the gills and skin. They are commensals and rarely cause disease but are more likely to create disease in home aquariums where overcrowding exists or when the water quality is poor. Most trematode species that affect fish belong to either the *Dactylogyrus* spp. (gill flukes) or *Gyrodactylus* spp. *Gyrodactylus* are usually on the skin and rarely affect the gills.

Clinical signs. Fish show signs of gill dysfunction, rapid respiration or swimming near the surface or inactivity at the bottom of the tank and death. *Gyrodactylus* spp. inhabit the skin and cause behavioural changes, such as flashing, rubbing or clamped fins. Localised haemorrhages, excessive mucus and skin ulcerations may be evident with *Gyrodactylus*. The tails and fins may appear ragged and secondary bacterial infections are common.

Diagnosis. Definitive diagnosis requires a biopsy of the gills or skin scrapings. A few species of trematodes are large enough to be seen with the unaided eye.

Treatment. Praziquantel — 2 mg/l in aquarium water or 10 mg/l as a 3 hour bath — will kill most external cestodes or trematodes. Formalin baths as described under *Ichthyrophthirius* can also be effective.

Prognosis. The prognosis is variable.

Cutaneous nodules

Description. Cutaneous nodules caused by protozoal parasites, such as *Myxobolus* spp., *Henneguya* spp. or *Myxidium* spp. are common. Neoplasia is a rare cause of nodules on fish. Cutaneous nodules may also be caused by a viral infection referred to as **lymphocystis**.

Clinical signs. Parasitic organisms cause nodules or cysts in the skin and gills. The nodules vary in size and do not appear to cause the fish any discomfort. They are often considered an incidental finding at necropsy examination. Lymphocystis is easily recognised by proliferative nodular/warty growths on the skin and fins that vary from pinhead size to very extensive granular masses covering a large portion of the body. Lesions are white, grey or pink. The gills are only rarely involved. This disease is associated with stress. Lesions may rupture and leave a light-coloured scar at the site.

Diagnosis. Diagnosis of parasitic nodules can be made from the gross appearance. Microscopic examination of skin scraping material will have large numbers of characteristic spores with two polar capsules. Diagnosis of lymphocystis relies on recognition of the gross lesions. Skin biopsies for histopathological examination will have enlarged connective tissue cells with intracytoplasmic inclusions. Virus isolation is difficult and usually not necessary.

Treatment. No treatment is recommended for either parasitic nodules or lymphocystis.

Prognosis. The prognosis is poor.

Cutaneous haemorrhages

Description. Bacterial skin diseases of fish are transmitted orally, through abraded skin or via damaged gills. Some bacterial infections occur after damage to the skin from parasitic infestations. Outbreaks are often preceded by environmental changes or stress. The most common bacterial skin diseases of fish are caused by *Aeromonas* spp., *Pseudomonas fluorescens*, *Vibrio* *anguillarum*, *Streptococcus* spp., *Flexibacter* spp. and *Mycobacterium* spp.

Clinical signs. The most common sign of a systemic or cutaneous bacterial infection is cutaneous haemorrhages. Bacterial infections may cause localised skin haemorrhages, ulcers, injected fins and discoloured skin. Erythema progresses along the base of the fins and around the mouth.

Diagnosis. Definitive diagnosis requires cultures of the skin; it cannot be based on clinical signs alone. A moribund fish should be submitted to a diagnostic laboratory to be sacrificed for culture. Alternatively, the fish can be sacrificed in the hospital and the kidney submitted for culture. Impression smears of visceral granulomas, if present, should be Gram stained and acid-fast stained for presumptive diagnosis of *Streptococcus* spp. or *Mycobacterium* spp.

Treatment. Treatment should be based upon culture and sensitivity. The route of delivery chosen will depend on the species, the aquarium system and the drug selected. Bacterial dermatitis without septicaemia may respond to local topical therapy. The fish can be quickly netted and the lesions swabbed with a disinfectant, such as povidone-iodine, chlorhexidine or a topical antibiotic cream. Treatments need to be done daily. Treatment of severe bacterial infections of several fish is better accomplished with baths or dips. Information on antibiotics and delivery systems can be found in the bibliography.

Prognosis. The prognosis is guarded.

Fin rot

Description. Fin rot caused by *Flexibacter columnaris* can infect most freshwater fish. Necrosis of the fins can occur in progressive septicaemia regardless of the strain of bacteria.

Clinical signs. Fin rot is usually preceded by some type of stress. The disease is usually localised to gills, fins and tail. The gills may be necrotic and bleached. The lesions on the body appear as grey-white foci that develop into ulcers. The fins may ulcerate and have a pink or yellow colour.

Diagnosis. A presumptive diagnosis of *Flexibacter* can be made by skin scrapings or squash preparations of the fin; long, filamentous, Gram-negative rods will be seen. Definitive diagnosis is made by bacterial culture.

Treatment. Treatment should be based upon culture and sensitivity. Recommended therapy for small numbers of fish include baths and dips. Oral antibiotic therapy with oxytetracycline has been effective.

Prognosis. The prognosis is guarded.

Cutaneous fungal infections

Description. The most common causes of cutaneous fungal infections in fish are the Oomycetes which includes *Saprolegnia* and related species. These organisms affect freshwater fish and are usually associated with poor environmental conditions coupled with damage to the skin, fins, or tail.

Clinical signs. Superficial fungal infections in fish appear as cottony growths on the skin and gills that grow in a radially symmetrical pattern. The mycelia trap debris and lesions may appear almost any colour. These fungal organisms are opportunistic and usually invade wounds and colonise dead fish. Systemic infections do not occur.

Diagnosis. Definitive diagnosis is made via fungal culture and microscopic examination of the fungal hyphae. The hyphae are broad and aseptate.

Treatment. A variety of antifungal agents can be used, including formaldehyde (see above under white spot disease), malachite green (0.2 mg/l as a 1 hour bath) and methylene blue (3 mg/l as a bath for up to 5 days). Individual wounds can be swabbed with 10% povidone–iodine or other disinfectants.

Prognosis. The prognosis is variable.

22

Skin Diseases of Amphibians

JOANNE PAUL-MURPHY and KAREN MORIELLO

Frogs, toads, and salamanders are not common pets but they are increasing in the pet population and are also commonly used in schools' basic biology classes. Surprising little is known about the medical diseases of these species compared with reptiles, fish and birds. These animals have a short life span, are very sensitive to pollution and toxins and are often restricted to moist habitats.

Amphibians are ectothermic and the skin is the most important organ for many species. It is a respiratory surface for oxygen exchange and is responsible for respiratory, osmoregulatory and electrolyte balance. Proper hydration is a major consideration for these pets. The skin acts to camouflage the animals in the wild. The skin is shed in pieces or one large piece and is usually eaten.

Environment

Since amphibians are extremely dependent upon appropriate habitat to survive it should come as no surprise that the pet's environment is key to its health. The husbandry requirements will vary with the species and may be quite specific. In general, these animals are best maintained in an aquarium or terrarium with a lid to maintain humidity, temperature, and appropriate photoperiod and to minimise escapes. Terrestrial species need a leaf, soil or sphagnum moss substrate and access to water. Aquatic species need to be kept in an aquarium with a constant source of water that is filtered mechanically or biologically or changed regularly. The water source for both terrestrial and aquatic species should be either deionised or distilled; these species are very susceptible to metal and chemical toxins.

All species require hiding places and some will burrow into soft substrates. The tanks should be cleaned regularly and disinfected with boiling water; chemical disinfectants should be avoided due to the potential for toxicity. Dilute chlorine bleach can be used if rinsed very thoroughly. Temperature requirements vary with the species: temperate species requiring 15–23°C and tropical species require 24–30°C. Temperatures may need to be even lower during periods of hibernation.

Nutrition

Adult amphibians are carnivores. Immature amphibians can be carnivores, omnivores, or herbivores. Carnivorous species usually eat only live moving prey which may include night-crawlers, earthworms, crickets, fruit flies, mealworms, *Tubifex* worms, newborn mice or small fish. All food should be fresh and mineral and vitamin supplements should be added to the diet. Commercial amphibian foods are available and can be part of a varied diet. Owners should investigate the specific food requirements of the species they own.

History Taking and Physical Examination

It is difficult to make a diagnosis without examining the patient and clients should be instructed to bring the animal to the clinician for examination. The amphibian should be brought in its own tank, if possible, otherwise a small transport tank can be used. Care should be taken to protect the patient from dehydration and major fluctuations in body temperature.

The patient's environment should be examined closely since many problems relate to poor husbandry. The owner should be questioned about the length of time the patient has been owned, the husbandry, water sources, diet, temperature, number of amphibians owned, and any new additions to the tank. The animal should be observed in its tank before any handling. Unusual postures and skin colour changes or congestion should be noted.

DIFFERENTIAL DIAGNOSIS OF SKIN DISEASES OF AMPHIBIANS	
Skin haemorrhages	Bacterial infections Gas bubble disease Poor water quality Chemical toxins
Skin ulcers	Bacterial infections Fungal infections Capillariasis Trauma Chemical toxins
Skin nodules	Fungal infections Parasitic infestations Capillariasis Mycobacteriosis Neoplasia Trematode cercariae
Black spots	Trematode cercariae Chromomycosis
Yellow-white nodules	Xanthomas

Fig. 22.1 Differential diagnosis of skin diseases of amphibians.

Examine amphibians gently and quickly, wearing moistened latex gloves, to avoid unnecessary stress. The skin glands are very secretory and certain species have irritating or toxic secretions. Most animals require two hands cupped for safe restraint. Soft nets help lift aquatic species from the water. Healthy species resent and resist restraint; an easily handled amphibian is a sign of illness. Normal skin is moist and tacky, but not excessively mucoid. The skin should be carefully examined for ulcerations, haemorrhages, swellings, masses or cysts. Amphibians normally slough their skin (ecdysis) and eat it. Evaluate body condition by grading the skeletal prominences especially in the area of the urostyle. Low body weight may indicate dehydration. The eyes should be prominent and moist and the corneas should be clear. Heart and respiratory rates vary with species.

Diagnostic Sampling

Skin Scrapings

A mucus sample can be obtained by gently scraping the skin with a cover-slip. Wet mounts can be prepared for microscopic examination by placing the coverslip on a moistened glass microscope slide. After direct examination, a drop of new methylene blue stain should be added and the microscopic examination repeated looking for protozoans, bacteria, and fungi.

Skin Biopsy

Skin biopsies are easily performed and are indicated when focal or nodular lesions are present. It is very important to request an acid-fast stain, in addition to routine H&E stains. A 27 gauge needle is used to infiltrate the subcutaneous area around the lesion with a small volume of dilute lidocaine (2 mg/ml). Aggressive administration of lidocaine may cause systemic anaesthesia or death. Small iris scissors can be used to obtain the skin biopsy and to assure minimum penetration of instruments into the underlying body wall. Due to the thin nature of amphibian skin, the sample should be placed immediately into tissue cassettes or mounted on a small piece of tongue depressor to prevent curling of the specimen.

Gill Biopsy

This procedure is as described in *Chapter 21* (Diseases of Fish).

Cultures

Moist miniature sterile swabs work well for obtaining material from superficial ulcers for bacterial and fungal culture. One swab should be submitted for each culture to ensure that adequate samples are obtained by the reference laboratory. In frogs, lymph fluid is the best sample source for identification of septicaemic bacterial infections. To obtain a specimen, hold the frog vertically and milk the lymph into the hindlegs until the lymph distends the skin. A sample is obtained by aspirating the fluid with a 25 or 27 gauge needle. The sample should be submitted for culture and cytological examination.

Selected Skin Diseases of Amphibians (see Fig. 22.1)

Bacterial infections

Description. Bacterial infections of the skin are a common cause of death in amphibians. Infections are usually associated with stress; newly acquired animals are particularly at risk. Poor husbandry is also a risk factor. The organisms that are most commonly isolated are Gram-negative bacteria: *Aeromonas*, *Pseudomonas*, *Citrobacter*, *Proteus*, *Salmonella*, *Mima*, and *Acinetobacter* spp.

Clinical signs. Most commonly, amphibians with skin disease are found dead. In less severe cases, the skin loses its bright colour, and becomes congested; skin haemorrhages are present on the legs, feet and ventrum — thus the name of **red leg disease** (Plate 24). Ulcerations of the skin may develop on the limbs. Loss of digits and limbs may also occur. *Pseudomonas* infections frequently cause skin sloughing. Infected animals are often anorexic and lethargic, they have diarrhoea, and may be anaemic. Some animals have ascites.

Diagnosis. Definitive diagnosis requires culturing of the causative agent. This can be done by culturing the skin or by culturing lymph, or ascitic fluid if present. In some cases definitive diagnosis is made at necropsy.

Treatment. Infected animals should be isolated and the environment thoroughly cleaned. Initial treatment with chloramphenicol succinate (50 mg/kg SC, IM, IP q 24 hrs) or enrofloxacin (5 mg/kg SC or IM q 24 hrs), or amikacin (2.5 to 5.0 mg/kg SC IM, IP q 24 hrs) is recommended until results of the culture and sensitivity are available. Antibiotic sensitivity testing is highly recommended due to risk of plasmid transfer of resistance common to many of these bacteria. Increasing the salinity of the water (0.05%) may also be useful in addition to antimicrobial therapy. Bathing for 5 minutes in 0·5% sodium chloride for several days may be helpful.

Prognosis. The prognosis is guarded.

Tuberculosis

Description. Chronic subcutaneous mycobacteriosis is common in anurans. The organisms are found in soil and water and infect amphibians through skin wounds. *Mycobacterium xenopi*, *M. marinum* and *M. rane* are most commonly isolated. This disease occurs most often in stressed or compromised individuals but enzootics may occur in poorly managed collections.

Clinical signs. Skin lesions are well-circumscribed indurated nodules or ulcers which expand slowly. Death is caused by the loss of osmoregulatory functions of the skin.

Diagnosis. Dermal mycobacteriosis nodules need to be differentiated from tumours or cysts. Skin scrapings or impression smears from ulcerated lesions should be examined with an acid-fast stain. Unfixed slides should be submitted to the reference laboratory. Biopsy specimens of nodules should always be examined with an acid-fast stain as well since amphibian heterophils in the granulomas have acid-fast granules in addition to the mycobacterium. Cultures from the skin with swabs is not useful in the diagnosis; mycobacterial organisms are ubiquitous and isolation may indicate infection or an insignificant growth. Definitive diagnosis requires demonstration of the organism invading tissue.

Treatment. There is no treatment for this disease but it can be controlled by maintaining a healthy environment.

Prognosis. The prognosis is grave and this disease has zoonotic potential; people may develop dermal lesions.

Fungal infections

Description. Amphibians are prone to developing opportunistic fungal infections of the skin due to trauma and poor hygiene. Opportunistic organisms include but are not limited to *Fonsecaea*, *Cladiosporium*, *Mucor*, *Basidobolus* and *Nigrosporum* spps. *Saprolegnia* is a common isolate from aquatic amphibians.

Clinical signs. Infections are usually associated with pre-existing skin damage. Most of the superficial fungal organisms produce cottony growth on the skin and gills. Some of the pigmented fungi (e.g. *Cladosporium*) can also cause dermal nodules and ulcers in the skin. Some of the pigmented fungi may also cause black spots on the skin. If the fungal infection goes unrecognised, the animal will often develop anorexia and infection of deeper organs-granulomas.

Diagnosis. Definitive diagnosis can often be made via wet mounts looking for fungal elements. A more common diagnostic aid is a fungal culture. It is important not to culture these lesions on DTM; the antibacterial and antifungal agents added to the medium may inhibit the growth of these opportunistic saprophytes.

Treatment. Itraconazole or ketoconazole (10 mg/kg *per os* daily may) be effective. Fungal mats should be manually removed from the skin. Topical application, i.e. spot therapy, with mercurochrome merthiolate may be beneficial. Whole body dips with methylene blue (4 mg/l) or benzalkonium chloride (2 mg/l) for 1 hour daily are used in severe cases.

Prognosis. The prognosis is variable.

Capillariasis

Description. Capillariasis is a parasitic infection caused by *Pseudocapillaroides xenopi*. This infection is most common in clawed frogs (*Xenopus*).

Clinical signs. Infected frogs show darkening and scaling of the skin, especially on the back. This rapidly develops into desquamation, ulceration, anorexia and death. In some individuals, nodules will also develop.

Diagnosis. Definitive diagnosis is made by finding the nematode (2–4 mm in length) on skin scrapings or in the sloughed skin.

Treatment. Ivermectin (0.2–0.4 mg/kg percutaneously, orally or SC) is curative. The tank needs to be disinfected concurrently.

Prognosis. Good if recognised early in the disease process.

Protozoal infections

Description. Aquatic amphibians and larvae are susceptible to external parasites such as *Costia*, *Tricodina* and *Oodinium*, much like fish. Salamanders and frogs may develop cysts in the skin from sporozoans such as *Dermocystidium* and *Dermosporidium*.

Clinical signs. Generalised signs of skin irritation and increased mucus secretion occur when aquatic species are affected by integumentary protozoans. Anurans and salamanders affected by dermal protozoans will have numerous cysts in the skin. A systemic infection can be very debilitating.

Diagnosis. Definitive diagnosis is by skin scrapings examined microscopically as wet mounts. See section under fish (*Chapter 21*).

Treatment. Aquatic amphibians with skin parasites are treated similarly to fish; salt baths (2.5% NaCl for 2 hours) or copper salts can be tried. Due to species sensitivity to heavy metals, treat only a few animals initially before proceeding with an entire collection. Protozoal cysts in frogs and salamanders may be eliminated by elevating the temperature to 25°C for several days.

Prognosis. The prognosis is variable and depends upon the severity of the lesions.

Gas bubble disease

Description. Gas bubble disease is caused by exposure to water that is supersaturated with air. It occurs when the total dissolved gas pressure is greater than the atmospheric gas. Leaks in the filtration system are the major cause. Aquatic amphibians are very susceptible under these conditions.

Clinical signs. Affected animals are depressed; the skin is hyperaemic and skin haemorrhages are common. Subcutaneous emphysema may be present in the webs of the feet.

Diagnosis. Definitive diagnosis is made by clinical signs.

Treatment. Early recognition of signs and correction of the husbandry are curative. Animals with secondary bacterial infections may require antibiotic therapy.

Prognosis. Good if the disease is recognised early.

Poor water quality and toxins

Description. Water quality is critical to the life of all amphibians. These animals are extremely sensitive to chlorine, ammonia, pesticides and copper, lead and other metals. Petechial haemorrhages can progress rapidly to skin ulcerations. High levels of ammonia and nitrite can cause the skin and/or gills to slough. Iodine-based disinfectants are very toxic to small species.

Clinical signs. The clinical signs may be difficult to separate from infectious skin diseases of amphibians. In general, lethargy, skin haemorrhages, ulcers, sloughing of the skin and internal organs may occur.

Diagnosis. Definitive diagnosis is difficult as many affected individuals may have secondary infections. A careful history and examination of the tank are the key when suspecting toxins and poor water quality.

Treatment. Supportive care with fluids, food and antibiotics are necessary. This condition is more easily prevented than treated. The tank should be carefully cleaned with boiling water and rinsed thoroughly. Water sources should be limited to distilled or deionised water.

Prognosis. The prognosis is variable.

Nodules/plaques in the skin

Description. The most common cause of nodules or plaques in the skin is xanthomatosis. This is a skin disease frequently associated with hypercholesterolaemia in adult Cuban tree frogs. It is associated with improper nutrition: xanthomatous develops in animals with abnormal fat metabolism or abnormal cholesterol in the diet.

Clinical signs. Xanthomas appear clinically as small yellow-white nodules or coalescing plaques. The development of the nodules is slow. Some frogs develop disseminated lesions and corneal lipidosis.

Diagnosis. Definitive diagnosis requires skin biopsy. Histologically, xanthomas are characterised by foamy macrophages laden with lipid and cholesterol clefts.

Treatment. No effective treatment has been reported.

Prognosis. The prognosis is variable. Xanthamatous lesions progress with age.

23

Skin Diseases of Reptiles

JOANNE PAUL-MURPHY and KAREN MORIELLO

Reptiles are popular pets and commonly found in school classrooms as teaching animals. The most common reptiles kept as companion animals are snakes and iguanas although other types of lizards (such as chameleons) and chelonians are becoming more popular.

The vast majority of reptiles have adapted to a more terrestrial life-style and their skin is very much different from that of other animals', it is dry and mostly aglandular. However, many lizards have femoral glands and pores on the ventral surface of the thighs and crocodilians have scent glands in the cloaca and inner jaw.

Except for the shell of chelonians, the epidermis of reptiles is relatively soft and overlies a dermis of loose connective tissue. The keratinised epidermis is folded grossly into scales or scutes. Crocodilians and some lizards have bony plates in the dermis under the scales; turtles and tortoises have a shell which is composed of an outer keratinised epidermis overlying dermal bone. Squamata (snakes and lizards) periodically shed the outer layer of keratinised skin and this is called **ecdysis**. Snakes shed their skin in one piece while lizard skin is shed in several pieces. The rate of growth determines the frequency of ecdysis. Chelonians and crocodilians moult in a piecemeal fashion, but the chelonian shell is not shed.

Skin diseases in reptiles may be caused by poor husbandry or primary cutaneous infectious diseases or they may be signs of systemic illness. The most important diagnostic aids are careful review of husbandry practices, physical examination and skin biopsies.

Environment

There are over 6000 species of reptile, each adapted to a specific niche in nature, and it is necessary to understand the natural ecology and husbandry of the species in question. However, some general husbandry points will be mentioned.

Most of these animals are terrestrial or arboreal and are best housed in terrariums and cages that are escape-proof and easily cleaned. Common substrates include newspaper, wood chips, indoor–outdoor carpet and alfalfa pellets. Avoid highly resinous wood chips, such as cedar, that may be toxic. Avoid granular substrates such as gravel, cat litter and fine wood shavings since these are difficult to clean, they hold moisture and they may be ingested while the animal is feeding. A hide-box should be provided in all cages. Large flat containers of water should be available for humidity and a place to soak. Drip systems are necessary for certain arboreal lizards and snakes that will not drink from containers.

All reptiles are ectotherms. They have a preferred optimum temperature zone (POTZ) and their physiological and immune system are directly dependent upon this temperature range. Most reptiles do well at a range of 26–33°C; the temperature of the tank habitat should be adjusted for the species in question. The heat source may vary depending on the reptile's habitat — whether it is terrestrial or arboreal. When using bulbs or heat tapes, it is essential that animals should not be able to come into direct contact with the source, as burns are a common result. Herbivorous reptiles also require ultraviolet light in the range of 290–320 nm to activate vitamin D precursors in the skin. Unfiltered sunlight provides the best effects and specific requirements for artificial lights are still being investigated. The optimum humidity for most reptiles is 50–60%; however, desert species thrive best at 10% and some tropical reptiles may need daily misting.

Nutritional recommendations are difficult to summarise because reptiles may be frugivores, insectivores, omnivores, herbivores or carnivores. Additionally, many of the recommended diets have been contrived empirically and probably have little or no resemblance to the natural diet. Nevertheless, some effort should be made to investigate the natural ecology and diet, and a diet that most closely resembles the natural diet should be fed. Carnivorous snakes and lizards do well on whole-animal diets, i.e. rodents or fish, and it is recommended that these should be fed dead. Feeding live rodents risks the reptile being attacked and bitten by its intended prey.

History and Physical Examination

A definitive diagnosis cannot be made without examining the patient; clients must be willing to transport their reptiles to the veterinary hospital when necessary. All reptile patients, like other animals in the waiting room, should be adequately restrained and confined in a container, e.g. tank, secure pillowcase or box. Unless absolutely necessary, lizards and snakes that are currently in a cycle of ecdysis should not be manually restrained for more than short periods. During ecdysis, the skin is very fragile and manual restraint can result in a premature shed.

The history should focus on husbandry practices. A complete physical examination should be preceded by observing the patient in its container or unrestrained in the examination room to note responsive behaviour, respiration and posture. Reptiles should not be restrained by the owner during the examination. Small delicate lizards often have very fragile skin that can tear during restraint and so caution must be exercised. Inhalation anaesthesia with isoflurane will allow a complete examination of these animals. The physical examination should include recording of the body weight and an examination of all body systems and orifices, especially the oral cavity, nares and cloaca. The skin should be examined carefully both ventrally and dorsally. The skin between the scales in the axillary and inguinal regions should be examined for ectoparasites. 'Spectacles', (the scales covering the eyes of snakes and some lizards) should be clear and smooth. Mites may be found in the area betweens the spectacles and surrounding scales. The tips of the ventral scales and scutes should be carefully inspected for haemorrhage or necrosis. The tympanic membrane of chelonians is a common site for abscesses and is easily inspected. Hydration can sometimes be assessed by skin turgour. The skin should be palpated for masses and nodules.

Selected Skin Diseases of Pet Reptiles (see Fig. 23.1)

Dysecdysis

Description. The most commonly encountered skin disease in snakes and lizards is dysecdysis, an abnormal moult. Under good conditions, snakes entering a shed cycle will become anorectic; the spectacles and skin become milky white-blue (Plates 25

DIFFERENTIAL DIAGNOSIS OF SKIN DISEASES OF COMMON PET REPTILES	
Scaling of the skin	Humidity problems Hypovitaminosis A Hypervitaminosis A Fungal infections *Dermatophilus congolensis* infection Retained skin
Ulcerations of the skin or shell	Septicaemic cutaneous ulcerative disease of chelonians Cutaneous ulcerations secondary to bacterial sepsis Cutaneous ulcerations secondary to burns Spirorchid trematode infestation
Cutaneous masses or nodules	Mycobacterial infections Aerobic and anaerobic bacterial granulomas Opportunistic fungal infections Fibropapillomas Poxvirus infections Parasite infestations Neoplasia
Pigmentary changes	Grey patch disease (Herpes virus infection)
Traumatic skin lesions	Fractured or cracked shells Abrasions Bite wounds Burns

FIG. 23.1 Differential diagnosis of skin diseases of common pet reptiles.

and 26). Snakes should not be handled during this period to avoid tearing the unshed skin and damaging the soft new skin underneath. After a period of 4–7 days, the eyes and skin become clear and the snake begins to rub on rough surfaces. The skin detaches from the eyes, nostrils and mouth and the snake can move out of the old skin. Most lizards shed their skin in large pieces. In captivity, dysecdysis can be due to inappropriate humidity, inappropriate temperature, lack of abrasive materials in the cage, ectoparasitism, systemic disease or endocrine disease. The most common aetiology is poor husbandry with inappropriate humidity, temperature or lack of rubbing surfaces.

Clinical signs. Reptile skin will appear dry and the animal may be dehydrated when humidity is low. Retained spectacles often occur in snakes with dysecdysis, and may be the primary complaint at presentation. If small pieces of skin are retained on the appendages or tail tip, they can become constricting bands leading to avascular necrosis of the underlying tissue. Lizards can lose digits. Retained pieces of skin provide a nidus for parasitism or microbial infection.

Diagnosis. Diagnosis of dysecdysis is made by clinical examination and a thorough review of husbandry practices.

Treatment. Treatment should be conservative at first. Soak the reptile in warm, shallow water for 1–2 hours daily for 2–3 days and provide appropriate substrate in the cage for rubbing. If this is not sufficient, the retained skin can be gently removed immediately following a warm soak, using moist gauze pads or forceps. Special attention should be given to distal appendages in lizards. Removing retained spectacles must be done with caution. Following a warm bath, place several drops of warm saline on the eyes. This conservative therapy should be continued until shedding has occurred, and the retained spectacles are often shed at that time. If unsuccessful, more aggressive treatment may be indicated; fine-tipped ophthalmic forceps are used to grasp an exposed edge of the retained cap and it is gently lifted off. Excess force can damage the cornea if the skin is tightly adhered or if the subspectacular space has collapsed. It also becomes difficult if several eyecaps are adhered

together. Application of acetylcystine to the eye may assist in softening and lubricating the retained spectacle. Changes in husbandry practices can be the most important part of treatment and prevention.

Prognosis. The prognosis is excellent for snakes and lizards with retained skins. The prognosis is variable for retained spectacles and depends upon the chronicity of the problem.

Hypovitaminosis A

Description. Hypovitaminosis A is a nutritional disease that is common in young aquatic turtles. It causes epithelial hyperplasia and squamous metaplasia of epithelialised and glandular tissues. The skin and mucous membranes are often visibly affected along with respiratory, ocular, gastrointestinal and genitourinary tissues. Secondary microbial infections occur due to alterations in the epithelium.

Clinical signs. Affected animals have conjunctivitis, blepharitis, palpebral oedema, anasarca and lichenified skin. Overgrowths of the mandibular and maxillary mouthparts may occur.

Diagnosis. The history usually indicates an inadequate diet and the clinical signs are enough for diagnosis. Biopsy of affected tissues would histologically confirm squamous metaplasia, but this is usually unnecessary. Secondary ocular and respiratory infections may require culture of the conjunctiva or choanal opening respectively.

Treatment. Clinical signs rapidly regress with an appropriate diet and temporary supplementation. Additions of fresh dark greens high in beta-carotene will improve the diet. Clinically affected turtles should receive supplemental vitamin A. Oral supplementation depends upon the severity and can range from 50 to 10,000 IU/kg. Parenteral treatment should be avoided due to toxicity of hypervitaminosis A. Conjunctivitis will respond well to appropriate topical antibiotics. Chronic respiratory infections are aided by improving the diet but systemic antibiotics are a useful adjunct.

Prognosis. The prognosis is excellent but chronic cases require a long period for recovery.

Hypervitaminosis A

Description. Vitamin A toxicity is usually an iatrogenic problem that occurs when tortoises are treated with parenteral vitamin A. Historically, injections of vitamin A have been given empirically when treating respiratory or ocular diseases. Terrestrial chelonians are herbivores so their diet usually provides sufficient levels of beta-carotene and other carotenoids.

Clinical signs. Initially the skin becomes scaly and dry, then the epidermis is sloughed from the limbs and head. The underlying dermis appears erythematous and inflamed and often becomes invaded by opportunistic bacteria and fungi in the environment. Extensive skin sloughing can lead to dehydration. The skin is very sensitive and the animal appears irritable.

Treatment. Supportive care should include a warm, clean environment; the cage should be disinfected daily. Oral fluid therapy is recommended for dehydration and electrolyte imbalance. Artificial skin products and bandages may protect the dermis, keep it moist and encourage regeneration of the epidermis.

Prognosis. Early recognition of the problem gives a better prognosis. Tortoises with severe skin-loss may die despite aggressive therapy.

Superficial fungal infections

Description. Superficial fungal infections caused by opportunistic pathogens such as *Fusarium*, *Trichosporon*, *Geotrichum*, *Penicillium*, *Oospora* and *Trichoderma* have been observed in lizards, snakes and turtles. Phycomycosis (*Mucor* spp., *Basidobolus* spp.,) can involve the skin of reptiles or invade the dermal plates of chelonians. These organisms may cause necrosis of surrounding tissues due to infiltration of adjacent blood vessels. Damp and unsanitary environments predispose the animal to fungal infections of the skin.

Clinical signs. Superficial fungal infections commonly appear as thickened yellow-brown hyperkeratotic plaques, multifocal necrotising lesions or occasionally as granulomas. *Geotrichum* can cause pustules in the skin of snakes and lizards.

Fusarium has been frequently isolated from cutaneous and ocular ulcers, granulomas, and other reptiles.

Diagnosis. Crusts/plaques should be inoculated on both plain Sabouraud's media and blood agar to ensure that the pathogen is rapidly identified. Fungal cultures are best incubated at 20–24°C. Wood's lamp examination will not be useful. Subcutaneous caseous nodules can be lanced and the exudate examined microscopically with Gram stain, lactophenol cotton blue and acid-fast stains. A sample of the exudate should be submitted for culture. Biopsies of focal lesions are easily obtained for culture and histopathological examination. A surgical preparation of the skin will decrease contamination of the cultures. The lesion should be infiltrated with 2% lidocaine. It is important to correlate the histopathology and the cultures. At least one biopsy specimen should be cultured; the reference laboratory should be instructed to grind the specimen for culture.

Treatment. Most superficial fungal infections are due to excessive humidity and poor hygiene. Rapid correction of both of these problems is strongly indicated. The thermal gradient should be appropriate for the species' POTZ. Most topical antifungal agents used in small animal medicine are not effective against these particular fungal pathogens. The crusts should be removed and/or the granulomas surgically removed if not too numerous. Topical chlortrimazole may be effective if applied 2–3 times daily for 3–4 weeks. Ketoconazole or itraconazole (15 mg/kg) may also be used. Superficial mycotic infections may respond to daily soaking in dilute iodine solution for 20–30 minutes.

The animal's environment should be carefully cleaned with boiling water. Most environmental fungicides are only effective against the plate form of the fungus, i.e. mycelium, and not the form present in the environment. The only environmental disinfectant tested by one of the authors that was 100% effective (i.e. killed all organisms after one application) was concentrated household bleach; this is a caustic substance to use in the environment of these animals and must be thoroughly rinsed from the cage surfaces. However, almost all fungal pathogens are killed with boiling water.

Prognosis. The prognosis is good if the condition is recognised early and predisposing conditions are corrected.

Ulcerative and/or septicaemic infections of the skin

Description. Gram-negative bacteria are the most common cause of bacterial skin diseases in reptiles. Most bacterial infections of the skin occur when the animal has been thermally stressed and/or injured or burned. The immune system of reptiles is temperature dependent. Bacteria that invade the skin are present in the environment and in the intestinal tract; most bacteria causing these lesions are secondary invaders. The most commonly isolated organisms are *Aeromonas* spp., *Citrobacter* spp., *Pseudomonas* spp. and *Serratia* spp. In some cases, staphylococcal and streptococcal organisms have also been isolated.

Blister disease denotes a condition of necrotic dermatitis occurring in snakes and lizards associated with moist, unsanitary conditions. Bacterial septicaemia in lizards and snakes may initially present as haemorrhages of the scales, skin and mucous membranes. An ulcerative skin disease unique to chelonians — septicaemic cutaneous ulcerative disease or SCUD — has been described; it is seen most commonly in freshwater turtles, and *Citrobacter* spp. and *Serratia* spp. are believed to be synergistically involved in the disease (Plate 27).

Less specific superficial erosions and ulcerations of chelonian shells are often termed shell rot. This is a slowly progressive, chronic shell ulceration due to poor husbandry conditions. *Benechae chitinovora* is a common isolate from these lesions. Ulcerative skin lesions on the shells of turtles can also be caused by migrating spirorchid trematodes.

Reticulated pythons can have necrotic skin lesions associated with migrating filaroid nematodes. Ectoparasites, such as mites and ticks, can cause focal ulcerations.

Clinical signs. The dermatitis has a dry, brown necrotic appearance but the scales and underlying skin may be moist. Invading bacteria hasten epidermal necrosis; lesions may enlarge and become erythemic or ulcerated. The ventral body surface, feet and tail are common sites for lesions. Thermal burns may be the cause of the initial injury. Blister disease initially appears as tiny vesicles on the ventral surface of the snake or lizard. These enlarge and progress rapidly to moist deep ulcers.

The first signs of septicaemia may be very subtle with only scales and crusting noted on the skin. In some cases the progression of lesions may be quite rapid. Obvious lesions that should be recognised as signs of sepsis are necrotising and haemorrhagic skin, especially on the ventral surface of snakes. In many cases, the skin will slough. Depending upon the location of the infection, digits or limbs may slough.

In SCUD, the skin of the legs and shell becomes ulcerated and necrotic; turtles are lethargic and anorectic. Chronic ulcerations of the chelonian shell are dark-rimmed and associated with loose, peeling scutes of both the plastron and carapace. In turtles infested with trematodes, the eggs of the parasites become lodged in small vessels causing infarcts and necrosis of the shell and skin due to vascular occlusion.

Diagnosis. Diagnosis is made on the basis of clinical signs, cytology, and bacterial culture and sensitivity. It is important to use a reference laboratory that is familiar with the isolation of bacteria from reptiles. Remember many of the organisms that can cause sepsis in these species are opportunistic secondary invaders that may be classified as contaminants. MIC values should be obtained, whenever possible. Diagnostic samples can be obtained by taking culture swabs of ulcerated lesions, aspirates of fluid from vesicles or biopsies of the material (as for fungal infections). Affected scales can be removed with scissors or a scalpel blade. In cases of suspected septicaemia, a definitive diagnosis is made by blood culture.

Treatment. Affected individuals should be isolated in a hospital cage or tank. The ambient temperature should be optimal for the species; many animals that are infected have been kept at suboptimal temperatures. Environmental temperature affects the reptile immune system as well as the uptake and distribution of systemic antibiotics. Care should be taken not to increase the ambient temperature above what is recommended for the species; small reptiles can rapidly dehydrate. Deep lesions can be soaked and gently debrided. Sterile lavage fluid or normal saline should be used. Topical antibiotics that are useful in Gram-negative infections include silver sulfphadiazine cream and mupirocin ointment. Affected individuals can be soaked a dilute solution of 2% chlorhexidine (16 ml 4 1 distilled water) twice daily until the lesions are healed. Systemic antibiotics are recommended in most cases and a bacteriocidal antimicrobial should be selected based upon the culture and sensitivity results.

Intramuscular administration is recommended, using the cranial portion of the reptile's body.

Migrating parasites causing skin lesions need to be surgically removed or killed with a parasiticidal drug, usually ivermectin (200 μg/kg IM or SC). Ivermectin is toxic to chelonians and the drug of choice in these animals is praziquantel (8 to 20 mg/kg IM), and then repeated in 2 weeks.

Prognosis. The prognosis is variable depending upon the severity of the infection.

Nodular skin lesions

Description. There is a wide range of aetiological causes of nodules in reptiles. Nodules can be due to bacterial or fungal infections, foreign bodies, migrating parasites (*Paratrichosoma*, cestodes, trematodes, ticks/tick bites), viral infections (fibropapilloma, poxvirus infection, papillomas) and neoplasia (squamous cell carcinoma, fibrosarcoma, malignant melanoma, chromatophoroma, iridophoroma). Yet the most common nodule in the reptile is the bacterial abscess. Granuloma formation is the normal reptilian response to inflammation. *Dermatophilus congolensis* is an unusual filamentous bacterium that infects the skin of lizards; it is usually associated with stress, moisture and poorly ventilated environments.

Clinical signs. Masses may or may not be associated with changes in the overlying skin. Migrating parasites may be observed moving in the subcutaneous tissue or may even be palpable under the skin. Tumours and infectious processes may appear indistinguishable, with exudation and inflammation of the skin readily visible. Reptile abscesses are caseated, dry and white-yellow in colour, and are often well encapsulated.

Diagnosis. Definitive diagnosis cannot be based upon clinical examination alone. Reptiles present-

ing with masses should be carefully examined. Subcutaneously migrating parasites may be observed to move. Impression smears of exudate should be examined microscopically. Most masses require skin biopsy and histological examination of the tissue. Bacterial culture and sensitivity should be performed when impression smears or histological changes are suggestive of sepsis or an abscess. Well-encapsulated masses, such as abscesses, can be infiltrated subcutaneously with 2% lidocaine for excision and should be excised with the capsule intact. Culture samples should be taken from the lining of the pocket, not the core of the granuloma.

Treatment. Treatment depends upon the aetiology. Parasitic infestations should be treated with a systemic parasiticide and/or surgical removal of the parasite. Neoplastic masses may be surgically excised, although this depends upon the extent of the tumour. Orthovoltage and injectable cis-platinum have also been tried. Infectious agents are often difficult to treat with antibiotics because the granulomatous nature of the infection tends to wall off the infectious agent from the antibiotics; surgical excision of localised granulomatous infections is often the best therapeutic approach. If excision is incomplete or the abscess was lanced, the region should be curetted and flushed. Daily flushing with dilute disinfectants helps prevent recurrence. Topical application of mupirocin ointment is helpful.

D. congolensis infection is best treated by eliminating the underlying cause: excessive moisture. Lesions should be gently soaked off of the patient's skin, which should then be allowed to dry. Treatment with systemic antibiotics may not be necessary but this organism is very sensitive to broad spectrum antibiotics.

Prognosis. The prognosis is variable.

Grey patch disease

Description. Grey patch disease is a viral infection of the skin that affects chelonians. The causative agent morphologically resembles a Herpes virus. This disease is seen most commonly in young green turtle hatchlings between the ages of 56 and 90 days. Severe epizootics have occurred in the summer under crowded, unsanitary conditions.

Clinical signs. Skin lesions begin as small circular papular eruptions that coalesce into spreading patches.

Diagnosis. Diagnosis is based on clinical signs, skin biopsy and possibly viral isolation. The epidermal cells contain characteristic intranuclear inclusion bodies.

Treatment. There is no specific therapy. Affected animals should be isolated, ambient temperatures should be optimal and scrupulous hygienic practices should be employed. This virus is easily spread in aquatic turtles. Many of the affected animals will have secondary bacterial infections; cultures and sensitivities should be performed and appropriate antibiotic therapy should be selected based upon these findings.

Prognosis. The prognosis is variable.

Poxvirus infection

Description. Poxvirus infection in crocodiles, caiman and tegu produces multifocal lesions on the skin.

Clinical signs. Caiman pox occurs over the entire body as circular grey-white lesions, but these are concentrated around the face. Lesions may also occur in the oral cavity. Pox lesions in tegus are brown papules on the skin.

Diagnosis. Biopsy specimens should be obtained.

Large eosinophilic inclusion bodies can be identified histologically within epidermal cells.

Treatment. There is no treatment. Lesions tend to resolve spontaneously.

Prognosis. The prognosis is good.

Fractured shells

Description. Fractures in the chelonian shell occur because of trauma and are relatively common.

Clinical signs. Fractures of the shell are usually obvious and may be secondarily infected.

Diagnosis. Clinical signs are usually sufficient; however, radiographs may be necessary in some cases to determine the extent of the injury. Three radiographic views are recommended.

Treatment. Infected lesions should be flushed, debrided and cleaned prior to repair of the fracture. Systemic antibiotics should be initiated prior to wound cleaning. The fracture fragments should be returned to their original site and stabilised with wires, if necessary. Large defects or highly contaminated wounds require several days of wound care to establish a clean granulation bed before the shell is sealed. Defects can be covered with a fibreglass patch and epoxy resin or methylmethacrylate resins. The reader is referred to the bibliography for more information.

Prognosis. The prognosis is often very good.

24

Skin Diseases of Pet Birds

JOANNE PAUL-MURPHY and KAREN MORIELLO

Birds are common companion animals and there is a marked increase in the number of birds kept as pets each year. Importation of birds has been restricted in the US and the production of birds for the pet trade should encourage veterinarians to work closely with aviculturists, as well as individual owners. Maintenance of good health relies on proper husbandry, nutrition and an understanding of normal physiology and behaviour.

The skin of birds consists of scales, a few specialised glands, beak, cere, claws, foot pads, feathers, and other specialised structures. The skin is very thin compared with other species and does not contain sweat glands. Specialised glands include the **uropygial gland** (not present in all species), glands in the external ear canal and glands around the vent. The feather follicle is analogous to the hair follicle but is more complex. Feather follicles are arranged in feather tracts or **pterylae** and the areas of skin between the tracts are called **apteria** (sing. apterium). The basal portion of the feather is the **calamus**; the main shaft is the **rachis**. Birds have ten different types of feathers but, simplistically, these can be divided into two groups: large (flight or contour feathers) and small (semiplume, down, powder down, filoplumes, bristles and semi-bristles). Small feathers provide insulation, water-proofing and flotation.

Similar to shedding in mammals, birds 'shed' or moult feathers. This cyclical process occurs in most species once a year following the breeding season; however, it may occur throughout the year in some species. During a moult, 'old' feathers are pushed out by the growth of new ones and this is analogous to the process by which fur-bearing animals shed hairs. The moult usually follows a regular pattern and is progressive so that not all feathers are shed at once. Moulting is physiologically demanding in birds and there is a marked increase in their basal metabolic rate and nutritional needs, particularly their protein requirement since feathers are primarily protein.

History and Physical Examination

As with most special species, the history is critical to the diagnostic process. This is especially true with skin diseases of birds, since many problems may be related to diet, husbandry and/or behavioural problems. Additionally, the bird's environment should be examined; when possible, the owner should bring the bird in its cage for the examination. The cage should not be cleaned for at least 24–48 hours prior to the examination. The following are a few examples of the types of questions to pursue:

- How long has the owner had this bird?
- Where was the bird obtained from?
- What type of food is offered? What does the bird actually eat? Has this changed recently?
- What type of water is used and what type of container is it in?
- How often is the food and water changed?
- How often is the cage changed?
- Does the bird come out of the cage? Does it fly?
- How long has the bird been moulting or when was the last moult?
- Has the owner used any pesticides or toxic compounds in the house?
- Have new birds been brought into the house?
- Are other birds affected?
- How long has the bird been ill? How long has the skin disease been present?
- Have any other birds died?
- Has the owner used any medications on the bird? If so, what was the response?
- Has the bird's personality or behaviour changed?
- Are there any changes in the bird's preening activity?
- Is the bird breeding or sexually active?
- Where is the cage located?
- Are there other birds in its cage?

It is beyond the scope of this chapter to describe in detail the elements of a thorough physical examination in birds. The reader is referred to several excellent references in the reading list. Examine the bird at rest in its cage and note any grooming, rubbing or feather-ruffling behaviours. The dermatological examination of an avian patient should include a careful examination of the skin, feathers, cere, the vent, and uropygial gland. A magnifying loop can aid examination, especially in small patients.

- The cere, legs and feet should be examined for crusting or excessive scaling and discolourations.
- The feathers should be examined for evidence of self-mutilation (discoloured feathers, frayed ends, broken feathers).
- Stress bars may indicate a temporary stressful event or illness.
- Feather colour is determined by pigments and structured colour; lack of appropriate colour may indicate a dietary deficiency such as lysine, choline, riboflavin, folic acid or iron. Effects of specific nutritional deficiencies vary with the species of bird.
- Uropygial secretions can add sheen to feathers.

The structure of the feather should be examined:

- Stunted, clubbed or immature feathers may be a sign of a viral infection.
- Enlarged feather follicles may be sign of bacterial or fungal infection.

Diagnostic Tests

Cytology

Cutaneous and subcutaneous lesions tend to be very accessible for cytological examination. Samples can be obtained by pressing a slide directly on to an exudative lesion or gently scraping a lesion for material. Avian skin is very thin (3–5 cells thick) so caution is advised when scraping with a blade. Aspiration of samples from subcutaneous masses can be informative but caseous material does not aspirate well.

Feather Pulp

Dermatitis and folliculitis can be assessed by cytological examination of the feather pulp material. A growing feather in the affected area can be

DIFFERENTIAL DIAGNOSIS OF SELECTED SKIN AND FEATHER DISEASES OF BIRDS	
Skin	
Discoloration of the face	Bruises Liver disease
Scaling or crusting	Chronic ulcerative dermatitis Frost-bite Low humidity *Cnemidocoptes* mite infestation Poxvirus Insect-bites Cutaneous papillomatosis
Deformed beaks	Psittacine feather and beak disease Tumours *Cnemidocoptes* mite infestation Liver disease Malocclusion Trauma
Nodular masses	Gout Feather cysts Skin tumours Uropygial gland tumours Granulomatous dermatitis Foreign body granulomas
Feathers	
Feather-loss	Folliculitis Altered moult/failure to moult Hypothyroidism Feather picking Administration of thyroxine
Abnormal feathers	Stress bars or stripes Nutritional deficiency Heavy metal intoxication (lead) Viral infections Poor housing/trauma Feather chewing

Fig. 24.1 Differential diagnosis of selected skin and feather diseases of birds.

removed from its follicle and the pulp material impressed on a slide. Samples can be Gram-stained and screened for evidence of infectious agents such as bacteria or fungal elements, or intranuclear inclusions that occur with viral feather dystrophies.

Feather Biopsy

This term applies to the excision of the skin and follicle surrounding a feather and the feather left within the follicle. Growing feathers with evidence of pulp still present should be selected for biopsy. Often a small patch of 7–8 contour feathers can be identified to represent the feather dysplasia under investigation. Incise the skin deep to the subcutaneous layer with an elliptical shape. The skin edges tend to widen once the sample is removed and can be opposed with absorbable or nonabsorbable suture or a thin layer of tissue glue.

Selected Skin Diseases of Birds

Bruises

Description. The featherless facial skin of birds is very delicate and can be easily damaged from minor blunt trauma. Digital pressure on the facial skin while restraining a bird, especially macaws, can result in bruising. Pet birds that are allowed to fly free in the home are susceptible to injuries. Transient erythema or facial patches can be a normal response to excitement in some species.

Clinical signs. Bruises first appear as dark red discolourations on the face for the first 24 hours. Gradually, the bruise will change to a green colour as the biliverdin infuses into the subcutaneous tissues.

Diagnosis. Diagnosis is usually made on clinical signs and history.

Treatment. No treatment is necessary unless other injuries are present.

Prognosis. The prognosis is good.

Cnemidocoptes mite infestation (scaly face mites)

Description. *Cnemidocoptes* spp. mites infest the cere and facial area of birds, especially budgerigars and canaries (Fig. 24.2), but the problem has also been reported in finches, cockatiels, cockatoos, *Neophema* spp., Amazon parrots and ringneck parakeets. In canaries, the legs are often infested and this is called 'tassle-foot'. These mites spend their entire life cycle on the host and are highly contagious. Young birds tend to be clinically affected more frequently.

Clinical signs. Early lesions appear as a powdery white line at the junction of the cere and the beak. As the infection progresses, the keratin layer of the beak becomes covered with a tan-coloured powdery scale and crust. The crust is often visibly perforated with small holes where the mites have burrowed. As the infestation becomes generalised, the vent and the scaled portion of the legs and feet may become involved. If left untreated, the beak and toes may become deformed. Birds are not usually pruritic, but lameness may be present if the legs are severely involved.

Diagnosis. Gross appearance can be diagnostic. Finding the sarcoptiform mite on skin scrapings or potassium hydroxide (KOH) preparations is definitive.

Treatment. Ivermectin is the treatment of choice. In small birds such as canaries and budgerigars, one small drop of 1% bovine ivermectin is placed on the skin over the right jugular vein. In birds with a body weight greater than 80 g, a measured dose of 0.2 mg/kg administered SC, IM or *per os* can be used. Treatment should be repeated in 2 weeks. All birds in contact with the infected bird should be treated. Although the authors have not experienced toxicities, we are aware of anecdotal reports of deaths in small birds due to this treatment.

Prognosis. The prognosis is excellent.

Nutritional and environmental causes of scaling

Description. Protein deficiencies in birds may cause feather disorders and may also cause scaling of the beak and legs. This is similar to seborrhoea in dogs caused by a protein deficiency. The duration of the problem will influence the severity of the lesions. Birds with nutritionally related exfoliative skin diseases of long duration will often have other accompanying feather disorders. Vitamin A deficiency can cause hyperkeratosis on the plantar surface of the feet and may be an underlying cause of pododermatitis. In addition, birds housed in environments with

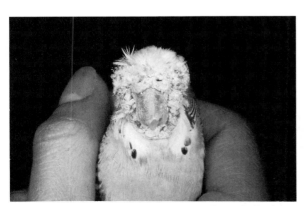

FIG. 24.2 *Cnemidocoptes* mite infestation in a budgerigars. Slide Courtesy of Dr Julie Langenberg, International Crane Foundation, Wisconsin.

low humidity may also develop scaling of the legs and cere. Older birds may develop increased proliferation and prominence of the scales on their legs. The cere of adult budgerigars (most frequently females) can become hyperkeratotic but the aetiology is unknown.

Clinical signs. Fine scaling and/or crusting of the cere and legs is the most obvious sign, but apterium skin will be dry and flaking, as well. If the dietary or environmental problem has been long-standing, the affected areas may be erythematous. The plantar surface of the feet may be sensitive to the touch. Feathers should be carefully examined for signs of stress bars and abnormal feather growth.

Diagnosis. Skin scrapings should be performed to rule out mites. A careful dietary history should be obtained; nutritional deficiencies are one of the most common causes for skin and feather problems in birds. The bird's environment, especially temperature and humidity, should be reviewed; remember that the bird's environment extends beyond its cage.

Treatment. Specific treatment depends upon the cause. Dietary changes are relatively easy to institute (see Discoloured feathers) but response to nutritional supplementation may not be obvious for several months. The humidity in the bird's cage area can be increased by daily water sprays or bathing/showering the bird. If necessary, the bird's legs and cere can be treated with humectant formulated for dogs and cats. After a hyperkeratotic cere is softened, the upper layers of keratin can be peeled away.

Prognosis. The prognosis is good to excellent. Recurrence of cere hyperkeratosis is common.

Avian poxvirus

Description. Avian pox occurs in numerous species and is caused by several strains of *Avipoxvirus*. Several syndromes are associated with this viral infection, but only the cutaneous manifestations will be described here. Transmission occurs when injured skin is exposed to the virus by direct contact, biting insects or a contaminated environment. It is highly contagious and often causes an epornithic in the same species housed together. Poxvirus can also remain latent in a flock for several years.

Clinical signs. The cutaneous dry form of pox is common, especially in passerines. Papular lesions form on the head, beak, eyelids, feet and other unfeathered areas of skin. Papules eventually become yellow-brown crusts. Ocular lesions, including crusts and secondary keratitis, are common with 'wet' pox in blue-fronted Amazon parrots, mynahs and several psittacine species.

Diagnosis. Skin scrapings or biopsy samples are diagnostic. Large eosinophilic cytoplasmic inclusion bodies, referred to as Bollinger bodies, are identified in the epithelium.

Treatment. No specific treatment is available but supportive care is often necessary. The skin should be kept clean and dry and ocular lesions treated. Antimicrobial therapy may be warranted in severe cases. Specific vaccines are available for some strains such as pigeon, canary and parrot poxvirus.

Prognosis. The outcome may vary with the species of bird and strain of virus, as well as the extent of the lesions. Individual birds may be symptomatic for 3–4 weeks. Recovered birds are protected for several months.

Dermatitis

Description. Inflammation and ulceration of the skin has been associated with wounds, abscesses, contact irritants, neoplasia, giardiasis, vitamin E deficiency or underlying metabolic disease. Commonly affected sites include the patagia (skin membranes where the wings joint the body), sternum, pericloacal region, legs and feet. Damaged skin may be primarily or secondarily infected with bacteria or fungus. Commonly isolated bacteria are *Staphylococcus* and *Streptococcus* spp.; fungal isolates are less common and quite variate. Amazon parrots are prone to a pruritic condition of the feet and legs that causes the bird to self-mutilate these areas. The aetiology is unknown.

Clinical signs. Chronically affected skin is inflamed, oedematous and/or ulcerated. The dermatitis may involve both skin and feather follicles. Transudation and exudation may be present. Cockatiels and lovebirds are commonly affected by giardiasis with an associated ulcerative dermatitis and feather-picking behaviour. These lesions are usually not pruritic. Sternal lesions can often be traced back to an earlier traumatic event, bruising, or devitalising of the skin. The Amazon parrot syndrome (most commonly in the yellow-naped Amazon parrot) initially appears as erythema of the foot or both feet and rapidly progresses to black discolouration of the skin. Self-mutilation often occurs before the early signs are noted.

Diagnosis. Evaluate the diet and the environment. Examine stool samples for *Giardia* by direct smear, ELISA or immunofluorescent tests. Culture exudative or ulcerated lesions for bacteria and superficial fungus. Biopsy of chronic non-responsive lesions may be useful. The feet of parrots with self-mutilation should be biopsied; look for an underlying cause. Bacterial and fungal elements have been associated with some of these cases.

Treatment. Make recommendations for a balanced diet. *Giardia* is treated with metronidazole; (10–30 mg/kg *per os* b.i.d.) for 10 days. Cases of *Giardia*-associated dermatitis have benefited from parenteral administration of vitamin E.

Exudative lesions should have the surrounding feathers removed; the lesions should be debrided and then flushed. Bacterial or fungal infections are treated with systemic antimicrobials as indicated by sensitivity testing. Use only water-soluble topical medications. Self-adherent wound dressings are recommended for deep infections. Surgical excision and primary closure of necrotic or non-healing wounds will speed recovery. Lesions that are being self-mutilated, especially in the wing patagia, will benefit from bandaging and placing and Elizabethan collar on the bird.

Amazon parrot foot necrosis is treated with systemic antimicrobial therapy based on culture and biopsy findings. In addition, strict hygiene and sanitation is indicated, plus some combination of an Elizabethan collar, neck brace, antihistamine, topical steroids or topical disinfectants.

Prognosis. Chronic ulcerative lesions may heal, but scar tissue in the patagia may become deforming and can lead to future irritation. Dermatitis of the distal extremities heals slowly. Amazon parrot foot necrosis may recur.

Cutaneous papillomatosis

Description. Small, proliferative wart-like growths have been described on unfeathered areas of some birds. Papillomavirus is associated with proliferative masses on the legs of finches. A papillomavirus was identified from proliferative lesions on the head and eyelids of an African grey parrot. Squamous papillomas occur on the feet of cockatoos associated with Herpes virus-like particles. Proliferative growths on feet, wings, uropygial gland, eyelids and skin around the beak occur in several psittacine species. A viral cause is suspected for these wart-like lesions, but has not been consistently demonstrated.

Clinical signs. Clinical signs commonly include a dry, slow-growing, proliferative growth on the skin. Growths on the feet and legs are hyperkeratotic. Lesions may have the appearance of a benign epithelial tumour.

Diagnosis. Excisional biopsy material should be examined histologically. Viral particles may be identified by electron microscopy. Viral culture is difficult and often inconclusive.

Treatment. Surgical removal is the treatment of choice.

Prognosis. The prognosis is good. Regrowth may recur if total excision was not accomplished.

Feather follicle cysts

Description. Feather cysts are most common in canaries and have been described in psittacines and mynahs. The pathogenesis is unknown, although there may be a genetic predisposition to develop cysts. Follicular cysts occur when the follicular orifice is obstructed. The growing feather does not emerge and continues to grow inside the follicle, enlarging in size and collecting keratin debris and caseous material.

Clinical signs. Feather cysts may occur anywhere on the bird's body, but are most common on the wings and back. They may be singular or multiple. In canaries, entire feather tracts may be involved. The cysts can rupture, ulcerate and become secondarily infected.

Diagnosis. The diagnosis is usually obvious from the clinical examination. The major differential diagnosis is a tumour; tumours of the feather follicle and skin are relatively uncommon.

Treatment. Treatment is by surgical excision of the feather follicle or affected feather tract.

Prognosis. The prognosis is excellent but care must be taken to prevent excessive haemorrhage during surgery. Affected birds should not be bred.

Lipoma/liposarcoma

Description. Lipomas are common skin tumours of pet birds, especially budgerigars and rose-breasted cockatoos. Lipomas may develop as early as 1 year of age. Obesity may predispose birds to lipomas, and a genetic influence is suspected in budgerigars. Liposarcomas are rare in birds, and may be locally invasive and metastatic.

Clinical signs. The most common sites for lipomas are in descending order of occurrence: sternum, wings, leg and abdomen. Birds often present with an obvious subcutaneous mass or the owner observes abdominal distention. Depending upon the location of the lipoma, the bird may or may not be able to fly or breathe normally. The skin over the lipoma may be xanthomatous (yellow and thickened due to infiltration of the skin with foamy macrophages) or thin and friable. Lipomas tend to be well encapsulated in the subcutis. Necrosis may occur in the center of large lipomas, or the surface may be traumatised. A thorough review of the diet is important. An additional physical finding may be an enlarged liver, often associated with hepatic lipidosis. Liposarcomas are firm on palpation, not well-encapsulated and are lightly vascular. Common sites include the sternum and the uropygial gland area.

Diagnosis. A fine needle aspirate can provide the cytological diagnosis. The aspirated material from a lipoma appears greasy and, when stained, lipocytes are the dominant cell type. Fat droplets may fill the background. Lipomas at the thoracic inlet must be differentiated from goitres. Biopsy for histological diagnosis is necessary for liposarcoma.

Treatment. Birds should undergo dietary changes to reduce fat intake and provide a balanced diet. Small, recently developed lipomas may respond to dietary management and exercise alone. Large or necrotic lipomas may need surgical removal if possible. The mass is often well vascularised, so caution is necessary. Liposarcomas are difficult to excise. There are a few anecdotal reports of birds with lipomas that responded to thyroxine therapy but its nonspecific use is not recommended. A TSH-response test can identify birds with hypothyroidism.

Prognosis. The prognosis is variable. Liposarcoma carries a poor prognosis. Dietary improvement may help to shrink the tumour as an aid to surgical excision.

Xanthoma/xanthomatosis

Description. Xanthoma means 'yellow mass' and is an accumulation of lipid-laden macrophages, giant cells and free cholesterol. The aetiology is unknown, but high-fat diets have been suspected.

Clinical signs. Xanthomas can occur anywhere on the skin and they frequently overlie lipomas. A xanthoma may appear as a featherless area with diffuse, friable, yellow thickening of the skin or well-defined subcutaneous nodules.

Diagnosis. A fine needle aspirate can provide the cytological diagnosis. Macrophages (filled with fat, multinucleated giant cells) and cholesterol crystals are present. Histological examination of a skin biopsy would appear similar but the crystals dissolve when alcohol fixatives are used.

Treatment. Xanthomas are a problem when they are very large or if the bird begins to mutilate the area. Surgical excision is recommended when necessary. Large, diffuse xanthomas may not be resectable but have responded to irradiation and hyperthermia. Partial amputation of an extremity has also been recommended for non-resectable xanthomas.

Tumours of the uropygial gland

Description. The uropygial gland is found on the caudal dorsal area of the back near the tail head.

This gland secretes oils used for preening and is not present in all species of birds. The uropygial gland may become impacted and infected, and is the site of several tumours. Squamous papillomas, squamous cell carcinomas, liposarcomas, adenomas and adenocarcinomas can occur in this area.

Clinical signs. Skin tumours of the uropygial gland are usually noticed when the bird is seen 'picking' at this area. Blood and discharge may be noted in the cage if the mass has ulcerated. If the gland's function is severely impaired, the bird's feathers may appear unkempt.

Diagnosis. The diagnosis of a tumour is usually made by clinical examination and biopsy for histological examination of tissue. In some cases, an impression smear of the mass may be useful.

Treatment. The treatment of choice is surgical excision if the tumour can be completely resected. Radiographs are indicated to identify possible metastasis or local invasion into the bone.

Prognosis. The prognosis is variable. Removal of the gland has few clinical side-effects.

Discoloured feathers

Description. A case of liver disease or heavy metal poisoning may present with abnormally coloured feathers and skin. Achromia — the lack of pigmentation — has been produced in poultry by specific dietary deficiencies (lysine, folic acid). Few dietary trials have been conducted on psittacine species, but those done with cockatiels demonstrated abnormal feather colouration when choline or riboflavin were withheld (Plate 28). Specific dietary deficiencies or excesses may have different effects with different species.

Brown or black feather tips may appear in mature green feathers due to superficial wearing of the keratin to reveal the melanin pigment within the feather.

Clinical signs. Signs of nutritional deficiencies include pale feather colouration, yellow instead of green and, in addition, the presence of stress bars. Birds with underlying liver disease may be initially presented by the owner for poor plumage long before more obvious signs of liver disease are evident. Elevated levels of biliverdin can affect skin and light-coloured feathers by staining them yellow or a greenish tinge. Feather discolouration may also occur with heavy-metal poisoning.

Diagnosis. Definitive diagnosis of a nutritionally related disease of the feathers is often difficult. In most cases, the diagnosis is presumptive, based upon a response to diet improvement. When birds are presented with discoloured feathers, the owner should be carefully questioned about feeding practices; what foods are offered and what the bird actually consumes, water sources, water containers, and the bird's activities. Birds that are allowed to roam free in the house may have access to toxins that are not readily apparent during the routine interviews. Stress bars can also be associated with changes in feeding habits or schedules and may support the diagnosis. Heavy-metal poisoning is diagnosed by blood analysis. Brown or black feather edges are associated with excessive wear and the owner should be asked when the previous moult occurred. If the bird has not moulted during the past 12 months, metabolic or endocrine disorders need to be investigated.

Treatment. If the specific dietary needs of the species are known, these should be reviewed and the diet improved. Most commonly, however, owners of pet birds are under the misguided assumption that bird seed alone is a balanced diet. Additionally, owners may store bird food improperly and allow seeds to get rancid or mouldy. Birds require a balanced diet and for many companion bird species this is best met by a formulated diet. A combination of formulated diets (75%) supplemented with fresh vegetables and fruits (25%) appears to keep most birds in good condition. When hepatic disease is diagnosed, the specific aetiology needs to be treated when possible.

Prognosis. The prognosis is usually good for nutritional problems. However, it is important to inform owners that colour is permanent in existing feathers; colour abnormalities will not resolve until a new feather replaces the old discoloured feather. In cases of corrected hepatic disease, affected feathers may return to the normal colour without a moult.

Husbandry causes of poor feather conditions

Description. Poor husbandry practices are a common cause of poor feather condition in companion birds. Inadequate diet, poor housing, inappropriate humidity and problems with cage mates result in poor feather condition.

Clinical signs. Affected birds may present with frayed feathers, discoloured feathers (discussed above) stress bars, bleeding feathers and broken feathers. Often, several of these conditions will coexist.

Diagnosis. A thorough history and examination of the bird in its cage is necessary. Attention to husbandry details cannot be emphasised enough. Signs of malnutrition and feather changes have been discussed. Birds in cages that are too small will often have broken or bleeding feathers. If the tail feathers are damaged, the location of the perches should be examined; the tail feathers may be sitting in a water dish or rubbing against the cage all day. Birds in large cages should be observed for stereotypic behaviour such as circling and climbing the cage, which causes repetitive damage. Improper wing clipping may be the cause of the bird 'crashing' into surfaces when it tries to fly. 'Stress bars' represent a previous episode that has caused the developing feathers to be incomplete in a single band. If several bars are found on a feather, it indicates recurrent stressful events.

Treatment. If malnutrition is suspected, a formulated diet plus a good source of fresh, dark green and yellow vegetables should be recommended. Too much supplementation may dilute the nutrients provided in a balanced pelleted feed. If the damage is due to malnutrition, it may take 8–12 months of dietary improvement before normal feathers are produced. The size of the cage should be examined: it should be large enough so that the bird's feathers are not constantly rubbing up against the walls of the cage. If the rubbing is due to stereotypic behaviours, then behaviour modification (as discussed for feather picking) may be needed. Daily water sprays should be added to the bird's routine to help increase humidity and encourage grooming. Pulling out old feathers from these birds is not recommended, as the new feathers do not look much better than the older ones.

Prognosis. The prognosis is good, if the underlying cause can be identified and husbandry improvements can be made.

Feather dystrophy/dysplasia

Two major viral diseases of pet birds affect the growth of feathers: psittacine beak and feather disease (PBFD) and polyomavirus infection (previously termed papovavirus). The feather lesions may appear grossly similar when caused by either virus. 'French moult' is a generic term referring to abnormal feathers, as seen with polyomavirus or PBFD.

Stress bars

Stress bars are pale or translucent horizontal lines across the feather and they represent a defect in the formation of barbs and barbules. They may indicate illness, malnutrition of a temporary stressful event — for example capture, acute trauma, heat, cold, food deprivation — or may be associated with changes in feeding habits or schedules.

Psittacine beak and feather disease

Description. PBFD is caused by a small DNA virus recently placed in the family Circoviridae. It causes feather dystrophy and generally affects young birds. It has been observed in over 40 species of birds, but was first described and is most prevalent in cockatoos (Fig 24.3a,b). The virus has been recovered from faeces, crop material and feather dust, which can all contaminate the environment. Vertical transmission of the virus is also suspected. Asymptomatic adults that produce clinically affected offspring should be suspected as carriers.

Clinical signs. PBFD is most often a disease of immature birds, but adults also can develop clinical signs (Plate 29). The history often includes progressive feather-loss and replacement with dystrophic feathers (retained feather sheaths, clubbed feathers, blood within the feather shaft and constrictions of the feather shaft). All feathers may be infected. When birds are infected as neonates, abnormal feathers are noticed when the first down feathers are replaced. Feathers may have circumferential constrictions along the shaft. Birds that maintain a chronic infection with PBFD have more affected feathers with each moult. In some species the beak becomes affected as the disease progresses: overgrowth, irregular growth, necrosis and longitudinal

(a)

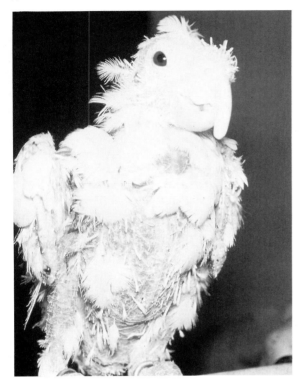

(b)

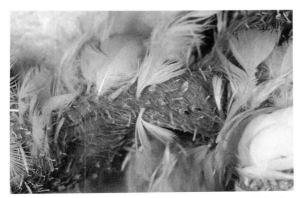

FIG. 24.3 (a) Cockatoo with psittacine beak and feather disease; (b) view of abnormal feather development. Slide Courtesy of Dr Julie Langenberg, International Crane Foundation, Wisconsin.

splitting are common. Affected lovebirds may have nodules in their skin.

Diagnosis. PBFD should be suspected when a psittacine has progressive feather-loss and deformed feathers. Skin biopsy of at least three to four feather follicles can assist the diagnosis (Plate 29). Basophilic, intracytoplasmic inclusion bodies in the pulp or epithelium is diagnostic. Intranuclear inclusions may also be present but are not conclusive. Sometimes, intranuclear inclusions in the pulp and feather follicles can be demonstrated by an impression smear and this is a useful pre-purchase test for clinically normal adult birds.

Specific and sensitive DNA probes are available and can be used on biopsy samples or blood samples to detect PBFD virus. The DNA probe test using whole blood (not coagulated) is recommended to identify subclinical infections in birds with normal feather appearance. Normal-appearing birds that test positive should be retested in 90 days. If the sample is still positive, the bird is a latent carrier. If negative, it can be assumed the bird has been exposed and has eliminated the virus.

Treatment. No treatment is available. Birds with only feather lesions may require supportive care if secondary diseases occur. Beak and nail lesions are thought to be painful for the bird. Euthanasia is recommended for debilitated birds. A carrier bird should be isolated from other birds, especially neonates.

Prognosis. The prognosis is poor and infected birds should be isolated.

Polyomavirus

Description. Polyomavirus is a DNA virus in the family Papovaviridae. Budgerigar fledgling disease is an acute generalised infection caused by a polyomavirus and providing a range of signs in neonatal budgerigars (1–8 weeks) from acute death to abnormal feather formation. Other psittacine species are affected by polyomavirus, but infections tend to be systemic and feather abnormalities are rare.

Clinical signs. Budgerigars that survive the acute phase of the virus infection may have dystrophic feathers. Some birds show only malformed feathers, without previous signs of illness. Primary and tail feathers are dystrophic, and down feathers may be absent along the back and abdomen. These feather lesions may resolve after several months.

Diagnosis. The gross appearance of abnormal feathers caused by polyomavirus can look similar to PBFD. Histologically, a biopsy will contain basophilic intranuclear inclusion bodies. A definitive diagnosis requires identification of the virus using a sensitive and specific DNA probe for polyomavirus. Viral neutralisation can be used if virus is cultured. Serology is also available to identify exposed birds with antibodies. Budgerigars that are carriers can be identified by sustained high titres to polyomavirus. The best sample to detect viral shedding by birds is a cloacal swab tested by the viral-specific DNA probe.

Treatment. There is no specific treatment. Birds with clinical systemic signs do not respond well to supportive care.

Prognosis. Birds with only feather lesions may resolve to normal plumage after several months. Carriers of polyomavirus can intermittently shed virus in excrement and feather dust. These birds can be maintained as pets if kept isolated to prevent exposure of other birds, especially neonates.

Feather picking

Description. Feather picking is a generic term used to describe a bird's plucking and self-mutilation of its feathers or skin in captivity. The signs may vary from mild to severe, with progressive damage to the feather follicle. 'Feather picking' generally refers to birds with a behavioural problem but it is important to remember that this term describes a clinical sign and that behavioural feather picking is only one cause. Feather picking may also be a manifestation of internal disease or a response to chronic dermatitis.

Clinical signs. Feather-loss caused by 'feather picking' has a characteristic distribution. Normal feathering is present on the head but damaged or missing feathers are present in all areas that the bird can reach with its beak. If the feather picking is being done by another bird, then feathers around the head and neck are also affected.

Diagnosis. The underlying cause of feather picking can be difficult to determine. It is important to remember that the diagnosis of behavioural or psychogenic feather picking should be considered a diagnosis of exclusion. Examination of a feather picking bird needs to be approached systematically. A complete history and review of husbandry practices may yield important information. The physical examination needs to be thorough. Evidence of infectious causes of feather-loss need to be investigated. This may require skin scrapings, impression smears, feather pulp culture and cytology and skin biopsies. Birds presented for chronic feather picking may have subclinical internal disease; faecal Gram's staining, faecal parasite examination, complete blood count and serum biochemistry panel need to be performed. Many self-mutilating birds have evidence of liver disease or other organopathies for which radiographs or endoscopy are useful. Serum electrophoresis to identify inflammatory conditions may be beneficial.

Treatment. Treatment depends upon the underlying cause of the feather picking; specific diseases should be treated accordingly. The treatment and management of birds with psychogenic feather picking are similar to and as difficult as those of the cat with psychogenic licking. Behaviour modification, diet correction and environmental stimulation may help birds with psychogenic feather picking. Enlarged cages, toys, more social interaction from owners, adequate sleep (cover the cage or move to a quiet environment for 8–12 hours), eliminating exposure to cigarette smoke and providing routine exposure to sunlight may assist positive behaviour changes. The diet should be carefully reviewed and improved. Dietary variety with vegetables and fruit will help to enrich the bird's environment. Some birds may benefit from the companionship of a cage mate; this does not always work and the new bird may be overpreened, as well. Sexual frustration can lead to self-mutilation and this can be resolved when given breeding opportunities. When feather picking is determined to be psychological and is nonresponsive to environmental enrichment, then drug therapy may be attempted but is not always successful. Behaviour-modifying drugs such as tricyclic antidepressants, haloperidol and naltrexone hydrochloride have been suggested. Antihistamines such as hydroxyzine hydrochloride have also been tried.

Treatment with hormones such as thyroxine, testosterone and medroxyprogesterone has also been reported. Every agent has undesirable side-effects, so the risks must be evaluated along with potential benefits. The use of Elizabethan collars is controversial among avian practitioners; these collars may interfere with the bird's ability to groom normally, eat and drink. A collar may interrupt the behaviour but it does not address the underlying problem.

Prognosis. The prognosis for birds with psychogenic feather picking is variable. Even when an inciting cause is identified and treated, feather picking can be a habit difficult to break. Chronic mutilation can damage the follicles so that feather development is impossible.

25

Skin Diseases of Small Mammals

JOANNE PAUL-MURPHY and KAREN MORIELLO

Small mammals (rodents, rabbits, hedgehogs, chinchillas and ferrets) are becoming increasingly popular as pets. They are also commonly found in school classrooms as teaching animals. In their natural environment, most of these species spend a large portion of their day searching for food, burrowing and escaping predators. When housed in captivity with *ad libitum* feeding and no threat of predators, these animals have little to do each day in their relatively sterile environment. Because of this, it is important to determine whether the animal's skin disease is being caused by spontaneous disease or by habitat. Self-mutilation or aggression are common causes of skin lesions in some rodents. Poor sanitation, over-crowding, leaky water bottles, and poor nutrition are all potential causes of skin disease.

History

It is critical to obtain carefully as much information as possible about the husbandry practices of owners with small mammals. With the possible exception of ferrets, most small animals kept as pets are 'for the children' and often not much thought was given to the decision to obtain the pet; it is common for owners of small animals to know little about the housing, feeding and care of the animal in question. If possible, the animal should be brought in its cage for veterinary examination.

In addition to the routine clinical history questions owner's should be asked:

- How long have they owned the animal? (The life expectancy of these animals is not very long. Recently acquired animals from pet shops or breeders would be more likely to have infectious/contagious skin diseases.)
- How many animals are housed together or are allowed even partial contact with each other?

(Over crowding leads to aggression, increases the need for sanitation, may be the cause of nutritional diseases, etc.)
- How is the animal housed? How is the cage cleaned and with what chemicals? Does the bedding get wet from the water bottle? Where is the cage kept? What is the temperature of the cage?
- What are the feeding practices?
- What other animals is the animal exposed to in the home?
- Does a pet rodent roam free in the home?
- What toys or other 'activities' does the animal have in the cage?

Physical Examination

Physical examination techniques and procedures in these species are not very different from those used to examine dogs and cats.

It is important to be familiar with proper techniques for restraint, both to protect the examiner from injury and to protect the pet from injury. It is important to be familiar with the normal anatomical structures in these species that can occasionally be associated with skin diseases. **Gerbils** have a ventral marking gland or scent gland that is tan-yellow in appearance. **Hamsters** have a flank gland that is costovertebral in location; this gland is more prominent in males and appears as a black/brown thickening of the skin. In **guinea pigs**, there are two areas with prominent accumulations of sebaceous glands — the dorsal sacral area and in the perineal and genital area, particularly in males. **Rabbits** have scent glands located in blind pouches that are lateral to the anogenital line. All of the dermal sebaceous glands in a **ferret** are scent glands; however, there are two perianal glands that are very prominent.

DIFFERENTIAL DIAGNOSIS OF SKIN DISEASES OF SMALL MAMMALS

Pruritus	Mite infestations Lice Fleas Dermatophytes Pinworms
Hair-loss	Ectoparasites Dermatophytes Behavioural causes Endocrine disorders Malnutrition
Aggression/self- mutilation	Behavioural causes of hair-loss Bite wounds
Scaling, crusting and matting of the hair coat	Mite infestations Bite wounds Seborrhoea, low humidity and ringtail Dermatophytosis
Subcutaneous nodules	Abscesses and granulomas Neoplasia Cuterebra fly larvae
Ulcerative skin lesions	Contact irritant reaction Bacterial infections Neoplasia Pododermatitis Treponema

FIG. 25.1 Differential diagnosis of skin diseases of small mammals.

Selected Skin Diseases of Small Mammals

Parasitic Skin Diseases

Lice infestations

Description. Lice infestations are uncommon in most small rodents with the exception of guinea pigs. Guinea pigs are common hosts for the biting louse *Gliricola porcelli*, and more rarely *Gyropus ovalis*. Lice can infest rats, mice and rabbits. The louse of rats and mice is the sucking louse, *Polyplax* spp.; and the rabbit louse is *Haemodipsus* spp. Lice infestations are usually associated with poor husbandry and overcrowding.

Clinical signs. Lice infestations in guinea pigs are very similar to those in other pets. Lice cause pruritus, hair-loss and excoriations. The first signs may be an unkempt hair coat. *Polyplax* spp. infestations can cause anaemia if severe.

Diagnosis. Lice are easily found by clinical examination alone. A hand-held magnifying lens may be helpful; alternatively, lice may be found after flea-combing of the coat.

Treatment. Biting lice can be treated with ivermectin (300–400 µg/kg SC). This treatment should be repeated in 2 or 3 weeks. Alternatively, the guinea pig can be treated with a pyrethrin flea spray. The flea spray should be thoroughly applied to the hair coat twice weekly for at least 4 weeks. Flea sprays labelled as safe to use on kittens are recommended. It is important to treat all guinea pigs in the household and to clean the environment thoroughly. Lice cannot live off the host for very long but there is a slight chance of reinfestation from the environment.

Prognosis. The prognosis is excellent. Lice are host-specific and are not a source of zoonotic disease, although *Haemodipsus* spp. are vectors of *Francisella tularensis* from rabbits to man.

Fleas

Description. Flea infestations can be a problem in rabbits, hedgehogs, ferrets and occasionally small rodents. In clinical practice, infestations with *Ctenocephalides* spp. are possible in any small mammal that lives in a home with dogs and cats.

Clinical signs. Flea infestations are very similar to those in other species. The fleas cause pruritus, hairloss, and self-excoriation. Flea-bite allergy dermatitis can occur, especially in ferrets.

Diagnosis. Fleas are easily found on physical examination or with the aid of a flea comb or hand lens.

Treatment. Flea-infested small mammals should be treated very similarly to flea-infested cats. These small mammals should not be dipped with flea dips. Pyrethrin or carbaryl based products labelled as safe for use in cats are recommended. Fleas need to be eradicated from the animal's environment.

Prognosis. The prognosis is excellent. It is important to remember that fleas can cause flea-bite anaemia in heavy infestations.

Mite infestations

Description. Mites are the most common ectoparasite of rodents. The various species of mite and their respective hosts are summarised in Fig. 25.2.

Clinical signs. Mite infestations in small mam-

ASCARIASIS OF SMALL MAMMALS	
Species	**Parasite**
Rabbits	*Cheyletiella* spp. *Sarcoptes scabiei* *Notedres cati* (fur mites) *Listrophus gibbus* *Psoroptes cuniculi* (ear mite) *Demodex* spp. (rare)
Rats and mice	*Myobia musculi* *Myocoptes musculinus* *Myocoptes rombusti* (fur mites) *Radfordia affinis* and *ensifera* *Notedres* spp. (ear mites)
Guinea pigs	*Trixaxarus caviae* *Chirodiscoides caviae*
Hamsters and gerbils	*Demodex criceti* *Demodex aurati*
Hedgehogs	*Chorioptes* spp.
Ferrets	*Sarcoptes scabiei* *Otodectes cynotis*

FIG. 25.2 Ascariasis of small mammals.

mals cause hair-loss, pruritus, scaling and excoriations. The severity of the pruritus can vary from mild to severe. Weight-loss and debilitation are possible in long-standing heavy infestations. Sarcoptic mange in ferrets can affect primarily the feet and nail bed or they may have a more generalised form with alopecia. Both forms are very pruritic. Hedgehogs may lose spines from chronic mite infestations. Demodicosis is uncommon in young animals and it is most likely seen in older animals. Demodicosis is often associated with some underlying disease, as in hamsters with adrenal tumours. Hamsters may have mixed infections with two species of *Demodex*: one looks like the *Demodex* mite of dogs, while *D. criceti* is less typical in appearance. Ear mite infestations can be asymptomatic or they may be associated with crusting, exudate and pruritus. Rabbits may develop aural haematomas and head tilts secondary to ear mite infestations (Plate 30).

Diagnosis. Uniformly, mite infestations are diagnosed via wide, deep skin scrapings.

Treatment. With the exception of demodicosis, mite infestations in rabbits and rodents are best treated with 300–400 µg/kg of ivermectin SC repeated at weekly or biweekly intervals for three treatments. Mice can be treated topically with a drop of 1% ivermectin at a dose of 0.2 mg/kg. All

animals should be treated. The environment should be cleaned to prevent fomite transmission.

When treating ear mites, remove the crusting debris from the ears. In rabbits, ear cleaning can be difficult and irritating to the animal. One to two drops of ivermectin at 0.4 µg/kg placed directly in the ears is an effective treatment. Ferrets also respond well to direct application of ivermectin in the ears. A micropipette is necessary to deliver the small volume (approximately 5 µl for a 25 g mouse). Topical treatment alone with traditional ear mite medications may not be successful because owners may have difficulty applying the medication and it might not penetrate the thick crusted debris. Feline flea products are safe to use in ferrets and rabbits. Treating the body with a flea powder or spray can assist in reducing mite populations.

Treatment of demodicosis is difficult. Amitraz dip can be used but it may be possible to treat demodicosis with ivermectin. Dogs with demodicosis have responded to daily ivermectin (200–600 µg/kg for at least 30–60 days) and the same protocol may be useful in other species.

Prognosis. The prognosis is excellent. It is important to remind owners that some mite infestations are zoonoses, such as *Sarcoptes* (rabbits and ferrets) and *Cheyletiella* (rabbits and ferrets), and that lice from wild rabbits may transmit *Francisella tularensis*.

Pinworms

Description. Pinworms are species-specific. Rabbits and mice, rats and other rodents are commonly infested.

Clinical signs. Clinical signs of oxyurid infestation are rare, except in mice in which intense anal and perianal pruritus can occur. Self-mutilation of the tail head may be evident.

Diagnosis. Definitive diagnosis is made via faecal examination or by pressing cellophane tape to the perineal area and then pressing the tape on to a glass microscope slide.

Treatment. Pinworm infestations can be treated with ivermectin (300 µg/kg *per os* or SC), thiabendazole (100 mg/kg) every 7 days for four doses or with mebendazole (40 mg/kg *per os*) for two treatments 7 days apart.

Prognosis. The prognosis is excellent.

Hair-Loss

Dermatophytosis

Description. Dermatophytosis is an uncommon problem in young rodents, hedgehogs, rabbits and ferrets. The most common cause is *Trichophyton* spp. but *Microsporum canis* has been isolated from rabbits and ferrets.

Clinical signs. Hair-loss and scaling are the most common clinical signs. Initial lesions are found around the head and feet. Pruritus is variable. Rabbits can be asymptomatically infected with *Trichophyton* spp.

Diagnosis. Definitive diagnosis is made via fungal culture.

Treatment. Dermatophytosis is a self-limiting disease; most healthy animals will self-cure. The purpose of treatment is to limit contagion to people and other animals and to speed recovery. The decision to treat the animal will depend upon the severity of the lesions, the number of animals to be treated and ability of the owner to medicate the animal. Griseofulvin (25–50 mg/kg *per os*) once daily until mycological cure is the standard treatment of choice. Itraconazole (10 mg/kg *per os*) once daily for 15 days will abort the infection and is an alternative therapy when large numbers of animals are involved. Lime sulphur sponge-on dips (4 ounces/gallon or 25 g/l) are reported to be helpful, but usually topical agents as sole therapies are ineffective.

Prognosis. The prognosis is excellent. Dermatophytosis is a zoonotic disease and transmission is a public health concern.

Behavioural causes of hair-loss (see Self-mutilation/aggression)

Endocrine causes of hair-loss

Description. Endocrinopathies or suspect endocrine causes of hair-loss are recognised in hamsters, guinea pigs, and ferrets. Hamsters have been reported to have signs suggestive of hyperadrenocorticism. These signs are believed to be due to a functional adenoma or adenocarcinoma of the adrenal gland or a pituitary adenoma. Female guinea pigs may lose hair during late gestation. Aged female guinea pigs may be affected with a reproductive hormone disorder. Signs are believed to be due to ageing changes in the ovary and possible production of increased or altered reproductive hormones.

Hyperoestrogenism and adrenal gland hyperplasia or neoplasia are well recognised in ferrets (Plate 31). The exact pathogenesis of adrenal gland hyperplasia in ferrets is unclear; this disease is not hyperadrenocorticism. There is no increase in serum cortisol nor are adrenal tests abnormal. The clinical signs may be due to the abnormal production of reproductive hormones. Some authors have speculated that the increase in incidence of adrenal tumours may be associated with early neutering practices. Generalised alopecia of the ferret may occur with neoplasia of the reproductive tract. Ferrets will also show seasonal symmetrical hair-loss of the tail only.

Clinical signs. Hamsters, particularly the long-haired breed, may develop a bilaterally symmetrical alopecia of the caudal trunk and lumbosacral area. The skin becomes hyperpigmented and thin and is non-pruritic. Guinea pigs will show non-inflammatory, non-pruritic, bilaterally symmetrical alopecia of the lumbosacral area. Female ferrets that have not been neutered or bred will enter into a prolonged oestrus; this state of hyperoestrogenism will result in pale mucous membranes (anaemia), a swollen vulva, petechial haemorrhages, anorexia, melaena, depression and symmetrical alopecia.

Another syndrome that is recognised in ferrets is adrenal gland disease. Adrenal gland hyperplasia or neoplasia usually starts in ferrets at around 3 years of age and two-thirds of affected ferrets are females. Almost all these ferrets have been neutered at or around 6 weeks of age. The first sign is usually hair-loss. Alopecia may initially be a seasonal condition in the late winter and early spring. The hair may regrow in the summer and this cycle is repeated in the next winter and spring. Hair-loss eventually continues and involves the tail, lumbosacral area, ventrum and trunk. The endocrine alopecia may also be sudden and persistent. The hair easily epilates with traction and the skin may be mildly inflamed, pruritic and scaly. The vulva is enlarged in 90% of affected female ferrets and there may be mucoid discharge. Abdominal palpation may occasionally reveal a mass just cranial to the left kidney, but often the adrenal enlargement is not gross enough to be detected by palpation or ultrasound.

Seasonal alopecia of breeding and neutered ferrets has been recognised. Affected ferrets will have a thinning of the coat in the spring. Tail alopecia of ferrets is usually seasonal and comedones can appear.

Diagnosis. Diagnosis of endocrine-related hair-loss in small mammals can be difficult and validated serum assays are not always readily available. Diagnostic tests for hamsters and guinea pigs are not reported; most clinical cases of endocrine-related diseases have been reported as presumptive diagnosis or are diagnosed upon necropsy. The dexamethasone suppression test or ACTH response test does not aid the diagnosis of ferret adrenal hyperplasia or neoplasia.

Since many female ferrets are neutered at a young age, hyperoestrogenism is relatively uncommon. The history of an intact female ferret exhibiting signs of anaemia and prolonged oestrus is usually sufficient for making a diagnosis.

Surgically neutered ferrets with signs of adrenal gland disease can be challenging diagnostically. Adrenal gland function tests are normal in these animals. Complete blood counts and serum chemistry panels are usually normal. Abdominal radiographs and abdominal ultrasound are most useful for diagnosing an enlarged adrenal gland. Elevated serum levels of adrenal androgens or oestradiol can be an indication of adrenal corticol neoplasia. Spayed females presented with an enlarged vulva and early signs of symmetrical alopecia may have either an adrenal gland tumour or an ovarian remnant. A trial of human chorionic gonadotropin (1000 units) or GNRH (20 µg) administered twice at 2-week intervals may be helpful. If the vulvar enlargement is due to an ovarian remnant, the treatment will decrease the size of the vulva.

Treatment. Surgical removal of the ovaries is the treatment of choice in guinea pigs with suspect ovarian disease causing hair-loss. Hamsters with suspect adrenal tumours have responded to oral metyrapone (8 mg daily) mixed in corn syrup.

Seasonal alopecia of the ferret is usually self-limiting but often recurrent. Surgical removal of the adrenal gland or ovariohysterectomy in ferrets are the respective treatments of choice for adrenal gland disease or hyperoestrogenism.

Prognosis. The prognosis is variable.

Self-Mutilation/Aggression

Hair-loss

Description. Aggression and self-mutilation are very common causes of hair-loss in small mammals. Female animals may pull hair from their abdomens to line nests, or alternatively they may pull hair from pups at or around the time of weaning. Dominant mice, rats, gerbils, and guinea pigs commonly 'barber' or chew off the hair of subordinant members in the group. Animals with poor housing may have 'bald' noses due to constant trauma with cage bars, water dishes, etc.

Chinchillas will release a patch of fur if handled roughly or from fighting. This 'fur slip' leaves a smooth area of hairless skin.

Clinical signs. Behavioural causes of hair-loss usually occur in groups of animals. Close examination of the group will usually show that the largest and/or most dominant member is free of hair-loss and lesser members of the group have areas of hair-loss. Overcrowding is an inciting condition in laboratory rodents but is less common with companion animals.

'Barbering' tends to occur around the head, back and tail; close examination of the hairs will show that individual hairs are blunted. Bite wounds and other signs of trauma may be found.

Diagnosis. Definitive diagnosis may be difficult in some cases. Skin scrapings for mites and a dermatophyte culture(s) should be performed. The diagnosis is much easier to make if all of the animals in a group can be examined; the dominant animal or adult is free of hair-loss. In many species, the female is most aggressive and dominant.

Abrasions or hair-loss on the face of a solitary animal suggest self-mutilation from lack of bedding and/or appropriate housing.

Treatment. Treatment is relatively easy. The most dominant animal should be separated from the group; young animals should be separated from adults at the time of weaning; male animals are usually aggressive and should be separated or castrated. Reduction of day length and light intensity may help to reduce social stress.

Prognosis. The prognosis is excellent. Chinchillas may take several months to regrow hair-loss due to 'fur-slip'.

Bite wounds

Description. Bite wounds are very common in many small mammals that are housed in groups. Bite wounds are usually the result of aggression and dominance activities. Male mice are extremely aggressive if allowed to interact. In ferret breeding behaviour neck biting is a normal activity.

Clinical signs. Bite wounds may present with a variety of clinical signs ranging from matting of the hair coat from exudate and blood to clinically obvious abscesses. Depending upon the severity of the signs, the victim may or may not be clinically ill.

Diagnosis. Diagnosis is usually obvious with exudate and/or puncture wounds readily apparent. Impression smears of the exudate and Grams stain are usually sufficient to diagnose a bite wound. *Streptococcus* spp. and *Staphylococcus* spp. are frequently identified by culture of an abscess.

Treatment. The hair from the area immediately surrounding the wound should be clipped and the wound cleaned and debrided. Depending upon the severity of the lesion, systemic antibiotic therapy may be indicated. Corrections of underlying housing conditions to reduce aggression is indicated.

Prognosis. The prognosis is good.

Scaling Diseases

Seborrhoeic skin disease

Description. Non-infectious, non-contagious seborrhoeic skin diseases in small mammals are either the result of low humidity or are due to the normal accumulation of sebum on the hair coat of species with specialised glands. Humidity is a critical factor in the housing of small mammals. If the relative humidity is below optimum for many species, the hair and skin will dehydrate and exfoliation will occur. Alternatively, a rough unkept hair coat may be a sign of too high humidity in the cage, possibly from a leaky water bottle. Rats will commonly be affected by a condition called 'ringtail' if the relative humidity is less than 30%, the environmental temperature is high or frostbite has occurred. Ischaemia develops due to damage to the microcirculation.

Clinical signs. Dry scaling of the skin and hair coat are seen clinically. Rats with ringtail present with annular constrictions of the tail. Gangrene of the tail and sloughing will occur in advanced cases. Oily matted hairs, especially in male animals, are highly suggestive of normal sebum discharge from a scent gland.

Diagnosis. A wide range of infectious and contagious skin diseases can cause scaling in small mammals. Skin scrapings should be performed to look for parasites; a dermatophyte culture should be performed. The feeding practices of the owner should be carefully examined; low protein and dietary fats can be a cause of scaling. The location of oily seborrhoea in an area with known accumulations of sebaceous glands is diagnostic of normal scent-gland accumulations.

Treatment. Treatment is not necessary for increased sebum production in areas of scent glands. If necessary, castration can be considered since testosterone will increase sebum production. Ringtail is treated by amputation of the necrotic portion of the tail. In cases of seborrhoea due to low humidity, management practices should be improved. The relative humidity should be maintained at 50%, especially for neonates. Many people commonly keep small mammals near forced-air heating vents to keep them warm or have heat lamps over their cages. Moving the cage to a different location and increasing the humidity in the home is helpful.

Prognosis. The prognosis is good.

Nodules

Abscesses and granulomas

Description. Abscesses and granulomas are common causes of lumps in small mammals. In young animals, it is much more likely for a lump to be an abscess or granuloma than a tumour. Hamsters have cheek pouches and many emergency lumps are impacted cheek pouches or just pouches stuffed with food. Oral abscesses are common in guinea pigs and rabbits that chew bedding or wood. Abscesses in rodents, especially gerbils, can be deep and extensive. In mice most lumps are usually tumours.

Subcutaneous abscesses may be single or multiple in rabbits and occur spontaneously or be related to trauma. *Pasteurella multocida* is a common bacterial isolate, but *Staphylococcus aureus*, *Pseudomonas* and *Bacteroides* are also reported. Abscesses along the lower mandible often have bone involvement.

Clinical signs. Abscesses and granulomas in small mammals are relatively common, especially in animals housed in a group, and are not clinically different from lesions presenting in dogs and cats. Rabbits and guinea pigs are commonly affected by cervical lymphadenitis. Often a thick caseous material is present. Hedgehogs may develop lymphadenitis with subcutaneous granulomas caused by *Mycobacterium* spp.

Diagnosis. Fine needle aspirates, impression smears and occasionally biopsy are necessary to make a definitive diagnosis. A 22 gauge needle may be necessary to aspirate the thick purulent material commonly found in rodent and rabbit abscesses. Radiographs are recommended when involvement of the bone or joints is suspected. Rabbit abscesses do not drain well and surgical excision is the recommended treatment. Complete excision may be impaired by purulent material dissecting through fascial planes. Culture and sensitivity can be very helpful since antibiotic therapy may require a term of 3–6 weeks.

Treatment. In most cases of abscesses and granulomas, surgical drainage is the treatment of choice. Oral antibiotics will minimise the spread of the infection to other areas and may help to resolve the infection post-operatively. Choice of antibiotics should be based upon culture and sensitivity as well as the species' sensitivity to antibiotics. Impacted cheek pouches should be emptied with forceps and swabs, then flushed with saline.

Prognosis. The prognosis is variable for a complete cure and depends upon the extent of the lesions. Abscesses in rabbits have a high rate of recurrence. Pasteurellosis can involve chronic formation of new abscesses in multiple locations.

Tumours

Description. Many different types of tumours have been recognised in small mammals; however, cutaneous tumours are relatively uncommon, except in ferrets and old gerbils (Plate 32).

Clinical signs. Because of the small size of many of these species, it is important to examine carefully any animal presented for a 'skin tumour'. Many tumours of the internal organs will be close to the body surface and may mimic a primary skin tumour. Depending upon the type, tumours may be haired or hairless, ulcerated, crusted and painful. Figure 25.3 summarises the most commonly recognised skin tumours of small mammals.

Diagnosis. It is important to differentiate between an infectious cause of a mass and a tumour. Fine needle aspirates and impression smears may be diagnostic but skin biopsy is more reliable.

Treatment. Treatment depends upon the tumour but in most cases surgical excision is the only viable treatment. Surgical excision may not be practical or possible, depending upon the biology of the tumour.

Prognosis. The prognosis is variable.

Cuterebriasis

Description. *Cuterebra* fly larvae develop in the subcutaneous tissue, forming a large swelling. This is a common problem of rabbits housed outside during warmer months.

Clinical signs. The larvae can be seen through an obvious air-hole in the subcutaneous mass. Purulent exudate may be present.

COMMON SKIN TUMOURS OF SMALL MAMMALS		
Species	**Tumour type**	**Clinical signs/comments**

Ferrets	Mastocytomas and mast cell tumour
	Sebaceous gland adenoma/
	  adenocarcinoma
	Squamous cell carcinoma
		Raised, red, mildly pruritic
		May be ulcerated, occurs around
		  prepuce of males
		Usually ulcerated, nodular or malignant

Mice	Mammary tumour
	
	Squamous cell carcinoma
		Malignant, surgical excision is difficult,
		  may be infectious (viral) in origin.
		  Affects both males and females
		Malignant, difficult to excise

Guinea pigs	Trichofolliculomas
	
	Mammary tumour
		Benign, surgical excision is curative,
		  may be multiple
		Usually benign fibroadenomas, rarely
		  malignant adenocarcinomas

Gerbils	Squamous cell carcinoma
	Adenoma and adenocarcinoma
	
	Melanoma
		Can occur anywhere
		Most commonly develop in area of the
		  ventral scent gland
		Most common near ears, base of tail
		  and feet

Hamsters	Papilloma; keratoacanthoma;
	  hemangioma; squamous cell
	  carcinoma; basal cell carcinoma
		Incidence of skin tumours is very low

Rabbits	Papilloma Lipoma	Benign neoplasms Benign neoplasms

Rats	Papilloma
	Squamous cell carcinoma
	Mammary gland tumour
		Prognosis for mammary fibroadenomas
		  is good if excised early. Often recur at
		  different sites

Hedgehogs	Papilloma Squamous cell carcinoma	Benign neoplasms Low incidence

Fig. 25.3 Common skin tumours of small mammals.

Diagnosis. Diagnosis is based upon visualising the larvae through the air-hole.

Treatment. Using local anaesthetics, such as a lidocaine block, enlarge the air-hole and remove the single larva. Flush the fistula with saline.

Prognosis. The prognosis is excellent.

Ulcerative Skin Lesions

Irritant contact reactions

Description. Irritant reactions are caused by a chemical insult against the skin. In small mammals the most common causes are soiled bedding (urine/faecal scald) and contact with a disinfectant. Irritant reactions usually occur rapidly, but they are concentration-dependent and it may take repeated exposure to the irritant before clinical signs are present.

Gerbils secrete porphyrins from the Harderian gland which can be irritating to the skin around the eyes and nose.

Clinical signs. The clinical signs of an irritant reaction will occur in the area where the skin has contacted the chemical. In most cases, the animal's feet and ventrum are affected. The area will be erythematous, exudative and often painful. Lacrimal porphyrins of gerbils cause an alopecia, dermatitis and irritation around the nose, hence the term 'sore nose'.

Diagnosis. Diagnosis is made by clinical signs and history of exposure to harsh chemicals and poor housing. Lesions may be secondarily infected and it may be difficult to separate the irritant reaction from secondary skin infections.

Treatment. Treatment requires a thorough cleaning of the animal's environment, improved sanitation and the use of bedding that is non-irritating and non-adherent to open wounds. Gerbils may benefit from a sand area for bathing to aid in self-cleaning.

The specific wounds should be gently cleansed with a mild antibacterial scrub, e.g. chlorhexidine. Topical antibacterial ointments, e.g. mupricin ointment, may be helpful. Systemic antibiotics may be necessary.

Prognosis. The prognosis is excellent.

Ulcerated pododermatitis

Description. 'Sore hocks' is a husbandry disease of rabbits and guinea pigs. Affected rabbits are usually large breeds, housed on wire, or have thin fur lining the hind foot pads. Rabbits that are constantly thumping with the hind feet are also prone to this problem. Wire-bottom cages are the most common cause of guinea pig pododermatitis.

Clinical signs. The hocks become inflamed, swollen, painful with secondary ulceration and infections. The most common isolate is *Staphylococcus* spp. Guinea pigs may develop calluses on the feet.

Diagnosis. Sore hocks are diagnosed via clinical examination and history.

Treatment. Treatment is challenging. The housing must be changed to coated grids, soft clean bedding, or other more supportive flooring. The feet should be debrided, flushed and treated with both topical and systemic antibiotics. Protective bandages are ideal, if the rabbit tolerates their presence.

Prognosis. The prognosis is variable. Affected rabbits should not be used for breeding: body size and thickness of the plantar surface of the feet are genetically determined.

Treponema

Description. *Treponema* is a venereal disease of rabbits that can occasionally cause skin lesions in areas other than on the genitals. This infection is caused by the spirochaete *Treponema cuniculi*. During grooming, rabbits will spread the infection to their face, nose and ears.

Clinical signs. Early lesions begin as vesicles that rapidly progress to macules and then scabbed ulcers.

Diagnosis. Definitive diagnosis is made via biopsy and serology; the organism is very difficult to culture. From active lesions the spirochaete can be seen with dark field preparations.

Treatment. The treatment of choice is penicillin (40,000 IU kg/day IM for 5 days) or benzathin penicillin G and procaine penicillin G (42,000–84,000 U/kg SC once weekly for three treatments). All exposed rabbits require treatment.

Prognosis. The prognosis is good.

26

Skin Diseases of Pet Pigs

KAREN MORIELLO

The most common porcine kept as a pet is the miniature or Vietnamese pot-bellied pig. The scope of this book does not allow for a detailed discussion of the breed's similarities and peculiarities relative to commercial pigs, but there is an excellent summary article of these topics, in other references.

History

As with all species, a complete history is often the key to making a diagnosis. Many people who obtain miniature pigs for pets do so as a status symbol and know little more about these pigs than what they look like. When presented with the pet pig for the first time, one is often at a loss. It is best just to consider these pigs to be strange-looking dogs. Just as in canine practice, the owners should be asked what diet is offered to the pig and what it eats, where it is housed, what the vaccination history is, what the owners have applied to the skin, whether it itches, how many animals are affected, etc?

Physical Examination

The physical examination of a pet pig can be quite challenging. These animals are usually very docile — except when they are transported or examined! Owners should be encouraged to harness train their pigs. Small pigs can be examined and handled like puppies but larger pigs are more difficult to examine. The key to a complete examination is to make sure that the pig has secure footing on a rug, towel or blanket. If the pig is small enough, it can be lifted on to a table. Pot-bellied pigs should **never** be lifted by their legs as is done with domestic commercial pigs; pot-bellied pigs' legs are easily dislocated and back injuries are possible. (A small animal practitioner would never lift a dog by its legs because of the possibility of injury.) Many pigs are best examined in lateral recumbency.

After appropriate restraint, the skin can be examined.

Selected Skin Diseases of Pet Pigs (Fig. 26.1)

Sarcoptic infestation

Description. Scabies in pigs is caused by *Sarcoptes scabei* var. *suis*. This mite is highly contagious and is the most common cause of pruritus in pigs. Most pigs are infested from the sow, which can be an asymptomatic carrier.

Clinical signs. Pruritus is the most common clinical sign associated with scabies in pigs. The pruritus is usually intense and will result in excoriations, lichenification, secondary bacterial infections, scaling and hair-loss. In severe cases, marked lichenification of the skin may be seen.

Diagnosis. Definitive diagnosis is made via skin scrapings. If sarcoptic infestation is suspected, however, the pig should be treated.

Treatment. Ivermectin (200–400 µg/kg IM) every 2 weeks for two treatments is recommended. Topical lime sulphur dip is recommended as a concurrent therapy; lime sulphur is miticidal and antipruritic.

DIFFERENTIAL DIAGNOSIS OF SKIN DISEASES OF PET PIGS	
Pruritus	*Sarcoptes scabiei* Lice
Scaling and crusting	Ectoparasites Non-infectious causes of seborrhoea (over-bathing, low humidity, normal skin) Staphylococcal infections (greasy pig)
Discoloration	Septicaemia Streptococcal infections Erysipelas Sunburn

FIG. 26.1 Differential diagnosis of skin diseases of pet pigs.

Prognosis. The prognosis is excellent. This is a zoonotic disease.

Lice

Description. Lice infestations are another common cause of pruritus in pigs. They are caused by *Haematopinus suis*.

Clinical signs. The clinical signs are very similar to scabies, except that the severity of the pruritus may be less.

Diagnosis. Lice are readily diagnosed via visual examinations.

Treatment. See treatment for scabies.

Prognosis. The prognosis is excellent.

Excessive scaling

Description. Excessive scaling is a common presenting complaint in pot-bellied pigs. Baby pigs have dry scaly skin at about 1 week of age but this is a normal phenomenon and they will shed large sheets of epidermis. In mature pigs, scaly skin is a common problem that may be due to excessive bathing by owners or to living in excessively dry environments, or it may be normal. Dietary causes are a consideration, but most pig rations are balanced and are not deficient in zinc and trace minerals.

Clinical signs. Excessive scaling is easily found on clinical examinations and is most noticeable on dark coloured individuals. Large flakes of skin will be shed. The pig should be carefully examined to make sure that there are no signs of pruritus or self-trauma; ectoparasites are common causes of scaling. If there are adherent crusts, zinc deficiency should be considered.

Diagnosis. Skin scrapings should be obtained to look for mites. A fungal culture can be obtained; but dermatophytosis is relatively rare in swine and it presents as a circular spreading lesion with raised crusts at the margins. Skin biopsies may be the most useful tool to determine whether the scaling is caused by a nutritional deficiency. If there is a history of bathing or living in the home, it is very likely that the skin is dehydrated and excessively scaling because of environmental reasons.

Treatment. Treatment depends upon the diagnosis. It is difficult to discourage owners from bathing these pigs; owners are unwilling to accept the natural odour of the animals. If the owners insist on bathing, hypoallergenic shampoos formulated for use on dogs are recommended. Moisturising cream rinses may be beneficial.

Prognosis. The prognosis is variable.

Greasy pig disease

Description. Greasy pig disease, or exudative epidermitis, is caused by infection with *Staphylococcus hyicus*.

Clinical signs. Exudative epidermitis is most commonly seen in pigs less than 8 weeks of age but it may also be seen in older pigs. Affected individuals are covered in a greasy crust that consists of sebum, serum and exudate, matting the coat. The pigs rapidly dehydrate, are febrile and can easily die.

Diagnosis. Diagnosis is made via clinical signs. Impression smears of the exudate will show an inflammatory exudate and intracellular cocci. Culture of the bacteria is helpful in identifying which antibiotic is best for treatment. Skin biopsy may be needed in cases where the clinical diagnosis is less certain.

Treatment. Pending culture and sensitivity results, affected pigs should be treated with penicillin (5000 IU/kg IM for 3–5 days) or lincomycin (10 mg/kg), topical antibacterial scrubs with chlorhexidine and antibacterial creams.

Prognosis. The prognosis is guarded. Infected pigs are often stunted in growth and may die of secondary complications.

Infectious causes of skin discoloration

Description. There are many infectious agents that can cause discoloured skin in pigs. Widespread erythema is a sign of septicaemia from agents such as *Salmonella*. Focal discoloration can be caused by streptococci, staphylococci and erysipelas.

Clinical signs. Widespread erythema is highly suggestive of septicaemia. Erysipelas infection is rare because most pigs are vaccinated against this agent. Nevertheless, diamond-shaped patches of erythema are the classic signs. Multifocal patches or pustules with erythematous borders are suggestive of streptococcal and staphylococcal infections.

Diagnosis. Diagnosis is made by isolating the organisms. If intact pustules are present, these should be cultured. If the erythema is more widespread, a full-thickness skin biopsy should be submitted for culture.

Treatment. Treatment should be based upon culture and sensitivity.

Prognosis. The prognosis is variable.

V   Problem-Oriented Approach to Skin Diseases of Specialised Skin Structures

27

Canine and Feline Ear Disease

IAN MASON and CRAIG GRIFFIN

A number of diseases can affect the aural pinna, the ear canal and the middle and inner ear. Inflammation of the ear canal, otitis externa, is the most important because it is so common in clinical practice. The prevalence of otitis externa in dogs is estimated to be 4–20%; it is less common in cats, with approximately 2–7% affected.

A discussion of diseases of the inner ear is beyond the scope of a dermatology book. This chapter will concentrate on the causes, diagnosis and treatment of otitis externa and media.

Pinnal disorders are shown in Fig. 27.1 and are discussed elsewhere in the text as indicated in the figure.

Aetiology and Pathogenesis of Otitis Externa

Otitis externa in dogs and cats has a complex pathogenesis involving initiating, predisposing and perpetuating factors. Identifying these factors and understanding their individual roles in the development of otitis externa is extremely important. Ear disease should be investigated thoroughly, carefully and **promptly**. Failure to 'unravel' the sometimes numerous pathogenic factors soon after the onset of disease may allow irreversible changes to occur within the external auditory tube or may prevent the identification of the primary initiating cause, (or causes) as the influence of perpetuating factors increases and secondary pathological changes occur.

Management of otitis externa should centre on the identification and correction of the primary and predisposing causes rather than simply prescribing topical glucocorticoid and antimicrobial preparations with no other therapy. The latter approach is seldom successful.

The aetiological and pathogenic factors involved in the development of this disease are listed in Fig. 27.2. **Primary factors** directly induce otitis externa, whereas **predisposing factors** place the animal at risk for the development of the disease. **Perpetuating factors** prevent resolution of the problem. Clinicians should remember that the ear canal of the dog and cat, like all types of skin, is a fragile, integrated ecosystem. Primary, predisposing and perpetuating factors act in concert to allow changes to the local micro-environment, thus promoting the multiplication of pathogenic opportunist micro-organisms and the establishment of otitis externa.

Primary Factors

Parasites

Otodectes cynotis is responsible for 50% of cases of otitis externa in cats and 5–10% of cases in dogs (otoacariasis). It is thought that aural inflammation follows the development of hypersensitivity to antigens in the saliva of the parasite. Cats can develop immunity to the mite, preventing reinfestation of the ear canal. This may partly explain the higher incidence of otoacariasis in young cats. Immune animals may become asymptomatic carriers and a source of infestation to other pets.

Other parasites which can infest the ear canal include *Sarcoptes scabiei*, *Notoedres cati*, *Demodex canis* and *Demodex cati*. Usually lesions are present on the pinnae and other skin sites. However, demodectic otoacariasis has been recognised in dogs and cats in the absence of other skin signs.

Foreign bodies

Grass seeds, debris and accumulations of dried medicaments may irritate and inflame the integument of the ear canal. Otitis externa due to grass seeds is common during the summer months. It is usually, but not invariably, unilateral. Clinical signs are acute and severe.

DISEASES OF THE CANINE AND FELINE PINNA			
Category	Disease	Species affected	Refer to chapter
Infections	Pyoderma Dermatophytosis	Dog Dog, cat	10 7, 15

Ectoparasitism	Sarcoptic mange
	Notoedric mange
	Localised demodicosis
	Insect-bites
	   Stomoxys calcitrans (stable fly)
	   Simulium spp. (black flies)
		Dog
		Cat
		Dog, cat
			5
			13
			6, 15
			5

Hypersensitivity	Atopy Dietary hypersensitivity intolerance Contact allergy (e.g. topical medicament)	Dog, cat Dog, cat Dog, cat	5, 13
Immune-mediated diseases	Pemphigus foliaceus Pemphigus erythematosus Pemphigus vulgaris Bullous pemphigoid Discoid/systemic lupus erythematosus Vasculitis Drug eruption	Dog, cat Dog, cat Dog Dog, cat Dog Dog, cat	7, 8, 15, 17
Environmental diseases	Frost-bite Solar-induced	Dog, cat Dog, cat	8, 17
Neoplasia	Squamous cell carcinoma Histiocytoma	Dog, cat Dog	8, 11, 17, 18
Miscellaneous disorders	Zinc-responsive dermatosis Juvenile cellulitis Idiopathic pinnal (pattern) alopecia Lichenoid-psoriasiform dermatosis Aural haematomata	Dog Dog Dog Dog Dog, cat	11 6 7
Note: Some pinnal disorders (especially hypersensitivity and immune-mediated disorders) may also affect the external ear canal leading to otitis. The role of these disorders in the pathogenesis of otitis are discussed fully in this chapter.			

FIG. 27.1 Diseases of the canine and feline pinna.

Hypersensitivity

Hypersensitivity is regarded as the most common initiating cause of persistent and recurrent otitis externa in dogs (*Chapter 5*). Inflammation and pruritus resulting from these disorders can be localised to the skin of the ear canal.

Atopic dermatitis can present solely as pruritic otitis externa with no other sign of skin disease. It is usually bilateral but unilateral cases, or cases where one ear is more severely affected have been recognised. At least 50% of dogs with atopic dermatitis have otitis concomitantly.

Although food allergy is much less common than atopy, it too can lead to otitis. One study reported that 18% of cats and 30% of dogs with food allergy also had otitis.

Contact allergy is a rare cause of otitis externa unless it is iatrogenic (medicament) induced. In such instances it may be regarded as a perpetuating factor, as discussed later. Animals may become sensitised to constituents of topical medicaments such as neomycin and propylene glycol. This phenomenon is much more common than most clinicians realise.

Keratinisation disorders and endocrinopathies

The skin lining the ear canal contains many sebaceous glands and modified sweat glands (**ceruminous glands**). Increased numbers of ceruminous glands may be associated with an increased susceptibility to otitis externa. Disorders of keratinisation and endocrine diseases may lead to quantitative and qualitative changes in the numbers and secretions of these glands. Certain of these secretions, especially essential fatty acids, may be pro-inflammatory. However, they also can provide a source of nutrient to pathogenic yeasts and bacteria and can change climatic conditions within the ear to favour bacterial multiplication. In the skin, keratinisation disor-

PATHOGENIC FACTORS IN CANINE AND FELINE OTITIS EXTERNA	

Primary factors	Parasites
	Foreign bodies
	Inflammatory skin disease
	  Hypersensitivity (atopy, food
	    hypersensitivity/intolerance, contact
	    allergy)
	  Keratinisation disorders (seborrhoea)
	  Endocrinopathies
	  Immune-mediated disorders
	Juvenile cellulitis

Predisposing factors	Conformation Climate Maceration of ear canal Iatrogenic factors Obstructive ear disease Systemic disease
Perpetuating factors	Bacteria Yeasts Otitis media Progressive pathological changes

FIG. 27.2 Pathogenic factors in canine and feline otitis externa.

ders lead to inflammation and pruritus; in the ear, they lead to otitis.

Immune-mediated disorders

Although these diseases predominantly affect the pinnae, it is possible for the lesions of systemic lupus erythematosus, pemphigus vulgaris and pemphigus foliaceus to extend down the ear canal to cause otitis externa (*Chapter 8* and *17*).

Juvenile cellulitis

Pups affected with juvenile cellulitis frequently have concomitant otitis externa with swelling, exudation and ulceration of the integument of the aural canal (*Chapter 11*).

Predisposing Factors

Conformation of the ear canal

Ear type has been shown to be an important risk factor in the development of otitis externa. The pendulous pinnae of breeds such as Cocker Spaniels leads to reduced evaporation of secretions from ear glands and inhibits heat dissipation. Resultant increases in temperature and relative humidity within the ear canal facilitate overgrowth of commensal yeasts and bacteria and the establishment of otitis

externa. The erect pinnae of cats may partly explain the low incidence of ear disease within this species. Conversely, German Shepherd Dogs with erect pinnae are prone to otitis externa despite the apparently favourable ear conformation of most individuals within this breed; this is likely to reflect the prevalence of primary causes of otitis externa, especially allergies, in German Shepherd Dogs.

Some dogs such as Poodles and the terrier breeds have large amounts of hair within the external auditory meatus which impair ventilation and the egress of glandular secretions. This may predispose to the development of otitis. Vigorous manual removal of hairs from the ear may inflame the integument of the ear canal and also lead to ear disease. The use of chemical depilatory creams has been advocated but the authors **strongly recommend** that these are **not** used: as they are highly irritant to the ear canal and may initiate severe otitis externa.

Climate

Variations in ambient temperature, rainfall and relative humidity correlate directly with the prevalence of otitis externa. There appears to be a lag period of around 2 months between climatic change and its effect on the ear.

Maceration of the ear canal

Increased humidity within the ear canal resulting from poor ear conformation, climatic factors or simply frequent swimming may lead to maceration of the integument, impaired barrier function, multiplication of commensal organisms and otitis externa.

Iatrogenic factors

There are several means by which inappropriate treatment can lead to worsening of an existing case of otitis externa. These include:

- Use of cotton tipped swabs for removing exudate from the ear canal.
  - Induces inflammation.
  - Pushes wax and exudate further inside ear canal.

- Vigorous hair plucking and use of depilatory creams.
  — Induces inflammation and secondary infection.
- Use of inappropriate antiseptic solutions as ear cleaners (especially alcohol-based products).
  — Inflames and/or macerates the skin of the ear canal.
- Inappropriate use of topical antimicrobial preparations.
  — May lead to super-infection of the ear canal with opportunist, Gram-negative bacteria.
  — May accumulate in the ear canal, restrict ventilation by narrowing the effective lumen and change the local micro-environment, leading to the development of opportunist infection.
  — May obscure the true extent of the disease and so delay investigation of the underlying cause.
  — May induce irritant, hypersensitivity or idiosyncratic reactions.

Obstructive ear disease

Restriction of the lumen of the external ear canal will alter the microclimate and predispose towards the establishment of infection and otitis. Obstructive factors include:

- Congenital atresia or stenosis (Shar Pei, Rottweiler).
- Proliferative inflammatory changes (usually a sequel to chronic otitis externa). This is particularly common and severe in American Cocker Spaniels.
- Neoplasia or hyperplasia (polyps).
- Accumulations of ear secretions and topical medicaments.

Systemic disease

Some systemic disorders may lead to immunosuppression and predispose to opportunist infection. Pyrexia associated with some diseases may alter the microclimate of the ear, affecting the microflora.

Perpetuating Factors

Bacteria

Commensal and potentially pathogenic bacteria may proliferate within an ear canal in which the microclimate has been altered by the factors previously discussed. Once microbial infection is established, inflammation is exacerbated and perpetuated. Bacteria involved include Gram-positive organisms (*Staphylococcus intermedius*, coagulase-negative staphylococci, alpha- and beta-haemolytic streptococci) and Gram-negatives (*Pseudomonas aeruginosa*, *Proteus mirabilis*, *Escherichia coli* and *Klebsiella* spp.). *Staphylococcus intermedius* is more commonly associated with acute infections while Gram-negative organisms, especially *Proteus mirabilis* and *Pseudomonas aeruginosa*, are cultured from chronically affected ears. Long-term antimicrobial therapy favours the development of infection with *Pseudomonas* and *Proteus*. These bacteria significantly contribute to inflammation and epidermal damage even though they are less commonly isolated that the Gram-positives.

Anaerobic bacteria have received little attention as factors in the pathogenesis of otitis externa. There is evidence that mixed aerobic and anaerobic infections are common and it is possible that anaerobes may be more important in the development of otitis externa than was previously thought.

Yeasts

Yeasts, usually *Malassezia pachydermatis*, play a similar role to bacteria in the development of otitis. *M. pachydermatis* is thought to be an inhabitant of the normal ear canal and an opportunistic invader of inflamed or macerated ears.

Otitis media

Extension of chronic otitis externa into the middle ear occurs in up to 50% of cases. In most instances the infection has extended from the external ear via a ruptured tympanic membrane. In some cases the tympanic membrane is intact but stretched and deflected by inflammation so that it invaginates into the middle ear, forming a false otitis media. Irrespective of whether or not the tympanum is intact, exudate within the middle ear is difficult or even impossible to remove without careful lavage. Such exudate contains pro-inflammatory toxins and forms a reservoir of bacteria which may be a source of reinfection for the external ear. Bacterial otitis media is an important cause of refractory, relapsing otitis externa.

Chronic inflammation

Epidermal and dermal hyperplasia result from chronic inflammation. Such proliferation is a major factor in the perpetuation of ear disease, leading to changes in the local micro-environment due to progressive luminal stenosis. These changes are exacerbated by the presence of an inflammatory infiltrate. Chronic inflammation within the ear canals also causes atrophy of the sebaceous glands and enlargement of the ceruminous glands. All of these factors favour microbial multiplication. Increases in microbial populations due to inflammation stimulate more of these changes so that a self-perpetuating cycle of disease is established.

Clinical Features

The clinical signs of otitis externa are well known to clinicians. Persistent or intermittent rubbing or scratching of the affected ear or ears is the most common complaint of owners. Head-shaking may occur and there may be pain on palpation of the ear. Odour, local self-trauma, pinnal erythema and oedema may be seen. Usually there is a ceruminous or suppurative exudate from affected ears along with an unpleasant odour. Occasionally, otitis externa may be associated with the formation of aural haematomata or local acute moist dermatitis.

Most cases of otitis media only present with signs of otitis externa. Head tilt, ataxia and Horner's syndrome, the expected signs of otitis media, only occur in advanced cases.

A Simple Problem-Oriented Approach to Otitis Externa and Media

The aim is to identify and treat primary, predisposing and perpetuating causes. The basic stages in diagnosis and therapy are:

1. Take full history and examine animal thoroughly.
2. Cytology of aural discharge.
3. Thoroughly clean and dry the ear canal.
4. Thoroughly examine the ear canal.
5. Proceed to other tests if necessary.
6. Address primary causes, using specific therapy.
7. Address predisposing and perpetuating factors.
8. Monitor progress carefully and regularly.

History and Examination

This will help the clinician to rank likely aetiological factors (*Chapter 2*). For example, evidence of contagion may lead to the suspicion that ear mites are involved. Skin disease affecting other sites may suggest that the underlying cause is a more generalised dermatological disorder such as a keratinisation defect or hypersensitivity. Sudden onset while at exercise may indicate that a grass-seed foreign body is present.

Cytology of Aural Discharge

This will facilitate the identification of micro-organisms and inflammatory cells:

- cocci — staphylococci, streptococci
- rods — *Pseudomonas*, *Proteus*
- yeasts — *Malassezia*, *Candida*

This valuable, simple and rapid technique is described in detail in *Chapter 3*. It is one of the most important stages in the investigation and management of otitis externa, yet it is used by few veterinarians. In early, uncomplicated cases, cytology is more valuable than bacterial culture and sensitivity. Culture and sensitivity should only be considered if toxic neutrophils and bacterial rods are present.

Cleaning and Drying the Ear Canal

This procedure is likely to be performed early in the approach to ear disease as it is usually necessary to clean the ears in order to allow thorough examination of the ear canal. There are several indications for removal of pus, cellular material, old medicaments, bacterial toxins, free fatty acids and other debris from the diseased ear canal:

- Debris prevents medicaments from reaching the skin of the aural canal and may prevent access of drugs to the micro-organisms present.
- Debris may inactivate some medicaments.
- Ear cleaning allows examination of the ear canal.

Care must be taken to flush the middle ear if debris in the tympanum is absent or invaginated. The middle ear may form a reservoir of infective material. Cleaning the external ear alone will not prevent recurrence of otitis externa from this source.

Chemical restraint

It is inevitable that some form of chemical restraint and analgesia will be required on both practical and welfare grounds. Otitis externa is a painful condition and cleaning of affected ears is impossible in an struggling patient. Failure to use such drugs will lead to an inadequate investigation, examination and treatment of the ear. Furthermore, many dogs which dislike veterinarians have previously had such unsympathetic handling. **Ear disease is painful!**

Local analgesia. In some cases, topical local anaesthetic solutions such as ophthalmic preparations containing proparacaine may be sufficient to allow cleaning and examination of inflamed ears. Two to five drops should be applied every 5 minutes for a total of three applications. This technique is ideal for the removal of large foreign bodies but is of limited value in severely affected and painful ears.

Sedation or general anaesthesia. There may be reluctance on the part of both owner and clinician to anaesthetise or sedate an animal simply to examine and clean the ears. However, it is often the most practical course of action and will spare the animal considerable immediate pain and discomfort as well as affording the best possible means for permanently resolving the ear disease.

Cleaning technique

There are four stages:

1. **Apply cerumolytic ear cleaning agents**. Suitable veterinary products are available in most countries. Typically they contain surfactants and detergents which emulsify wax and lipid. In theory, such products should not be applied to ears in which the tympanum is ruptured; however, in cases with very painful or waxy ears, it may be impossible to evaluate the tympanum without first cleaning the ear. As ear cleansers can be ototoxic, it is important to flush the middle ear thoroughly with sterile saline if it has become contaminated with ear cleanser during cleaning.

Ideally, ceruminolytic agents should be applied to the ears about 15 minutes before the induction of sedation or general anaesthesia. The external ear canal should be gently massaged percutaneously in order to mix the ear secretions with the cleansing agent.

2. **Flush the ear to remove dissolved ear debris**. Sterile saline warmed to blood temperature is ideal even if the tympanum is not intact.

Special rubber-bulb ear syringes are available. These are a highly effective means of cleaning the ear but are almost impossible to clean and sterilise after use. Alternatively a hypodermic syringe attached to flexible tubing (such as a cut-down canine urinary catheter or a gastric tube) may be used. The use of a syringe and tube is preferred to the use of the rubber-bulb ear syringe as the bulb syringe does not allow effective cleaning of the middle ear.

If a syringe and tube are used, the syringe should be of 5 ml capacity or less as excessive pressure on the tympanic membrane may be created with larger ones. If a rubber-bulb type syringe is used, care should be taken to ensure that there is a gap between the syringe and the wall of the ear canal otherwise back-flow is prevented and undue pressure may be applied to the tympanum. It can take 20 minutes to clean the ear canal thoroughly.

3. **Removal of residual fluid**. Fluid should be carefully removed from the now clean ear canal using a syringe with flexible tubing attached.

4. **Drying of ear canal**. Excessive moisture can lead to maceration of the ear canal and so promote multiplication of micro-organisms within the ear and recurrence of otitis (see previous discussion of aetiology and pathogenesis). Commercially prepared agents containing isopropyl alcohol with one of four acids (boric, benzoic, salicylic or acetic) should be placed in the ear canal; these will evaporate, thus having a drying effect. These substances are irritant and should be used with caution. Severely inflamed or ulcerated canals should not be treated with drying agents. It may be best simply to remove the fluid by suction using a syringe and tube or a rubber ear-cleaning bulb.

Examination of the Ear Canal

A thorough examination enables the identification of many primary, predisposing and perpetuating factors — for example foreign bodies, masses (tumours or inflammatory polyps), ear mites, chronic inflammatory changes. It also allows assessment of the severity of the problem, which will determine the nature and duration of therapy. Factors include the degree of inflammation, the presence of ulceration and the patency of the tympanum. If ulceration of the integument is present, the use of topical agents with a low pH or containing organic solvents is precluded due to the irritant nature of such substances. If the tympanum is not intact, the topical use of ototoxic substances such as the aminoglycoside group of antibiotics and many ceruminolytic agents is contra-indicated.

The patency of the tympanic membrane is difficult to establish. Often, a meniscus of aural exudate in the middle ear and external ear canal will resemble an intact tympanum. Alternatively, the tympanic membrane may be intact but invaginated into the middle ear by the aural exudate. In many instances, it is safest to assume that it has been ruptured rather than risk inducing iatrogenic ototoxicity.

It is preferable to examine the less severely affected ear first as there is less risk of contaminating one ear from the other. However, it is advised that speculae should be cleaned and placed in cold sterilisation fluid before use and that a fresh one be used for each ear.

Other Tests

These depend on the steps outlined above. If hypersensitivity or a defect in keratinisation is suspected investigate these problems as detailed elsewhere in the text (e.g. *Chapters 5, 7, 15*).

Therapy

Addressing Primary Causes Using Specific Therapy

Specific therapy for primary causes might include:

- Oral thyroxine supplementation for hypothyroidism
- Removal of foreign bodies
- Acaricidal therapy for otoacariasis

Topical Therapy

Many topical medicaments for the treatment of ear disease are available to the veterinary profession, and they include preparations suitable for reducing inflammation and killing any micro-organisms identified by cytology during investigation of otitis externa. In general, they contain several active principles such as glucocorticoids, antibiotics, antifungal agents and parasiticidal agents. Selection of an appropriate vehicle for these medicaments is almost as important as selecting the principles themselves. Many ear preparations have an oily or ointment base, so that they are suitable for ears which are dry, scaly and crusty. However, most ears affected with otitis externa are moist and exudative and the use of an occlusive vehicle is contra-indicated. In these instances, a preparation which is based in a lotion or solution is much more appropriate.

Glucocorticoids

Many different types and potencies of topical glucocorticoid are available. The clinician is advised to use a restricted range of these products and to be aware of the relative potencies of the products used. More potent agents (e.g. triamcinolone) can be used initially to control severe disease but less potent products, such as hydrocortisone, are advised for long-term maintenance therapy.

Most cases benefit from the topical use of glucocorticoids. They are antipruritic and their anti--inflammatory effects decrease exudation, swelling and glandular secretions. They reduce scarring and proliferative changes thereby promoting drainage and ventilation. However, potent topical glucocorticoids can be absorbed systemically and lead to elevation of liver enzymes and suppressed responses to stimulation with exogenous ACTH.

Antimicrobial agents

Products for aural use often contain antimicrobial agents along with glucocorticoids. These may be unnecessary as many cases of allergic ear disease can be managed with topical glucocorticoids alone. Antibacterial agents are indicated when infection is present. Selection of a suitable antimicrobial agent can be based on the results of cytology. The aminoglycosides (neomycin, polymyxin and gentamicin) and chloramphenicol are potent topical agents with good activity against the bacteria involved in otitis externa.

The use of topical antibacterial agents may lead to super-infection with resistant bacteria such as *Pseudomonas* spp. or the yeast *Malassezia*. The aminoglycosides can be ototoxic with prolonged use or when used in animals with ruptured tympanic membranes. Excessive granulation of the middle ear has been reported following the use of chloramphenicol.

Antiseptics

Povidone–iodine, chlorhexidine and acetic acid are all very helpful in the management of otitis externa complicated by bacterial infection. A 2% solution of acetic acid is highly effective against *Pseudomonas* within 1 minute of contact. Staphylococci and streptococci are killed within 5 minutes of contact with a 5% solution of acetic acid.

Strong concentrations of acetic acid (> 4%) may be irritant to the skin of the aural canal.

Antifungal agents

These agents are required in any case complicated by yeast (usually *Malassezia*) infection. Suitable agents include nystatin and miconazole.

Parasiticidal agents

These are indicated in otitis externa due to *Otodectes cynotis*. Suitable agents include pyrethrins and thiabendazole. All in-contact animals should be treated, whether affected by ear disease or not — untreated asymptomatic carriers form a potential source of reinfection. Treatment should continue for at least 3–4 weeks in order to allow sufficient time for eggs to hatch and susceptible larvae to be produced. It is also prudent to treat the coat with flea spray to kill parasites on the skin and limit reinfestation.

Systemic Therapy

Systemic therapy is indicated if otitis media is present or where such severe proliferative changes have occurred within the ear that topical therapy cannot be readily applied to all diseased tissue due to

---

MANAGEMENT AND TREATMENT OF *PSEUDOMONAS* INFECTION

- Keep the ear clean — daily flushing with water
- Most *Pseudomonas* spp. infections respond best to a combination of topical and systemic therapy

Topical antimicrobial therapy:
- gentamicin*
- amikacin* injectable applied undiluted (50 mg/ml) 3–5 drops/ear b.i.d. – t.i.d. and not mixed with other drugs
- neomycin combined with polymyxin* (requires clean ear at all treatments)
- tris-buffered EDTA, used for 15 minutes prior to an aminoglycocide
- acetic acid (50% white vinegar, 50% water), requires at least a 1 minute soak
- enrofloxacin (Baytril) injectable (diluted to 0.5–0.7% w/v with propylene glycol) or carbenicillin as ear drop (safety with a ruptured tympanic membrane is not known)
- Chlorhexidine 1%*
- Silver sulphadiazine 1% (or use silvadene cream diluted with an equal amount of water for 0.5% solution)

Systemic therapy:
- enrofloxacin
- gentamycin or amikacin (needs to be injected)
- carbenicillin

*These ingredients are known to be atotoxic if they reach the inner ear.

FIG. 27.3 Management and treatment of *Pseudomonas* infection.

---

stenosis of the canal. Systemic antimicrobial agents should be selected on the basis of cytology along with bacterial culture and sensitivity testing. In cases complicated with *Malassezia*, oral ketoconazole at 10 mg/kg daily may be of value.

Pseudomonas infection is a severe complication of otitis externa and may be extremely difficult to treat. Figure 27.3 lists treatment options for this bacterium.

Management of Otitis Media

Otitis media can be regarded as a bony-walled abscess requiring drainage. This can be facilitated by careful, thorough and regular ear flushing under general anaesthesia or, in advanced cases where there is radiological evidence of osteomyelitis, by bulla osteotomy.

Surgical correction of defects

In severe, advanced or neglected cases, medical treatment alone may be insufficient to control the problem. Anatomical defects and secondary changes leading to obstructive ear disease and chronic inflammatory change within the ear canal with poor ventilation and impaired drainage, may require surgical correction. This is particularly so in some cases of otitis media and in chronic cases of otitis externa where the ear canals are hyperproliferative and calcified. It is beyond the scope of this text to discuss the techniques of vertical wall resection, ear ablation and bulla osteotomy; the reader is referred to a surgery text. Ears that require surgery usually need total horizontal and vertical canal ablation. There is a high recurrence rate if all diseased ear canal tissue is not removed surgically.

Cases for surgery should be selected carefully. Surgery is not a substitute for a thorough diagnostic approach. Resection of the ears of atopic German Shepherd Dogs is counter-productive. The authors have seen many dogs with chronic dermatitis where radical aural surgery has been undertaken inappropriately with no benefit to the patient.

28

Anal Sac Disorders

IAN MASON

Anal sacs are probably vestigial structures in domestic carnivores. Expression of anal sac secretions occurs during defecation when the anal sphincter squeezes the glands against the faecal mass in the rectum. The anatomy and physiology of anal sacs is discussed in detail in *Chapter 1*. Anal sac disease is frequently encountered in small animal practice, but little is known of the aetiology and pathogenesis of anal sac disorders. Treatment is therefore empirical and depends largely on regular expression of the contents of these structures. This process is one with which small animal clinicians throughout the world are all too familiar. Anal sac disease tends to be recurrent and many pet dogs are subjected to regular ignominious veterinary interference.

Clinical Disease

Impaction, infection and abscessation of anal sacs are the disorders usually encountered. These are not discrete entities but probably represent a continuum of disease. The exact aetiology and pathogenesis of anal sac disease has yet to be elucidated. It is probable that the cause varies between cases and the development of anal sac disorders is multifactorial.

Retention of secretion may be idiopathic or due to:

- Anatomical factors.
- Soft motions (due to gastro-enteric disease or a low residue diet).
- Blockage of the anal sac ducts:
  — Primary (for example a poorly groomed long-haired dog with perianal faecal contamination may have blocked ducts due to inflammation, or simply due to the tightly adherent overlying faecal material).
  — Secondary (due to previous anal sac infection leading to thickening of the anal sac duct wall or the production of flocculent, purulent and or even granular material).

History

Signs of perianal discomfort, irritation or even pain usually stimulate pet owners to seek veterinary advice. **It is important at this stage to realise that anal sac disease is not the only cause of perianal pruritus and self-trauma in dogs and cats.** The classic presentation is that of an animal which frequently drags or rubs the perianal area on the ground. In some instances, such behaviour releases some of the secretion and

POSTULATED CAUSES OF ANAL SAC DISEASE	
Factor	**Example**
Genetic	This group of disorders is more common in certain breeds such as Miniature and Toy Poodles, Chihuahuas and Spaniels
Anatomical	Smaller breeds are predisposed
Retention of secretion	This is probably the major inciting factor leading to distension of the anal sacs, thinning of the epithelium, pain and, in many instances, rupture. Stasis of sac contents predisposes to secondary infection
Bacterial infection	Normal anal sacs have a micro-flora. Following retention of secretion, the local micro-climate may change leading to alteration of the number and types of bacteria present and favouring pathogens
Iatrogenic	The application of excessive pressure during manual emptying of anal sacs may lead to inflammation, damage to the sacs and ducts, retention of secretion and infection. **Excessive force should not be used when emptying anal sacs**

FIG. 28.1 Postulated causes of anal sac disease.

reduces the pain and discomfort. In other cases, the animal may constantly lick or chew at the area; this may lead to acute moist dermatitis (*Chapter 10*). Tenesmus, apparently painful defecation, tail chasing, discharge from the perianal area and self-trauma to the flanks and lumbarsacral area may all indicate that anal sac disease is present. Increased aggression may be encountered, especially if the rear half of the body is handled.

Physical Signs

On palpation of the perianal area, the anal sacs may be found to be enlarged and painful. Assessment of normal anal sac size is, to some extent, subjective; however, an anal sac can be considered to be enlarged if it is readily palpable through the perianal skin. Acute moist dermatitis, oedematous or even devitalised skin may be present locally. In

---

A SIMPLE, PROBLEM-ORIENTED APPROACH TO ANAL SAC DISEASE

Take Full History and Examine the Animal Thoroughly

This will enable other differential diagnoses to be eliminated and allow assessment of any predisposing, causal and perpetuating factors such as those given in Fig. 28.1. These steps will also allow the severity of the disorder to be evaluated and any abscessation or fistulation to be identified

Preliminary Investigations

*Examine the anal sac contents — the anal sacs should be gently expressed and the material examined microscopically. Nature of exudate:

• Thick, paste-like, brown or grey-brown. Occasionally inspissated and difficult to express. May appear ribbon like as it is expressed

Interpretation: Characteristic for anal sac impaction

• Purulent, blood-streaked, foul smelling

Interpretation: Acute infection

• Thin, watery, flocculent to creamy purulent

Interpretation: Chronic infection (in chronic infection, the sac walls feel thickened)

• Straw coloured to brownish liquid

Interpretation: Normal

• **Microscopical examination of stained anal sac secretions** may be helpful, especially in chronic cases. Infected sac secretions contain numerous bacteria and leucocytes and occasionally yeasts. Secretions from normal sacs contain epidermal and glandular cell debris, but few bacteria and leucocytes
• **Bacterial culture and sensitivity testing** is of limited value as the normal anal sacs have a micro flora that is similar to that of the rectum and large intestine. In cases of chronic infection, sensitivity testing may aid in the selection of suitable antimicrobial agents. Empirical therapy is usually effective (*Chapter 32*)

Initial Treatment

•Gently express anal sac contents and irrigate sacs with a mild antiseptic solution such as 0.5% chlorhexidine. This may be facilitated by inserting a naso-lachrymal cannula or tom cat catheter into the anal sac duct. With a cooperative patient, this can be performed in the conscious animal. **There are no indications for the cauterisation of infected anal sacs with irritant or caustic solutions such as phenol or silver nitrate. Such substances cause cellular damage and promote bacterial infection**
•Repeat treatment weekly until normal gland function is restored. Examination of secretions grossly and microscopically will enable recovery to be monitored
•After recovery, regular manual anal sac expression may be needed to prevent recurrence. The required frequency of this process varies between cases. In some instances, clients can be trained to do this
•If the anal sacs are impacted, then it may be impossible to remove the contents by manual expression. **Remember that excessive force should not be used.** The anal sac contents can be softened by irrigating the sacs with mineral oil or an aural cerumolytic agent. The sacs are massaged to mix the softening agent and then a further attempt to remove the contents is made. It is preferable to remove the contents gently and gradually over the course of several days than to remove all of the contents on one occasion by the use of undue force
•Severe infection may necessitate the use of antibiotic and glucocorticoid ointments (again instilled via a cannula) to reduce inflammation and infection. Systemic antimicrobial therapy is only indicated in the most severe cases
•Anal sac abscesses are managed as for any other abscess: poulticing of the unburst abscess to encourage it to 'point' followed by lancing. Sedation or anaesthesia may be required
•Burst or lanced abscesses should be flushed with an antiseptic solution such as 0.5% chlorhexidine and bathed regularly to ensure drainage. Systemic antimicrobial therapy is necessary in most cases as these lesions are often severe with pyrexia, pain and swelling
•Anal sac removal is indicated if the measures detailed above fail to prevent the continual recurrence of impaction, infection and abscessation. Surgery may be difficult. Failure to remove all of the sac will leave residual infection in the perianal area and a chronic draining abscess may result

FIG. 28.2 A simple, problem-oriented approach to anal sac disease.

advanced cases, a fistula from a burst anal sac abscess with a serosanguinous to mucopurulent discharge may be present. Acute anal sac abscessation can be an emergency presentation as the animal may experience severe pain.

Differential Diagnosis

Perineal discomfort, pruritus and pain may be associated with a number of disorders other than anal gland disease. These include food hypersensitivity, atopy and flea allergic dermatitis (*Chapter 5*); neoplasia (which may involve the anal sacs) (*Chapter 11*); anal furunculosis (*Chapter 10*) and behavioural disorders (anal licking in Toy and Miniature Poodles).

Failure to consider these other possible dermatoses may lead to inappropriate radical therapy such as anal sac removal.

29

Nail Disorders

IAN MASON

Diseases affecting the nails and nail-forming tissues are uncommon in clinical practice. However, when they do occur, they are painful and debilitating to the animal and a source of worry and frustration to owners and veterinarians.

Nail disease may occur in isolation or may be part of a more generalised skin disorder. Diseases may affect the nails themselves, the distal digit and/or the nail fold.

Nails are specialised keratinised epidermal structures derived from division of basal cells in the nail matrix (*Chapter 1*). In common with other epidermally derived structures, nail production is continuous. Therefore, at least in theory, nail growth is dependent on a balanced diet. Nail growth is relatively slow (around 2 mm per week) and so resolution of severe nail disorders may take several months.

Nomenclature of Nail Disorders

Paronychia

Paronychia is defined as inflammation of the nail-forming tissues or nail bed. One or more digits may be affected. Deformed nails may grow subsequent to paronychia; this is termed **onychogryposis**. Causes of paronychia include physical factors or trauma, bacteria, fungi and immune-mediated disorders (Fig. 29.1). Paronychia may be idiopathic. Pain, swelling and secondary bacterial infection are evident. Nails may be shed (**onychomadesis**).

Onychomycosis

Abnormal nail growth associated with dermatophyte infection is termed onychomycosis. It is usually associated with *Trichophyton* spp.

CAUSES OF NAIL DISEASE	
Factor	**Example**
Environmental trauma	Large (heavy) breeds, racing dogs, working dogs Inappropriate weight bearing (overlong nails) Over-zealous clipping[1] Prolonged immersion Road accidents and similar injuries Scaling, exposure to caustic agents Prolonged low environmental humidity
Infectious agents	Mites — *Demodex* spp. Hookworm — *Ancylostoma* spp., *Uncinaria ancyclostoma* Protozoa — *Leishmania* spp. Fungi — dermatophytes, *Candida* spp. Bacteria — various species, usually secondary opportunists Viruses — FIV, FeLV, cowpox, feline Herpes virus, feline calicivirus
Immune-mediated disorders[2]	Pemphigus group, especially pemphigus foliaceus Bullous pemphigoid Discoid and systemic lupus erythematosus
Systemic diseases	Any serious systemic disease which compromises nutrition or immune function (e.g. systemic lymphosarcoma) Endocrinopathy — especially hypothyroidism, diabetes mellitus, acromegaly, feline hyperthyroidism Superficial necrolytic dermatitis (hepatocutaneous syndrome)

[1] In the USA a particularly brutal form of nail clipping 'show clipping' is performed under general anaesthesia. This may subsequently lead to severe nail disease.
[2] Idiopathic glucocorticoid-responsive nail disease has been recognised; this is presumed to be immune-mediated in aetiology.

FIG. 29.1 Causes of nail disease.

A SIMPLE, PROBLEM-ORIENTED APPROACH TO NAIL DISORDERS	
Take History	
Environment	Prolonged exposure to wet floors; disinfectant irritants; poor kennel management; earth floors — hookworm
Trauma	Traffic or racing injury; pain and haemorrhage after nail clipping; overlong nails
Diet	Inadequate diet; malabsorption syndrome; low protein diets may lead to nail disease — the nail is mostly protein
Intercurrent disease	Systemic disease; immune-mediated disorders
Duration of disease	Short — isolated traumatic incident or accident
Examine Animal	
Overweight	Trauma
Poor foot conformation	Trauma
Evidence of intercurrent disease	Systemic or immune-mediated disease
Number of nails affected	One or few — neoplasia, trauma
	Several or all — systemic or immune-mediated disease
Preliminary Investigations	
• If appropriate, introduce a balanced, preferably commercial, diet for at least 3 months • Examine skin scrapings microscopically for evidence of *Demodex*, other ectoparasites and dermatophytes • Take scrapings of nail surface for fungal culture • If history compatible, examine faecal sample for hookworm eggs • If history compatible, take blood samples for investigation of systemic disease. Consider endocrine disease, hepatocutaneous syndrome and feline viruses such as FeLV and FIV • Smears of any exudate should be examined for bacteria, fungi and acantholytic cells	
Initial Treatment	
If no diagnosis is achieved from the above, then: • Induce general anaesthesia • Remove all loose nails by gentle traction • Inoculate bacteriological and fungal growth media with the proximal end of freshly removed nails • Gently clean and bandage feet • Administer high doses of oral, broad spectrum antibiotics for at least 6 weeks • Review choice of antibiotic and introduce antifungal therapy if appropriate once results of culture available	
Further Investigations and Treatments	
If the condition is still unimproved, then: • Biopsy • If no specific diagnosis is achieved and the diagnostic plan has been carefully followed, then empirical therapy with immunosuppressive doses of glucocorticoids is indicated (*Chapter 31*) • If there is no response to glucocorticoid therapy, or unacceptable side-effects develop, then radical excision of the distal digits of affected toes should be undertaken as described for biopsy	

FIG. 29.2 A simple, problem-oriented approach to nail disorders.

Onychomalacia

Production of soft nails is termed onychomalacia. This may be idiopathic, genetically determined or due to nutritional factors.

Onychorrhexis and onychoschizia

Onychorrhexis is defined as the production of brittle nails. Cracking and splitting of the nails is similar to onychorrhexis and is called onychoschizia. Both of these disorders may be caused by the same factors that cause onychomalacia.

Causes and Diagnosis

Examples of causes of nail disease are given in Fig. 29.1. Readers are advised to consult Sections II and III for more detail regarding the pathogenesis,

investigation and treatment of the systemic disorders listed in the two figures.

Biopsy

Biopsy is best accomplished under general anaesthesia. An elliptical skin incision is made around the distal portion of the distal digit P3. P3 is then sectioned and the nail is removed along with part of the distal digit and overlying skin. These specimens can be difficult to process so the histopathologist should be consulted **before** sampling. This technique is curative for the nail so treated. The incision should be sutured so that the suture line is parallel to the ground and the pad is pulled up over the front of the remnant of P3 to provide protection. If multiple nails are involved, the dewclaw (if affected) is easily removed for biopsy.

VI Therapeutics

30

Control of Ectoparasites

IAN MASON and KAREN MORIELLO

Management of Flea Allergic Dermatitis

Owner Education

Clients are often extremely reluctant to believe that flea allergy can be the cause of their pet's dermatitis. Unless a client can be convinced that flea allergic dermatitis is a possible cause, then it is unlikely that flea eradication will be undertaken with sufficient conviction to confirm the diagnosis and resolve the disease. There is no formula for handling such clients. Ideally fleas, flea excrement or both can be demonstrated to the client. A history of tapeworm (*Dipylidium caninum*) may also be employed as an argument in favour of a diagnosis of flea allergic dermatitis. A lesion map taken from a text book showing the distribution of typical lesions may convince some sceptics. A positive intradermal skin test result is very convincing, but a false-negative result may destroy the credibility of other arguments put forward in support of the diagnosis. It is advisable to discuss the high incidence of false-negative reactions *before* doing an intradermal skin test.

Many clients will argue that the problem cannot be flea-induced as they have not seen any fleas. The analogy of human midge *(Culicoides)* bites may help. People who have been bitten by midges rarely feel the bite at the time, nor do they see the insects, but the next day they know what has caused their lesions and would have little sympathy with anyone who told them, 'These can't be midge bites — you have no midges on your skin'. Another approach is to agree with the client that the problem is unlikely to be caused by fleas but then suggest: 'He's such a nice dog and you are quite clearly very fond of him. If we can't get a diagnosis here then we may have to treat him symptomatically, perhaps with steroids, for the rest of his life. Surely we don't want to do this before we've tried to rule out all of the possible causes? It will only involve you in a couple of months of flea control...' Or: 'Let's not spend lots of your money investigating uncommon diseases until we've ruled out fleas.'

When a client has been persuaded that flea eradication is worthwhile, the life cycle of the flea should be discussed in detail so that the reasons for the various stages given below become apparent. A detailed account of the flea life cycle is beyond the scope of this text and readers are referred to the bibliography.

Points to mention to owners include the following:

- While adult fleas live on dogs and cats, the other stages of the life cycle take place in the environment.
- Adult fleas are seldom seen on animals with skin disease because affected animals groom, lick and bite the skin excessively and remove evidence of these parasites with great effectiveness.
- Some stages of the life cycle in the environment are extremely difficult to kill: repeated applications of environmental insecticides may be needed. In some areas at certain times of the year, flea control may be impossible.

Flea Control

There are three facets to effective, comprehensive flea control: the animal, in-contact animals and the environment (Figs 30.1 and 30.2). In order for treatment to be successful all of these elements should be treated regularly with effective insecticides, following the manufacturer's instructions.

The author issues the instruction sheet shown as Fig. 30.3 to clients.

Treatment Recommendations for Generalised Demodicosis in Dogs

A whole-body clip of the hair coat is mandatory. This allows for a more complete penetration of the dip into the hair follicles. The hair coat should be kept very short throughout the treatment period.

FLEA CONTROL FOR DOGS AND CATS	
The Affected Animal and In-Contact Animals	
Sprays	Effective but need to be used frequently, especially during the warmer months. Some cats are impossible to treat
Dips	Labour-intensive but very effective. Many products are toxic to cats. It may be extremely difficult to dip cats anyway
Collars and powders	Limited effectiveness
Shampoos	Limited effectiveness as they are rinsed off and so have little residual effect. Unless environmental control is 100% effective (this is unlikely), then the unprotected animal will be returned to an infested environment after bathing
'Spot' products	Easy to administer and so an attractive option for fractious cats. However, some products are not licensed for cats and are toxic to them. Interval between applications is long. Some products are absorbed systemically while others are distributed throughout the outer layers of the epidermis. In either case it is unlikely that fleas are killed until they have fed and so hypersensitivity may still continue. May be of value for the treatment of lesion-free in-contact animals
Insect growth inhibitors	A recent development but possibly will become extremely useful in flea control in the future
The Environment	
Sprays	In the UK these are the most commonly used form of environmental flea control due to the unavailability of other products and formulations. They are effective, but labour-intensive and a potential environmental concern
Foggers	Suitable for use only when rooms are empty. They do not have the penetration of sprays
Sodium polyborate	A non-toxic safe treatment which only needs to be applied annually. Said to be highly effective. Currently not available in the UK

Note: Gardens may harbour flea populations at certain time of the year in warm, humid climates. Sunny exposed areas are unlikely to be infested, but if pets spend time lying under shrubs or in other shaded areas, then treatment of such areas with a non-toxic insecticide such as malathion may be of value. Free-living nematodes which feed on immature fleas are available for use in gardens in some countries.

All insecticidal agents should be used in strict accordance with the manufacturer's instructions and recommendations

FIG. 30.1 Flea control for dogs and cats.

If a deep pyoderma is present, the infection should be treated with a bacteriocidal, e.g. cephalexin (20 mg/kg *per os* t.i.d.) antibiotic for a minimum of 4–6 weeks, possibly longer.

Just before the application of a dip, the dog should be washed in a benzoyl peroxide shampoo. This removes dirt and debris from the skin and hair follicles. Towel the dog dry, then apply amitraz dip (diluted according to the manufacturer's recommendations) to the skin and coat for 10–15 minutes. Note that amitraz dip should be prepared fresh for each application: the solution will degrade once exposed to air, and the degraded products may be toxic. Do not divide the contents of the bottles.

The dip should be repeatedly poured over the dog and sponged into the skin and hair coat. The dog should be standing in a tub so that its feet soak in the dip. Do not rinse off the dip but allow the dog to air-dry.

Monitor the dog for adverse effects. The most commonly observed are pruritus, sedation and hypothermia. Other side-effects include anorexia, polyuria, polydipsia, vomiting, diarrhoea, ataxia, hyperexcitability, seizures, bloat, appetite stimulation and skin irritation. Yohimbine can be used to reverse severe adverse effects (0.03 mg/kg SC for pre-treatment, or 0.01 mg/kg IV for acute treatment).

Repeat whole-body applications of dips at weekly intervals. (Note that in some countries the manufacturer recommends bi-weekly dipping. Clinical trials have shown that weekly intervals are more effective but this is a non-label use of this drug in those countries.)

Monitor therapy every 2–4 weeks with skin scrapings from at least 4–6 areas. A response to therapy is indicated by a decrease in mite numbers, a shift from immature to mature life-cycle stages and a shift from live to dead mites. Dogs that are not responding to therapy will continue to develop new lesions and/or continue to have large numbers of live mites in all stages of growth. Therapy should be continued until skin-scrapes are negative at least twice at two consecutive hospital visits. The author initially treats all animals for 12–16 weeks before considering maintenance or alternative therapy.

SAMPLE FLEA CONTROL PROGRAMME

Animals

1. Bath all animals in a cleansing shampoo to remove debris, fleas and dirt

2. If the animal is heavily infested, an insecticidal dip should be applied to the skin. Cats are very sensitive to dips and only products labelled as safe for cats should be used. This may need to be repeated on a weekly basis in flea endemic regions

3. Alternatively, the pet can be sprayed with a flea spray labelled as safe for the particular species. This should be re-applied frequently; actual application rates may differ from recommendations by the manufacturer

4. Outdoor dogs, hunting dogs or outdoor cats may be difficult to treat. One alternative is the use of topically applied systemic antifungal drugs. Permethrin and fenthion (dogs only) are effective in controlling flea populations. These products are potentially toxic to cats and should not be used in this species. Outdoor cats may benefit from the application of foams and long-acting residual sprays with an insect growth hormone regulator and/or oral insect growth hormone treatments

Indoor Environmental Flea Control

1. The entire home should be thoroughly cleaned and vacuumed with a fresh vacuum cleaner bag. Fleas and flea larvae tend to crawl away from light and burrow into carpets. Special attention should be given to protected areas, e.g. under beds and couches. All furniture should be cleaned and thoroughly vacuumed. (Flea larvae live on organic debris in homes)

2. A spray with an insect growth hormone regulator should be applied thoroughly to all areas of the house. This should be repeated 2–3 weeks later to ensure that a thorough application of insecticide is present in the environment

3. 'Spot therapy' may be necessary, depending upon the flea burden. Extra attention should be given to areas where pets sleep, sun or frequent on a weekly basis. These 'hot spots' are sources of egg development and re-exposure

4. If the pet spends much time in the family car or van, the vehicle should be left in bright sun on a warm day with all of the windows closed for 3–4 hours. This should kill fleas and larvae that the pet may have deposited in the car. **DO NOT LEAVE PETS IN CARS IN THE SUMMER!**

Outdoor Environmental Flea Control

1. Fleas do not thrive in bright sunny areas; therefore attention should be directed at shady protected areas

2. Remove all mulch, leaves and other organic debris, especially in shaded areas

3. Replace decorative bark with stone

4. Shady areas under garden trees, shrubs or porches should be treated with a residual insecticide formulated for outdoor use. These are available at garden stores

5. A thorough search of the home's foundation and attic for areas where small mammals (e.g. mice) can live and enter should be made, and if found, sealed. Small mammals are believed to be the reservoirs of flea populations

FIG. 30.2 Sample flea control programme.

FLEA CONTROL: INSTRUCTION SHEET FOR CLIENTS

Flea-related problems are the commonest cause of skin disease in pets. Usually skin problems arise because the animal becomes allergic to saliva which the flea injects when it feeds. Not all animals within a household will develop flea allergy and so only one pet may show signs of skin disease (usually scratching). Some allergic animals are so sensitive to flea saliva that they only need to be bitten once a week to scratch persistently. For this reason it is unrealistic to assume that your pet does not have flea allergy simply because you do not see fleas on him or her. The only way to diagnose or disprove flea allergy is to eradicate them from the pet's environment

Fleas can spend part of their life cycle in the environment and on pets and so it is extremely important that thorough environmental decontamination is undertaken as part of a flea control programme. Lifelong flea control is very important in skin patients as fleas can flare up virtually any inflammatory skin disease. Moreover, household flea sprays have an effect on house-dust mites, allergy to which commonly causes problems in dogs and cats

The Affected Animals

Spray all cats and dogs in the house with topical insecticidal sprays every 7 days for the first month and then every 10 days for life

The Environment

Spray inside a new vacuum cleaner bag with an environmental insecticidal agent before fitting the bag to the machine, or place a flea collar within the bag of your vacuum cleaner
Vacuum all dust from any rooms to which pets have access
Spray the floors of each room with the environmental insecticidal agent, ensuring that the safety instructions on the can are adhered to. Pay particular attention to areas under beds, behind settees, under radiators and around skirting boards. Spray the pet's bedding. Cars should also be vacuumed and sprayed if appropriate
Repeat the above instructions 2–3 weeks later, then four times annually

FIG. 30.3 Flea control: Instruction sheet for clients.

FIG. 30.4 Experimental treatment for demodicosis.

EXPERIMENTAL TREATMENT FOR DEMODICOSIS	
Taktic (large animal amitraz 12.5%)	1 ml/100 mls of water applied to one half of the body every other day resulted in a remission rate of 79% in a small group of dogs with refractory demodicosis. The average treatment period was 3.7 months
Milbemycin oxime	0.5–0.82 mg/kg *per os* once daily for 90 days; if skin scrapes are still positive the dose is increased to 1.0–1.14 mg/kg *per os* once daily. Variable remission rates. Dogs may relapse when the drug is discontinued
Ivermectin	0.6 mg/kg *per os* or SC daily has been successful in a small number of dogs. Treatment periods ranged from 5 to 24 weeks
Double-strength amitraz	1 bottle diluted in 4l of water (double strength) has been beneficial in some patients anecdotally

If the dog is clinically normal but skin scrapings are still positive, the owner may elect to apply a monthly or bi-weekly dip. Dipping will maintain clinical normality in the patient. **Dogs with generalised demodicosis should not be bred and should be surgically neutered as soon as possible**.

Experimental Treatment for Demodicosis

Figure 30.4 summarises some newer therapies for refractory demodicosis in dogs. These therapies are considered experimental and mention of them does not constitute a recommendation or endorsement by the authors. They should be reserved for patients whose owners are considering euthanasia as the only alternative.

Scabies, Ear Mites and Cheyletiellosis

Treatment recommendations for mite and lice infestations are given in Fig. 30.5.

TREATMENT RECOMMENDATIONS FOR MITE AND LICE INFESTATIONS IN DOGS AND CATS		
Mite	**Treatment recommendations and options**	**Comments**
Ear mites	1. Clean ears thoroughly 2. Apply a miticide, e.g. pyrethrin, to both ears as directed by manufacturer for 30 days 3. Treat hair coat with a flea spray for 30 days	All in-contact animals should be treated in the household Reinfestation from hair coat is common; treat with flea spray In large kennels or catteries, ivermectin (200–400µg/kg *per os* or SC) every 2 weeks for three treatments is effective
Cheyletiella mites	1. Clip the hair coat of all long-haired animals 2. Bath animal in a cleansing shampoo 3. Apply a whole-body dip such as pyrethrin, lime sulphur or organophosphate. Repeat weekly for 5–6 weeks 4. Amitraz whole-body dip every 2 weeks for three treatments is curative. Do not use on cats 5. Ivermectin (200 µg/kg *per os* or SC) every 2 weeks for three treatments is effective	All in-contact animals should be treated Re-infestation from grooming establishments or boarding kennels is common The environment should be thoroughly cleaned and disinfected. Use a product formulated as a household spray for fleas. One application is usually effective Disinfect all possible fomities
Sarcoptes mites	1. Treat any concurrent superficial pyoderma 2. Ivermectin (200 µg/kg *per os* or SC) every 2 weeks for three treatments 3. Lime sulphur whole-body dips every week for five to six treatments 4. Some organophosphate dips are effective if used weekly for five to six treatments 5. Amitraz whole-body dips every 2 weeks for three treatments	Treat all in-contact dogs Disinfect the environment and spray with an environmental insecticide formulated for fleas If the dog is severely pruritic, lime sulphur is the most effective treatment because it is naturally antipruritic Corticosteroids should not be used unless mites have been demonstrated; do not use corticosteroids in a therapeutic trial
Lice	See *Cheyletiella* or *Sarcoptes* recommendations	Environmental control is not usually necessary Rinsing the hair coat with a 1:2 dilution of white vinegar and water will loosen nits attached to hairs
Notoedres	1. Ivermectin (200 µg/kg *per os* or SC) 2. Lime sulphur or pyrethrin whole-body dip every week for five to six treatments	Treat all in-contact cats

FIG. 30.5 Treatment recommendations for mite and lice infestations in dogs and cats.

31

Management of Inflammatory and Immune-Mediated Disease

IAN MASON and KAREN MORIELLO

Management of Canine and Feline Pruritus

Chapters 5 and *13* cover the diagnosis and treatment of canine and feline pruritus in detail. The principal purpose of this chapter is to give an account of the symptomatic management of pruritus in these species.

> Symptomatic therapy is not recommended in dermatology. It is essential that pruritus be thoroughly investigated and specific treatment implemented. Symptomatic therapy without thorough investigation denies the animal the chance of a permanent cure or resolution to its problem and may condemn it to lifelong glucocorticoid therapy.

There are a few specific indications for symptomatic control of pruritus:

- Where a diligent search for the underlying cause has been made but the problem is idiopathic.
- Where the underlying cause is known but no specific treatment is possible; the most common example is atopic dermatitis where exposure to allergens cannot be avoided. A discussion of the

---

MANAGEMENT OF FELINE AND CANINE PRURITUS

1. *Identify and treat the primary disease.* (*Chapters 5* and *13*). Examples include food allergy, contact allergy, flea allergic dermatitis and other ectoparasite disorders
2. *Control secondary pyoderma* (*Chapter 32*). Pyoderma may be a flare factor in canine pruritus
3. *Control fleas* (*Chapter 30*). Flea-bites may be a flare factor in pruritus
4. *Maintain good skin and coat care* — regular grooming, bathing, clipping etc. Ensure a good plane of nutrition **If the primary disease cannot be identified or specific therapy is impractical and if the above measures fail to control pruritus, then:**
5. *Symptomatic therapy*

FIG. 31.1 Management of feline and canine pruritus.

---

management of atopic dermatitis is presented later in this chapter.
- Where specific therapy is slow to take effect and unacceptable self-trauma supervenes.

Figure 31.1 briefly summarises the approach to pruritus control.

The following groups of drugs are used in the symptomatic management of pruritus in dogs and cats:

- Glucocorticoids
- Essential fatty acids
- Antihistamines and related drugs
- Topical therapy
- Miscellaneous treatments

In practice, a combination therapy protocol is formulated using a 'cocktail' of the above drugs and management factors tailored to the specific case. The formulation of such a treatment regimen is an art as well as a science and can be quite time-consuming for the clinician. The merits and disadvantages of these agents are shown in Fig. 31.2.

Glucocorticoids

The problems associated with the empirical use of glucocorticoids in dogs and cats are well documented. Clinicians can no longer justify the use of such drugs in pruritic animals unless a thorough diagnostic approach has been undertaken and conditions such as flea-bite hypersensitivity, dietary allergy/intolerance and ectoparasite infestations have been ruled out and other non-glucocorticoid therapies attempted. **Glucocorticoids should only be used as a last resort in the management of allergic patients.** No other form of treatment will surpass these drugs in the control of pruritus. However, their adverse

FIG. 31.2 Advantages and disadvantages of various drugs and treatments for the management of allergic skin disease.

ADVANTAGES AND DISADVANTAGES OF VARIOUS DRUGS AND TREATMENTS FOR THE MANAGEMENT OF ALLERGIC SKIN DISEASE		
Drug/treatment	**Advantages**	**Disadvantages**
Glucocorticoids	Highly effective, inexpensive	Potential side-effects including iatrogenic hyperadrenocorticism
Essential fatty acids	Safe	Expensive, slow onset of effect, helpful in only 24–40% of cases
Antihistamines	Safe	Helpful in a small number of cases
Topical therapy	Safe, rapid effect	Time-consuming, may be unsuitable for cats, effects wear off rapidly

effects limit their usefulness and have thereby spawned the sub-specialty of veterinary dermatology. Arguably these are the most abused drugs in veterinary medicine. It is outside the scope of this book to discuss the physiology and pharmacology of this group of medicaments; readers are referred to the Bibliography.

In view of the young age at which many animals develop hypersensitivity, the incurable nature of such conditions and the probability that chronic glucocorticoid therapy will lead to adverse effects, it is recommended that this form of therapy be reserved for those cases where no other treatment produces acceptable results. The only exception is the confirmed case of atopic dermatitis which is seasonal and readily responsive to modest doses of glucocorticoids given for less than 3–4 months each year. The other categories of medicaments listed above are much safer but are less likely to eliminate pruritus than are glucocorticoids. Despite this, a significant number of animals can be managed satisfactorily without glucocorticoids. Furthermore there may be synergism between non-steroidal drugs and glucocorticoids so that the dose of the latter may be reduced if they are used concomitantly.

There are a few simple rules that can be applied to the use of this valuable but potentially hazardous group of drugs:

- **Glucocorticoids should only be used as a last resort, where all other medicaments have failed to control the pruritus and, ideally, only in those cases where a specific diagnosis has been made.** The only exception is seasonal atopic dermatitis as discussed previously.
- **Systemic glucocorticoids should only be given orally.** Occasionally injectable use may be indicated (for example, the fractious cat belonging to

a frail and elderly owner) but oral therapy is preferred as the drug can be withdrawn if side-effects develop or if the animal develops another non-dermatological problem requiring medical or surgical treatment. (Imagine performing orthopaedic surgery following a road accident on an animal injected with a large dose of long-acting glucocorticoids 72 hours previously.) There is a role for topical glucocorticoids in trivial and localised disorders although animals may lick the medicament from the lesions and the overlying coat may make application messy and time-consuming.

- **Prednisone, prednisolone and methylprednisolone are the only drugs recommended for use** as their half-lives are short enough to render them suitable for alternate-day therapy.
- **Glucocorticoids should be administered as a single dose on alternate days.** It has been suggested that it may be preferable to treat dogs in the morning and cats in the evening to exploit the possible diurnal pattern of corticotrophin releasing factor, adrenocorticotrophic hormone and glucocorticoid activity although there are no convincing data in support of this. An initial dose of 1–2 mg/kg daily is suitable for induction of therapy but, once the condition is stable, the dose should be gradually tapered to find the minimum alternate-day dose which controls pruritus **without completely abolishing it**. The dose should be constantly re-evaluated. Some animals may only need glucocorticoid therapy twice weekly.

In general, cats will require, and will tolerate, higher doses of glucocorticoids than dogs.

- **Glucocorticoids are best used in combination with some of the other forms of therapy listed below**, as the concurrent use of such drugs and treatments may have a steroid-sparing effect.

Essential Fatty Acids

It has been suggested that there is a defect in the metabolism of *n6*-series essential fatty acids (EFAs) in some human patients with atopic dermatitis. Although there is no evidence to suggest that abnormalities in EFA metabolism exist in dogs and cats with atopy, there are data from double-blind, placebo-controlled cross-over studies which indicate that pruritus may be decreased in such animals by oral supplementation with EFA.

EFAs are precursors of potent short-lived molecules called **eicosanoids**. These are the prostaglandins, thromboxanes, leucotrienes and hydroxy-eicosatetraenoic acids (HETEs). Eicosanoids have a number of functions, some of which are beneficial to the animal and some harmful. They have a major role in the induction and modulation of inflammation and may be pro-inflammatory or, as is the case for the series 1 prostaglandins, anti-inflammatory. One of the mechanisms by which EFA therapy is thought to help in allergic skin disease is by altering the balance of eicosanoids in favour of anti-inflammatory substances. Oral administration of some EFAs, such as gamma-linolenic acid from evening primrose oil, may affect the biochemical pathways of eicosanoid production favouring the production of anti-inflammatory substances and inhibiting the production of those which promote inflammation. However, the mode of action of EFAs is likely to be more complex than this. It is possible that other mechanisms may be involved. For example, EFAs are involved in the maintenance of epidermal barriers and they influence cell wall receptors, particularly those of keratinocytes and leucocytes. The reader is referred to the Bibliography for more information on EFAs.

Although clinical signs can be completely controlled in some atopic animals using EFAs, more often it is necessary to augment their beneficial effects with other drugs such as glucocorticoids and antihistamines. Many clinicians have experienced poor results when managing atopy with EFAs; this is often because doses were inadequate or the treatment was not of sufficient duration, or both. Current recommendations are that the manufacturer's recommended dose be quadrupled and that the minimum treatment period be 8–12 weeks.

Antihistamines and Related Drugs

Antihistamines were regarded as ineffective in the management of pruritus because substances other than histamine (leucotrienes, thromboxanes, proteases and prostaglandins) were known to be mediators of inflammation in canine and feline skin. In recent years, however, there have been a number of reports of beneficial responses to antihistamine

ANTIHISTAMINE (H1 RECEPTOR ANTAGONISTS) TREATMENT OF CANINE AND FELINE PRURITUS					
	Agent	Body weight (kg)	Dose	Reported success rate (%)	Comments
Dogs	Clemastine	<10 10–25 >25	0.5 mg b.i.d. 1.0 mg b.i.d. 1.5 mg b.i.d.	30.0	Centrally-mediated effect Synergistic effect with EFAs
	Cyproheptadine		0.5–1.0 mg/kg b.i.d.	–	Serotonin antagonist
	Terfenadine		8.0 mg/kg b.i.d.	–	Serotonin antagonist
	Hydroxyzine		2.0 mg/kg t.i.d.	6.7	Stabilises mast cell membranes Centrally-active sedative effect
	Trimeprazine		1.0–2.0 mg/kg t.i.d.	3.3	Potentiates prednisone Centrally-mediated sedative effect
	Astemazole	<10 1–25 >25	2.5 mg once daily 5.0 mg once daily 1.5 mg once daily	3.3 (7 days only)	Binds irreversibly to H1 receptors Non-sedating Slow onset of action
Cats	Chlorpheniramine		2 mg/cat b.i.d.–t.i.d.	70	The success rate claimed in cats is extremely optimistic
NOTES: 1. None of these drugs is licensed for use in small animals in the UK or US. 2. Some of these drugs will potentiate essential fatty acids and glucocorticoids. 3. There are other drugs which are not included in this list in the interest of brevity. 4. In general use each drug for a week in turn and suggest that the client keeps a diary of response.					

FIG. 31.3 Antihistamine (H1 receptor antagonists) treatment of canine and feline pruritus.

therapy in pruritic dogs and cats, though no double-blind placebo-controlled studies have been conducted. There are two main groups of histamine receptor antagonist, H1 and H2, of which only the H1 antagonists appear to be of value in the management of allergic skin disease and pruritus. The reported benefits of this form of therapy might be explained, in part, by other actions of H1 receptor antagonists such as stabilisation of mast cell membranes, the induction of a centrally-mediated sedative effect, or antagonism of serotonin activity.

Figure 31.3 gives examples of products available in the UK along with reported success rates and doses. These drugs are not licensed for use in animals in the UK or the USA and so informed consent must be obtained from clients before use. Animals vary in their response to such drugs and it is not possible to predict which drug will be successful in a given case. One approach is to administer each drug in turn for 5–7 days and note any response. Subsequently the most effective product is used. Drowsiness, hyperexcitability and even increased pruritus have been reported as side-effects in up to 15% of dogs treated with antihistamines. There have been anecdotal reports of sudden deaths of dogs treated with chlorpheniramine and the use of this drug in this species is therefore not recommended.

In cats, chlorpheneramine was reported as successfully controlling pruritus in 19 of 26 (73%) cats. One of the authors of this book (ISM) has used this drug at the recommended dose (2 mg twice daily) but has not been able to achieve anywhere near this success rate. However, some individuals have shown a beneficial response and the drug does appear to potentiate the effects of glucocorticoids in cats. Other than chlorpheniramine, antihistamines are contraindicated in cats as they may lead to hyperexcitability.

Topical Non-Glucocorticoid Therapy

Shampoos, dips, sprays and rinses are a safe and often useful adjunct to the treatments discussed in this text. Their advantages are their safety and rapid onset of action but they have the disadvantages that they may be difficult to use and act for only a short time (usually only a few hours).

Where lesions are generalised, total body surface therapy with baths or rinses is required. This may be difficult with some cats, although some clinicians claim to be quite adept at bathing the feline.

The use of mild 'hypoallergenic' shampoos will be beneficial by removing allergens, debris, bacteria and their metabolites from the skin. The use of cool water alone or as part of the bathing process may also have a soothing effect that can last for several hours. Washing will hydrate the stratum corneum, thus raising the pruritic threshold. Occasionally bathing leads to increased pruritus; this is sometimes because hot water or an irritant shampoo constituent such as benzoyl peroxide has been used. It is recommended that hair driers are not used after bathing pruritic dogs.

There are several non-specific topical anti-pruritic agents. **Sulphur**, which is an ingredient of a number of medicated shampoos, is said to be one such substance. **Colloidal oatmeal** has been used for people with atopic eczema and leads to a fairly prolonged reduction in pruritus. The mechanism of action is unknown but it has been suggested that it persists on the skin surface after rinsing to act as an emollient (see below) and as a cleansing agent. The human products are difficult to use in dogs as the hair coat prevents access of the active principles to the skin. One colleague has reported that dogs may try to eat the oatmeal solution! Veterinary shampoos and cream rinses specifically formulated to avoid these disadvantages are available. Alternatively, oatmeal can be applied to the skin surface as a compress. A cupful of oatmeal is placed in a stocking and then soaked in cool water. The stocking is then applied to the inflamed skin for a few minutes.

Shampoos remove lipid from the skin surface, leading to loss of water and worsening of pruritus. Where prolonged shampoo therapy is required, an emollient or moisturiser should be used after rinsing. **Emollients** are usually oil- or wax-based and hydrate the stratum corneum by forming a barrier to evaporation. **Moisturisers** are oil-free and act by increasing the water content of the skin, often by raising the pH.

Local areas of pruritus such as the lesions of acute moist dermatitis ('wet eczema' or 'hot spots') may be soothed by the gentle application of ice wrapped in cloth, as has been recommended in human atopy.

Anecdotal evidence has indicated that a number of other substances may have a soothing effect on inflamed skin. Their mechanisms of action are unclear but it is possible that they may work simply by cooling the skin. Menthol is an example of these substances and it may also act via an effect on nerve endings. Another of these agents is *Hamamelis* extract (witch hazel). Sprays containing these substances alone or in combination with local anaesthetic or hydrocortisone are available to veterinarians.

Miscellaneous Treatments

There is anecdotal evidence that some other substances may have antipruritic effects in animal skin. These include aspirin, ivermectin, the tricyclic antidepressants and antimicrobial agents such as erythromycin and ketoconazole. These agents have been shown to have only marginal success in the management of canine pruritus although drugs which antagonise serotonin re-uptake (particularly the tricyclic antidepressant, clomipramine) may have a role in the management of psychogenic dermatoses such as acral lick dermatitis in dogs. None of these products is licensed for use in the management of allergic skin disease in dogs and cats in the UK or the USA. **Aspirin is not advised in cats.**

Combination Therapy

In anaesthesia and the chemotherapy of neoplasia, it has long been accepted that there is a role for combination therapy. The simultaneous use of a number of drugs which have additive or even synergistic effects will allow a reduction in the doses of each of the individual medicaments. This is of particular value where potentially dangerous drugs such as glucocorticoids or expensive drugs such as EFAs are used.

The concurrent administration of antihistamines, EFAs, and topical agents may be sufficient to control pruritus without the need for glucocorticoid therapy in some cases. The disadvantage is that such treatments may be too complex for some owners. Treatment should be kept as simple as possible; clear, preferably written, instructions should be given. The therapy should be tailored to the specific patient. Factors to consider include the severity of the disease, the susceptibility of the patient to the adverse effects of glucocorticoids therapy, the degree of commitment of the owner and the financial status of the owner. Such regimens should be constantly reviewed in response to changes in the animal's condition.

Management of Allergic Skin Disease

Ideally, allergic skin disease or hypersensitivity is managed by limiting or eliminating exposure of the animal to the causal allergen or allergens. Where this is not practical, or where the allergens cannot be identified, then pharmacological modification of the immune response is indicated.

Measures to Limit Exposure to Antigens

Clearly, the measures employed must relate to the nature of the causal antigen. Suggested measures are summarised in Fig. 31.4. It is the authors' experience that environmental control is of limited value in atopic dermatitis and is simply an adjunct to medical therapy. In most instances the effort expended in environmental control is not rewarded with a significant improvement in the animal's condition.

MEASURES TO LIMIT EXPOSURE TO ANTIGENS	
Antigen	**Suggested management**
Nutrients	Feed restricted diet
Contactants	Remove substances from environment
Flea saliva	Flea control
House dust, house dust mites and danders	Exclude the animal from bedrooms and other rooms immediately after vacuum cleaning. Do not permit the animal to sleep on stuffed bedding or upholstered furniture. Wash bedding in hot water (> 70°C)
Moulds	Avoid using dusty dog foods. Keep animal away from lawn cuttings and house plants
Pollens	Avoid access to fields. Keep lawn short. Rinse dogs after walking in long vegetation. Topical application of barrier cream

FIG. 31.4 Measures to limit exposure to antigens.

Measures to Modify Immune Response

In cases where exposure to antigens cannot be prevented (e.g. atopic dermatitis), modification of immune response is required. The medicaments discussed above (glucocorticoids, essential fatty acids, antihistamines and related drugs, topical therapy and miscellaneous treatments) can be successfully used alone or in combination therapy in atopy. In addition, there is a role for immunotherapy or hyposensitisation therapy.

Immunotherapy/Hyposensitisation

This form of therapy has been used in veterinary medicine, particularly in the USA, for a number of years. Currently it is not regarded as a suitable therapy for flea-bite hypersensitivity but is of undoubted value in the management of atopy in dogs and possibly in cats. Considerable commitment is required on the part of both owner and clinician and so cases should be very carefully selected for this type of treatment. The authors prefer to treat severely affected animals with pruritus which is present for a substantial proportion of the year. Ideally, such animals should belong to enthusiastic and compliant owners.

Although a great many protocols for immunotherapy have been described, they all have the following features in common. Gradually increasing concentrations of a mix of allergens are injected subcutaneously. The antigens are selected on the basis of positive intradermal skin test reactions or *in vitro* IgE assay. Most dermatologists use aqueous rather than alum precipitated allergens. The optimum dose and frequency of administration have yet to be determined. In general the manufacturers or importers of allergen solutions are willing to give advice regarding the hyposensitisation protocol.

Only one placebo-controlled double-blind study has been conducted; this was in Holland. Results demonstrated, unequivocally, that hyposensitisation therapy led to a significant improvement in around 60% of the antigen-treated group compared with 21% of the control group. Similar results have been reported in numerous uncon-

MANAGEMENT OF AUTOIMMUNE SKIN DISEASES IN DOGS AND CATS		
Disease	**Treatment options**	**Comments**
Discoid lupus erythematosus	1. Tetracycline and Niacinamide (<10 kg: 250 mg *per os* of each t.i.d.; >10kg: 500mg *per os* of each t.i.d.) 2. Oral vitamin E 400 IU *per os* t.i.d. 3. Topical betamethasone or fluocinolone daily until lesions regress 4. Prednisolone / prednisone 2–4 mg/kg *per os* initially, then in a decreasing alternate-day dose	Treatment 1 is treatment of choice if lesions are mild. Response usually seen in 4–6 weeks If lesions are severe and disfiguring, a more aggressive treatment with topical potent steroids or systemic prednisolone is indicated. Once lesions have regressed, alternative therapy is indicated
Pemphigus / pemphigoid	1. Induce remission with oral prednisolone or prednisone 2–4 mg/kg *per os* (dog) and 4–8 mg/kg *per os* (cat) daily or divided b.i.d. 'Remission' is defined as resolution of clinical signs and lack of new lesion development; may take 1–2 weeks 2. Begin an adjuvant glucocorticoid-sparing agent (a) azathioprine 2 mg/kg *per os* every other day (dogs only); (b) chlorambucil 0.2 mg/kg *per os* daily (cats); (c) gold salts 1 mg/kg IM weekly	Extremely rare that patient with autoimmune skin disease can be maintained on alternate-day prednisolone indefinitely. Patients either relapse and/or develop unacceptable adverse effects (polyuria, polydipsia, signs of iatrogenic hypercortisolemia, silent urinary tract infection, etc.) Adjuvant glucocorticoid sparing drugs generally take 2–3 weeks before being effective As soon as possible, the b.i.d. or daily glucocorticoid dose should be reduced to alternate-day therapy. May or may not be possible to eliminate the use of these drugs completely Haematology and biochemistry panel should be performed pre-treatment. Total WBC and PCV should be monitored as most adjuvant drugs affect bone marrow Urinalysis and urine culture should be performed every 4–6 months to screen for silent urinary tract infection
Systemic lupus erythematosus	See discoid lupus erythmatosus Therapy for this disease may be complicated if the patient is anaemic and/or thrombocytopenic	Avoid use of gold salts in these patients; may cause a glomerulonephritis and may complicate monitoring of SLE
Uveodermatological syndrome	See pemphigus / pemphigoid	

FIG. 31.5 Management of autoimmune skin diseases in dogs and cats.

trolled retrospective studies. Before embarking on this expensive and time-consuming form of therapy, owners should be warned that it is quite likely that their pet might not be helped and that it will take at least 6 months before failure can be assumed. Some patients may take a year before improvement is seen. If successful, treatment should be continued for life. In some instances 'improvement' simply means that the amounts of other medication are reduced. In the UK, no hyposensitisation preparations have a product licence for veterinary use.

The mechanism of action of hyposensitisation therapy is unknown; readers are referred to the bibliography for more details.

Management of Immune-Mediated Diseases

The clinical signs and diagnosis of auto-immune skin diseases (discoid lupus erythematosus, pemphigus/pemphigoid and systemic lupus erythematosus) are discussed in *Chapters 8* and *17*. Treatment options are given in Fig. 31.5.

Management of Feline Eosinophilic Disease

The aetiology, pathogenesis and diagnosis of this interesting group of disorders are described in detail in *Chapters 17* and *19*. The objective of the clinician when presented with a cat exhibiting an eosinophilic dermatosis is to identify the underlying cause (usually hypersensitivity or ectoparasitism) and treat specifically. This section covers the management of cases where a specific cause cannot be identified, although the management measures detailed here could be used as short-term supportive therapy in cases where a diagnosis has been made and the primary disorder is under treatment.

A number of medicaments, including glucocorticoids, antimicrobial agents, progestagens, immunomodulating agents and various forms of surgery (such as laser therapy, sharp surgical excision and cryosurgery), have been recommended for the management of these cases. Response varies between cases and it is impossible to anticipate which type of therapy will be efficacious. Therefore, it may be necessary to try various drugs sequentially and evaluate response. It is prudent to start with treatments that are associated with few side-effects before embarking on more aggressive therapy such as surgery or the use of immunomodulating drugs. A sensible regimen might be to start with systemic antimicrobial agents; if no beneficial response is seen, use glucocorticoids and then, if no response is seen, try immunomodulating agents or surgery. Progestagens such as megoestrol acetate are not recommended.

Antimicrobial Agents

There is clinical evidence that oral antimicrobial agents can induce partial or complete remission of some eosinophilic ulcers and collagenolytic granulomata. However, there are no controlled studies documenting these results.

These apparent responses may be due to antimicrobial activity although it is possible that there is some anti-inflammatory effect. Drugs used include trimethoprim-potentiated sulphonamides (30 mg/kg twice daily), cephalexin (25 mg/kg twice daily) and clavulanate-potentiated amoxycillin (12.5 mg/kg b.i.d.).

Glucocorticoids

Glucocorticoids have been used in the management of all three manifestations of eosinophilic skin disease. Injectable methylprednisolone (4 mg/kg IM) is the drug of choice. Irrespective of the animal's size, no cat should receive more than 20 mg in a single dose. Initially, injections should be given at fortnightly intervals until a beneficial response is seen; this typically takes two or three treatments. Once remission has been accomplished, maintenance injections every 2 months may be needed, but ideally treatment should be discontinued if possible.

Oral glucocorticoids such as prednisolone (5 mg/kg/day), methylprednisolone (4 mg/kg/day) or triamcinolone (0.5–0.75 mg/kg/day) have been advocated by some authors but anecdotal reports suggest that this form of therapy may be less effective than the use of injectable methylprednisolone. If lesions resolve, then the dose of oral glucocorticoid should be tapered to find the lowest alternate-day maintenance dose. In the case of triamcinolone, which has a longer half-life *in vivo* than the other oral glucocorticoids mentioned, it may be possible to treat twice weekly.

Immunomodulating Agents

Immunomodulating drugs should be used extremely cautiously in cats. Chlorambucil is relatively inexpensive and safe for use in this species at a dose of 0.1–0.2 mg/kg daily (this is approximately half a 2 mg tablet per cat per day). If a beneficial response is seen, the drug can be given on alternate days. Alternatively, oral levamisole (2 mg/kg on alternate days) or thiabendazole (5 mg/kg on alternate days) may lead to remission in the signs of eosinophilic dermatoses but **these drugs have been associated with serious side-effects such as bone marrow suppression and so cannot be recommended.**

Surgical Treatment

A discussion of surgical means of treating these disorders is beyond the scope of a medicine text. Recommended techniques include sharp surgery, cryosurgery, radiation and laser therapy.

Progestagens

Progestagens such as megoestrol acetate are no longer recommended in the management of feline skin disease. Numerous side-effects have been seen associated with the use of megoestrol acetate, including:

- Reproductive problems:
  defective spermatogenesis;
  pyometra;
  oestrus cycle abnormalities;
  mammary gland fibroadenomatous hyperplasia (may be irreversible after therapy ceases);
  mammary neoplasia.
- Endocrine disorders:
  diabetes mellitus (which may be transient or permanent after therapy ceases);
  adrenocortical suppression (which may persist for many weeks after therapy).
- Miscellaneous problems:
  behavioural changes (lethargy, aggression, increased docility);
  weight gain;
  polydipsia and lethargy.

The use of this drug should be reserved for cases that do not respond to other therapy and where the skin lesion are severe enough to warrant therapy. Induction dose is 2.5–5 mg/cat on alternate days. Maintenance can be accomplished with the same dose given every 7–14 days.

32

Management of Infectious Disorders

IAN MASON and KAREN MORIELLO

Antimicrobial Therapy in Canine Pyoderma

Once pyoderma has been recognised in a dog, meticulous efforts should be made to determine the underlying cause. This approach is discussed fully in *Chapter 10*. Antimicrobial therapy is used initially as supportive treatment in order to facilitate rapid healing of bacterial lesions while specific therapy is undertaken. A proportion of cases will be idiopathic and in such instances long-term strategic antibacterial therapy will be required. Unless the primary cause of pyoderma is identified and treated, there will be a recurrence once antimicrobial therapy is discontinued. Figures 32.1 and 32.2 summarises an approach to the management of pyoderma.

Systemic Therapy

The effective treatment of canine pyoderma with systemic antimicrobial agents depends on the use of the correct drug at the correct dose for a sufficiently long duration. Figure 32.2 shows suitable antimicrobial agents along with a list of doses and comments regarding the advantages and disadvantages of these drugs. The depth of infection should be established before therapy commences (*Chapter 10*) as this will determine the duration of therapy and may influence the selection of drug and the dose. In general, higher doses and longer courses of treatment are employed in deep pyoderma.

Bacterial culture and sensitivity testing may aid in the selection of the 'correct' drug but the value of such testing is controversial. Many veterinarians select systemic antimicrobial agents empirically as the prevalence of resistance to these drugs among strains of *Staphylococcus intermedius* is well documented. Furthermore, it is possible that the sensitivity profile of the strain isolated from the skin may not be representative of all the pathogenic staphylococci present. In some instances *in vitro* testing does not correlate with clinical results. Despite these limitations, sensitivity testing is indicated in deep, chronic or recurrent cases or in those instances where no clinical response is observed following empirical therapy.

Ideally the antimicrobial agent used in the management of canine pyoderma should inhibit pathogenic staphylococci in a bacteriostatic manner. If possible, the selected drug should be inexpensive, convenient to administer, easily absorbed and lead to few or no adverse effects. Narrow-spectrum drugs are preferred as they have little effect on the normal skin and gut microflora. In theory, bacteriostatic agents are only effective if the animal is not immunocompromised. In practice, it is often not possible to achieve these ideals and the use of bacteriostatic and broad-spectrum agents causes few problems. Bactericidal agents should be used in cases of deep pyoderma or where immunological defects are suspected.

MANAGEMENT OF CANINE PYODERMA

11. Identify underlying cause if possible
12. Initiate specific therapy
13. Make assessment of depth, extent and severity of infection
14. Administer appropriate systemic and/or topical medicaments
15. Monitor response carefully
16. In cases of superficial pyoderma, discontinue systemic therapy 10–20 days after resolution of bacterial lesions. Cases of deep pyoderma may need treatment for a month after resolution of lesions
17. Evaluate response to topical therapy alone. If favourable, gradually increase interval between applications
18. Where a primary cause has been identified and treated, it may be possible to discontinue antimicrobial therapy
19. Idiopathic cases will need long-term or even lifelong therapy
10. Glucocorticoids are contraindicated in almost all forms of pyoderma

FIG. 32.1 Management of canine pyoderma.

GENERAL TREATMENT RECOMMENDATIONS FOR CANINE PYODERMA	
Fold pyoderma	Topical antibacterial shampoos on a daily basis with or without the concurrent use of an antibacterial cream/ointment. Systemic antibiotics are beneficial, but should be limited to severe episodes. Some cases of fold pyoderma are aggravated by seborrhoea and secondary *Malassezia* dermatitis and may benefit from topical and/or systemic antifungal treatment (ketoconazole or itraconazole, 10 mg/kg *per os* daily). This may be a chronic problem and may require intermittent treatment
Pyotraumatic dermatitis in short-coated dog	Standard therapies are usually effective. Most cases have an underlying cause — fleas, ear infections, etc. The author always prescribes 3 weeks of oral antibiotics, topical antibacterial shampoo and a topical antibacterial ointment. The author does not use topical corticosteroids or astringents on the area. Elizabethan collars are beneficial
Pyotraumatic dermatitis in thick-coated dog	These are sometimes focal areas of deep pyoderma. After the lesion is clipped, it is common to notice satellite lesions of superficial pyoderma. Four to 6 weeks or oral antibiotics and topical antibacterial shampoos are recommended. Corticosteroids are contraindicated in all cases
Puppy impetigo	No therapy, topical antibacterial therapy alone for 2–3 weeks, or systemic therapy for 2–3 weeks
Superficial pyoderma (impetigo/folliculitis)	Topical antibacterial therapy for at least 2–3 weeks. Systemic antibiotics should be prescribed for at least 3–4 weeks; therapy should continue for at least 1 week past clinical cure
Generalised deep pyoderma	Same as for superficial pyoderma, except that systemic antibacterial therapy should be used for at least 4–6 weeks, possibly longer. Some cases of deep pyoderma can require up to 12 weeks of therapy. A bacteriocidal antibiotic should be used
Focal deep pyoderma	Same as for deep pyoderma. Topical antibacterial creams/ointments may be beneficial
Idiopathic recurrent pyoderma	See page 293

FIG. 32.2 General treatment recommendations for canine pyoderma.

Treatment may fail if bacterial resistance is present; if the micro-organism is protected by the production of enzymes such as the β-lactamases, or if the organism has adapted to survive within host cells such as macrophages and so is not exposed to the effects of the antimicrobial agent. Inadequate tissue concentrations may also lead to therapeutic failure. A drug which is readily adsorbed and penetrates well into skin should be selected and an adequate dose used. Unfortunately skin is one of the most difficult tissues in which to achieve high concentrations of antimicrobial drugs.

Doses should be calculated based on actual rather than estimated body weight. In general, doses are doubled for skin infections so that adequate tissue concentrations are more likely to be achieved. Treatment should continue until at least 10–20 days beyond the resolution of all bacterial lesions. In severe, chronic and deep pyoderma, treatment may need to continue for 2–3 months or longer.

Most coagulase-positive staphylococci produce β-lactamases (or penicillinases) and so antibiotics sensitive to these enzymes, such as **penicillin**, **ampicillin** and **amoxycillin**, are unlikely to be successful in the management of pyoderma and their use should be avoided. Some synthetic penicillins, such

as **oxacillin**, are resistant to β-lactamases and are highly effective. However, oxacillin is expensive and not licensed for use in animals. **Amoxycillin** has been combined with **clavulanic acid** which inhibits β-lactamase activity. Anecdotal reports indicate that, although almost all strains of *Staphylococcus intermedius* isolated from cases of pyoderma are sensitive to this drug *in vitro*, its clinical performance is disappointing.

The lincosamide antibiotics include **lincomycin** and **clindamycin**. These drugs, which penetrate readily into devitalised areas and fibrotic, purulent lesions, are very similar to the macrolide group which includes **erythromycin**. Resistance to one of these drugs may be associated with resistance to the others and clinicians should not switch from one of these drugs to another if the original drug is ineffective. In theory, bacteriostatic drugs such as erythromycin and lincomycin should be avoided in cases of deep pyoderma or where immunodeficiency is suspected.

Enrofloxacin has recently become available to veterinary surgeons in most countries. It is a broad-spectrum, bactericidal antimicrobial agent with a unique mode of action. It inhibits an enzyme, bacterial gyrase, which is responsible for maintenance of DNA configuration within bacterial cells and for DNA replication. As plasmid replication requires functional DNA gyrase, plasmid-mediated resistance has not been documented. Hence, resistance can only develop due to mutation, which is a much slower process. Enrofloxacin has been shown to be efficacious in canine pyoderma. However, it is not recommended for use in skeletally immature dogs because damage to articular cartilage and lameness can occur in such animals.

In the UK, **chloramphenicol** is seldom used in canine pyoderma despite being a cheap and often efficacious agent. The veterinary use of this drug is mentioned in the Royal College of Veterinary Surgeon's *Guide to Professional Conduct*. An investigation into the profession's use of antibiotics in 1968 led to the recommendation that veterinary surgeons should only 'use chloramphenicol as an exceptional measure reserved for special indications in order to reduce transferable drug resistance'. The basis for this advice was that, at the time, this was the drug of choice for treating *Salmonella typhii* in humans and that more widespread use of chloramphenicol might increase the number of strains of pathogenic salmonellae that were resistant to it.

Chloramphenicol has the disadvantage of being both broad-spectrum and bacteriostatic. Toxic reactions, particularly blood dyscrasias, have also been reported. The use of chloramphenicol cannot be recommended, particularly in the UK, whilst so many alternative agents are available.

In cases of deep pyoderma with chronic scarring, the presence of free hair-shaft keratin within the dermis and granuloma formation may make it impossible to achieve adequate tissue concentrations of those antimicrobials usually employed. **Rifampicin** is an agent previously used in human tuberculosis but it is also effective against staphylococci within cells and is useful in chronic granulomatous disease. One problem associated with its use is that bacterial resistance develops rapidly and so it must always be administered in combination with another antibiotic. Its major disadvantage is hepatotoxicity, with most cases developing elevations in serum alkaline phosphatase concentration following therapy. Other side-effects include thrombocytopenia, haemolytic anaemia and the development of gastrointestinal signs. It is not licensed for use in the UK and its use should be confined to those cases where euthanasia is being considered.

In summary, penicillin, ampicillin, amoxycillin and tetracyclines are usually ineffective in the management of this group of disorders. Good results are usually achieved with **erythromycin**, **lincomycin** and **trimethoprim-potentiated sulphonamides**, especially in those cases where antimicrobial therapy has not previously been used. The author uses either trimethoprim-potentiated sulphonamides or lincomycin as initial treatment in most cases of pyoderma unless the animal has previously failed to respond to these drugs or if deep pyoderma is present. There is evidence to suggest that potentiated sulphonamides should not be used in Dobermann Pinschers because drug-induced ocular and arthritic changes have been reported following their use in this breed. **Cephalexin** and **enrofloxacin** are expensive but highly effective. The author restricts the use of these drugs to severe cases of deep pyoderma, preferably where sensitivity data indicate that they are likely to be effective.

Cases of pyoderma which do not respond after 2 or 3 weeks of therapy should be reassessed with a view to investigating the case more fully. A number of other diseases, such as immune-mediated disorders and neoplasia, may resemble pyoderma. Re-evaluation of the diagnosis is likely to be much more rewarding than simply changing the antimicrobial agent.

Topical Therapy

Topical therapy is a useful adjunct to systemic treatment. In some cases of idiopathic recurrent pyoderma, it is sometimes possible to maintain dogs in remission by the use of topical agents alone, thereby avoiding the disadvantages of long term systemic therapy.

Local treatment

Pyoderma is seldom localised and local topical therapy is seldom satisfactory. Treatment of lesional areas alone may only lead to a short-term benefit before pathogenic bacteria recolonise the skin from adjacent untreated skin. Moreover, the canine skin surface is hairy and so the use of creams and ointments is messy and costly and therefore likely to be of limited benefit. There is also a tendency for dogs to lick medicaments from treated areas. Shampoos are used almost exclusively in the management of human scalp disorders; this is a situation analogous to canine dermatology.

Despite these reservations, there are limited indications for local topical therapy. Benzoyl peroxide gel is useful for infected calluses and canine acne. Mupiricin is a topical antibiotic used for localised bacterial dermatoses in humans. It is effective against Gram-positive cocci; it is bactericidal and is not systemically absorbed. In dogs, it penetrates well into the lesions of deep pyoderma, such as interdigital abscesses, and may be of value in their management. It should be applied twice daily. Indications include any localised pyoderma such as callus, chin and interdigital infection.

Shampoos

Shampoos are the most suitable topical agents in the majority of cases and currently a wide range of antibacterial shampoos are available. Figure 32.4 shows examples of commonly used agents. Almost irrespective of the active constituent, shampoos will benefit most dogs with pyoderma by hydrating the skin and removing crusts, scale and other surface debris which may form a nutrient source for bacteria. These effects help to restore the normal surface ecosystem and facilitate the re-establishment of the normal microflora. In addition, antimicrobial shampoos have a direct effect on cutaneous micro-organisms. The major disadvantage of shampoo therapy is the inconvenience to owners, particularly those with large or unruly dogs where

COMMONLY USED ANTIMICROBIAL AGENTS FOR THE TREATMENT OF PYODERMA IN DOGS				
Drug	Dose mg/kg	Advantages	Disadvantages	Comments
Cephalexin	20–30 b.i.d. or t.i.d.	Resistance is uncommon	Expensive	Best reserved for severe pyodermas
Clavulanic acid-potentiated amoxycillin	20–25 t.i.d.	*In vitro* resistance not reported	Expensive	Anecdotal reports cast doubt on efficacy *in vivo*
Clindamycin	5 b.i.d.	Good penetration into devitalised tissue	Bacteriostatic Cross-resistance with erythromycin and lincomycin	
Enrofloxacin	2.5–5 b.i.d.	Rapid bactericidal action Little bacterial resistance Good penetration into devitalised tissue	Can damage articular cartilage and cause lameness in young growing dogs Costly	Should not be used in skeletally immature dogs
Erythromycin	10–15 t.i.d.	Inexpensive May have an independent anti-inflammatory effect	Bacteriostatic Gastric irritant — may induce vomiting Needs to be administered three times daily Cross-resistance with lincomycin and clindamycin	
Lincomycin	15 t.i.d. (or 22 b.i.d.)	Can be given twice daily	Cross-resistance with erythomycin and clindamycin Bacteriostatic	Administer 1 hour before or after feeding
Oxacillin	20 t.i.d.	Resistance is rare	Not licensed for use in the UK Needs to be given three times daily Food interferes with absorption	Administer 1 hour before or after feeding
Trimethoprim-potentiated sulphonamide	30 b.i.d.	Relatively inexpensive	Idiosyncratic drug reactions (polyarthropathy, cutaneous drug eruptions, ocular lesions) Possible increase of bacterial drug resistance	Recent data suggest tissue concentrations are adequate at 30 mg/kg s.i.d.

FIG. 32.3 Commonly used antimicrobial agents for the treatment of pyoderma in dogs.

SHAMPOOS AND SURGICAL SCRUBS USED IN THE MANAGEMENT OF CANINE PYODERMA	
Active constituent	**Comments**
Benzoyl peroxide (2.5%)	Bactericidal Alters surface microenvironment (keratolytic, removes comedones) May be irritant and may dry skin. A humectant or emollient should be used if long-term therapy is proposed or if a scaling keratinisation disorder ('seborrhoea sicca') is present Potent degreasing agent. Useful in cases where pyoderma is accompanied by surface lipid May be irritating to inflamed skin especially in relatively glabrous areas Long residual action on surface bacteria
Chlorhexidine	Bactericidal Surgical scrub, available as 4% solution. Has activity against *Malassezia pachydermatis* at this concentration but best used at 0.5% for pyoderma Useful for local therapy, e.g. interdigital pyoderma Less effective bactericidal activity than benzoyl peroxide and less prolonged residual action
Ethyl lactate (10%)	Bactericidal Activity comparable with benzoyl peroxide but duration of effect not documented Less irritating and less drying than benzoyl peroxide Poor degreasing and follicular flushing activity Low irritancy
Poviodone-iodine	Bactericidal activity less than benzoyl peroxide, ethyl lactate and chlorhexidine Irritant Surgical scrub
Triclosan (0.5%)	Bactericidal activity less than the other substances in this table Useful if keratinisation disorders and excessive grease and scale are also present because it is formulated with sulphur and salicylic acid Low irritancy

FIG. 32.4 Shampoos and surgical scrubs used in the management of canine pyoderma.

shampooing may be impractical. It is important that dog owners are given clear instructions for the use of shampoos and are told how frequently to use the shampoo and for how long to leave it in contact with the skin before rinsing. Figure 32.5 shows a protocol appropriate for most antibacterial shampoos but the manufacturer's recommendations — particularly those relating to safety — should always be followed.

The frequency of shampoo usage depends on the depth and severity of the disease. In some instances, alternate-day or even daily treatment is needed, but most cases can be managed satisfactorily with treatment once or twice a week. When improvement is seen, the interval between baths can be gradually increased until a satisfactory maintenance interval is established.

A number of surgical scrubs have been used as antibacterial shampoos in dogs. These products are not properly formulated for use in this way and may lead to irritant, allergic or even toxic reactions in rare cases. Initially, these products were used because few specific licensed shampoos were available. However, there is now a large choice of antibacterial shampoos specifically formulated for use on canine skin (Fig. 32.4) and therefore there is little merit in using surgical scrubs. There is one exception: 4% chlorhexidine scrubs

have good activity against both bacteria and the yeast *Malassezia pachydermatis* (which has recently been implicated as a cause of pruritic dermatoses in dogs). This product is not licensed for use in dogs.

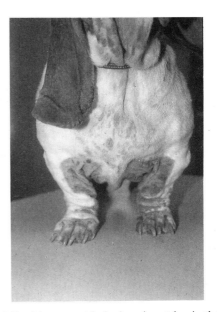

FIG. 32.5 Pruritic, symmetrical, alopecic patches in the axillae and leg folds of a Basset Hound due to *Malassezia* dermatitis. Slide courtesy of Richard Harvey.

Management of Idiopathic Recurrent Pyoderma

A diagnosis of idiopathic recurrent pyoderma is made on the basis of negative information. The underlying innate or adaptive immunological defects leading to this disorder have not been elucidated and so no diagnostic test has yet been developed. A diagnosis of idiopathic recurrent pyoderma can be made if:

- a thorough investigation of the case has been made and no underlying cause can be established; and
- if diseases which mimic pyoderma — such as neoplasia and some of the immune-mediated disorders — have been eliminated.

In this frustrating condition, the prognosis is guarded to poor because long-term (usually lifelong), antimicrobial therapy will be required. The prognosis varies between individual cases, with more extensive and deep pyodermas having a worse outlook. In many instances, euthanasia may be requested by the owner of a dog with this condition as the management may be expensive, particularly if antibiotics are used for prolonged periods in larger dogs. Treatment may also be extremely time-consuming if intensive topical therapy is undertaken.

The initial aim is to resolve the lesions rapidly. This is usually achieved with a combination of the systemic and topical agents previously discussed. Treatment should continue for at least 2–3 weeks after resolution of the lesions. In cases of severe pyoderma it may be prudent to continue treatment for even longer. Once the problem is in remission, a strategy to maintain this state is required. Often cases of superficial pyoderma can be maintained with the use of topical therapy alone. Benzoyl peroxide shampoos are the treatment of choice because of their prolonged effect on the cutaneous

---

PROCEDURE FOR SHAMPOO THERAPY

Wear suitable protective clothing and gloves
Wet entire body surface with warm water
Apply approximately half a teaspoonful of shampoo to the skin surface and gently massage to a lather
Repeat at an adjacent area so that the entire coat is lathered sequentially
Gently massage shampoo into the skin for 10 – 20 minutes before rinsing and drying thoroughly
Rinsing and drying of long-haired dogs may be facilitated by clipping

FIG. 32.6 Procedure for shampoo therapy.

---

microflora. In some dogs, irritant or allergic reactions may occur following the use of such products, in which case a less irritant shampoo such as an ethyl lactate based product, or one containing triclosan or chlorhexidine should be used. At first, baths should be administered two or three times weekly. If remission persists, the interval between baths can be gradually increased until the optimum treatment interval is determined by the owner. This may be as infrequently as monthly, but in most cases will be more often. In general, more frequent treatment will be required during the warmer times of the year and in warmer, more humid climates.

If topical therapy alone is insufficient to maintain a state of remission, then immunostimulation with some form of bacterial product, such as an autogenous vaccine or a purified staphylococcal extract may be required. Alternatively, long term antibiotic treatment is needed.

Chronic antibiotic therapy

Chronic systemic antibiotic therapy is a reasonable course of treatment if the dog does not respond to bacterins and shampoo therapy or if the owners want maximum relief from lesions. In the UK, bacterins are seldom used as they are not readily available; hence, long-term systemic antimicrobial therapy is often used.

Some antimicrobial agents are more suitable than others for such therapy. Use of trimethoprim-potentiated sulphonamides and the lincosamide or macrolide group usually leads to quite rapid development of drug resistance. Resistance is less likely to occur with drugs such as cephalexin, oxacillin, enrofloxacin and clavulanate-potentiated amoxycillin, but the use of such drugs may be prohibitively expensive. Several protocols have been suggested.

(a) *Full-dose chronic therapy.* The dog receives the full dose of medication on a daily basis, e.g. cephalexin 20 mg/kg t.i.d. This is continued indefinitely or as needed.

(b) *Full-dose pulse therapy.* The dog is treated for an appropriate period (4–6 weeks) until all signs of the pyoderma have resolved. (i) The dog then receives full-dose therapy two or three times per week; for example, cephalosporin 20 mg/kg t.i.d. on Tuesdays and Fridays or (ii) After initial stabilisation, the drug is used on a week-on/week-off basis. If there has been no relapse after, say, three cycles of such therapy, the off-treatment period is gradually increased to find the optimum maintenance interval.

(c) *Lose-dose chronic therapy*. The dog is treated for an appropriate period (4–6 weeks) until all signs of pyoderma have resolved. The drug is then given at 50% of the standard dose.

NOTE: Regardless of the protocol used, this form of management has a number of disadvantages, including the possibility that resistant bacterial strains may be encouraged and that adverse reactions may occur. Cost may also be a major consideration in some cases.

The authors are concerned that such regimens may encourage the development of antibiotic resistance bacterial strains but accept that in most instances there is little option. It is generally accepted that 'pulse therapy' is the most cost-effective means of managing these cases in the long-term.

Immunomodulation with bacterins

Bacterin therapy: Patients may benefit from commercially prepared or autogenous bacterin therapy. This therapy is expensive but if it is effective the dog may require significantly less antibiotics over the course of its life than with other treatment protocols. It is important to realise that dogs will require intermittent antibiotic therapy even with successful bacterin therapy.

Immunomodulation with bacterins is indicated as adjunct therapy in the treatment of dogs with idiopathic recurrent pyoderma. Autogenous bacterins are custom formulated from bacteria isolated from each patient while commercial preparations are made from *Staphylococcus aureus* or *Proprionibacterium acnes*.

The advantage of autogenous bacterins is that they are prepared from the specific bacteria that are involved in the patient's skin disease. The problem with these preparations is that there is no uniform preparation method and the higher risk of side-effects. Malaise, local inflammation and sterile abscesses are common side-effects from the use of authogenous bacterins. There are no controlled studies available to determine whether or not these products are superior to commercial preparations.

Commercially prepared bacterins have several advantages. They are readily available, they have a uniform content and are relative free of side-effects. In addition, the two most commonly used products, Staphage Lysate (SPL) and Immunoregulin, have been evaluated in clinical trials that demonstrated efficacy — 77–80% improvement over controls. It is important to have eliminated all potential underlying causes of pyoderma before initiating these therapies and to have good documentation of the dog's relapse cycle with respect to the pyoderma. If therapy is successful, it is continued indefinitely. Therapy should be considered beneficial if the dog has no relapses of pyoderma, less frequent relapses, or milder relapses.

Staphage Lysate: This product is administered subcutaneously. If an active pyoderma is present, the dog should receive 6–8 weeks of oral antibiotics (oxacillin or cephalosporin 20 mg/kg t.i.d.) as specific treatment for the existing pyoderma. At the same time as the oral antiobiotic therapy is initiated, SPL therapy is started. The client administers 0.5 ml SC of SPL twice weekly. SPL therapy should be continued at least 6–8 weeks beyond the discontinuation of antibiotic therapy. If the patient is going to benefit from SPL therapy, benefit will be seen in the latter half of the 12–16 week trial.

Immunoregulin: This product is administered intravenously. Antibiotics are administered as needed (1–12 weeks) to resolve any existing pyoderma. A veterinarian then administers 0.25–2.0 ml IV twice weekly for 2 weeks and then once weekly for 10 weeks. Immunoregulin therapy should be considered beneficial if the dog has no relapses of pyoderma, less frequent relapses, or milder relapses.

NOTE: The most common reason for bacterin failure is inappropriate use or premature use. With the exception of autogenous vaccines, immunostimulatory drugs are unlicensed or unavailable in the UK.

Relapse despite intensive topical therapy, either with or without the use of immunostimulants, indicates that long-term systemic antibacterial therapy is required.

Common reasons for treatment failure

The most common cause of recurrent pyodermas is inappropriate management of the patient. Approximately 50% of patients referred for the problem of recurrent pyoderma have an unidentified underlying cause for the pyoderma or pyoderma has been mistreated. The most common treatment errors observed are:

1. **The use of concurrent corticosteroids. Corticosteroids are always contraindicated in the treatment of canine pyoderma.**

Solution: Pruritus is a common complaint of clients with dogs pyoderma. Client education is extremely effective in minimising the request for 'something for the itching'. Intensely pruritic dogs may benefit from fatty acid supplements, antihistamines, frequent baths and lime sulphur dips. Pyoderma is often intrinsically pruritic — antimicrobial therapy alone may dramatically reduce pruritus.

2. **Inappropriate use of antibiotics.** Only a limited number of antibiotics are effective in the skin.

Solution: Choose an antibiotic that has known effectiveness against *S. intermedius* or base your choice of antibiotics on the results of a culture and sensitivity.

3. **Wrong dose**. Many patients are underdosed.

Solution: Weigh patients accurately and dispense medication based upon an actual per kg weight.

4. **Too short a course of therapy**. It is common to see antibiotics dispensed from only 10–14 days or changed after only 10–14 days of therapy. The skin receives approximately 4% of the cardiac output and the blood supply to hair follicles and the stratum corneum is poor when compared with other organs in the body. A dramatic improvement in clinical signs is usually not observed until after 14–21 days of therapy in severe cases.

Solution: Dispense a minimum of 21 days of antibiotics before re-examining patients. In severe cases of pyoderma or in recurrent cases, expect to treat patients for at least 4–6 weeks. Deep pyodermas may require up to 12 weeks of antibiotics before the infection is resolved.

GENERAL TREATMENT RECOMMENDATIONS FOR DERMATOPHYTOSIS IN DOGS AND CATS		
Treatment/option	**Rationale**	**Comments**
No treatment/self-cure	Self-curing disease in most healthy animals. In most cases lesions will spontaneously resolve within 60–100 days of infection	Reasonable option for outdoor animals with little or no human contact or when finances are limited Dermatophytosis is a zoonotic skin disease. Treatment will minimise contagion and speed recovery
Topical therapy with ointments/gels/creams	May be an adjuvant therapy in cases where no therapy is chosen. 'Spot therapy' will resolve clinical lesions but new lesions will continue to develop. No evidence to suggest that as a sole method of therapy, this resolves clinical infection any sooner than no therapy at all	Increases opportunity for clients to be exposed to dermatophyte and inadvertently become infected Miconazole or clortrimazole are treatments of choice but can be irritating to cats
Whole-body applications of topical antifungals	Recent studies show that many topical antifungals do not shorten the course of clinical infection. *In vitro* studies have shown that Captan, chlorhexidine solution used as a dip, 1:10 bleach, ketoconazole, chlorhexidine and miconazole shampoo are not fungicidal after one 5 minute application	Although agents do not significantly shorten the course of clinical infection, they may be useful in limiting environmental contamination. Use is optional and is dependent upon the client and the animal's tolerance
Clipping of hair coat	Has been recommended to decrease contagion and speed recovery. Clipping of hair coat may actually worsen infection in many cases	Recommended in severe generalised infections and in animals with long hair Clients should be warned that clinical lesions may worsen, temporarily Clipped animals should be treated with systemic antifungal agents
Systemic antifungal therapy	Treatment of choice, with either griseofulvin or itraconazole. These two therapies significantly shorten the course of clinical infection and result in a faster clinical cure than no treatment	Expensive, and owners must be aware of potential adverse effects. Idiosyncratic drug reactions are possible. Griseofulvin commonly results in gastrointestinal upset/irritation. Bone marrow suppression is the most life-threatening adverse effect. Itraconazole well tolerated in cats but anorexia has been observed. In dogs, idiosyncratic vasculitis has been observed
Fungal vaccines	Have not yet shown any efficacy in protection against challenge exposure. May be beneficial as adjuvant therapy	Experimental to date

FIG. 32.7 General treatment recommendations for dermatophytosis in dogs and cats.

PROTOCOLS FOR THE TREATMENT OF DERMATOPHYTOSIS	
Treatment	**Comments**
Clipping of hair coat	Optional in animals with mild infections or infected hairs from the margin of the lesion may be clipped Strongly recommended in animals with long hair or severe infections May temporarily worsen lesions If whole-body clipping is done, use systemic therapy
Local application of topical antifungal creams or ointments	Best avoided: Messy, may not significantly decrease infection course, and may give client a false sense of security
Sole topical therapy	Not recommended as sole therapy; concurrent systemic therapy is strongly recommended If used alone, may not significantly shorten course of infection Use of topical whole-body dips may decrease contagion Enilconazole (dogs only) or lime sulphur (1:16 or 1:32) is recommended. Lime sulphur may be irritating to the skin of cats, especially at higher concentration; has also been associated with toxicity and irritant reactions
Systemic therapy	Griseofulvin microsize 50 mg/kg *per os* once daily. Griseofulvin ultramicrosize 2.5 to 5.0 mg/kg *per os* once daily. Itraconazole 10 mg/kg *per os* once daily Therapy should be continued until mycological cure at least two negative fungal cultures at weekly intervals via the toothbrush fungal culture technique Most patients require minimum 8–10 weeks systemic therapy. Clinical cure will precede mycological cure by several weeks

FIG. 32.8 Protocols for the treatment of dermatophytosis.

Treatment Strategies for Dermatophytosis

Dermatophytosis is a self-limiting disease. Most healthy dogs and cats that do not receive treatment recover spontaneously within several months. Infections in long-haired animals will also resolve spontaneously, but they make take much longer. For example, the author monitored one group of Persian cats with endemic dermatophytosis. In this group, it took 3 years before infections resolved spontaneously.

There are several reasons to treat dermatophytosis in dogs and cats:

1. This disease is of zoonotic importance and every effort should be made to limit its spread to people, especially to debilitated individuals and children.
2. Treatment of an infected animal will minimise the risk of contagion to other animals.
3. Treatment will decrease contamination of the environment, which is an important consideration in multiple pet facilities.
4. Treatment will hasten recovery in an infected host.

Spontaneous recovery is dependent upon a healthy immune system in a healthy host. In many patients, this state of health is questionable.

Previous treatment recommendations have been based solely upon clinical experience and upon the extrapolation of *in vitro* drug testing to clinical patients. In general, treatment recommendations have included mandatory clipping of the hair coat and topical therapy as the cornerstones of antifungal treatment. In some countries systemic antifungal therapy was discouraged until it was clear that topical therapy has failed. The following treatment recommendations are based upon a series of controlled studies using an experimental model of dermatophytosis.

Clipping of the Hair Coat

The rationale for clipping of the hair coat is based upon the assumption that clipping will remove infected hairs, stimulate new hair growth and hasten recovery. However, clipping of the hair coat of infected cats sometimes leads to a worsening of signs within 7–10 days after clipping. The infection may worsen because of trauma or mechanical spread via the process of clipping and many animals develop widespread miliary dermatitis lesions over their body. These lesions may be Wood's lamp positive and fungal culture positive; microscopically, hairs plucked from these lesions may be positive for fungal spores and hyphae.

The value of clipping must be carefully weighed. In cats and dogs with limited clinically obvious lesions, it is probably better not to clip the entire hair coat. In order to limit contagion, only the infected hairs from around the periphery of the lesion should be clipped, with scissors. In animals with grossly obvious widespread clinical lesions, it is recommended that the entire hair coat is clipped to limit the spread of infected spores into the environment and limit contagion to people and other animals. Clipping is best done with scissors or a no. 10 clipper blade. The owner should be warned that the lesions may worsen after clipping.

In summary, clipping of the hair coat is optional and depends upon the severity of the infection. It is probably of value in animals with severe lesions, but it may do more harm than good in those with minimal lesions.

Topical Therapy

The author (KAM) has previously advocated the use of topical therapy as the sole treatment for dermatophytosis but now believes that it is inappropriate to use topical therapy alone. In one study, we compared the speed of recovery of four groups of kittens infected with *M. canis*. Three groups were treated topically and one group was untreated. At the end of 150 days of treatment, there was no difference among the groups; topical therapy had no effect on the outcome of the infection. During the study, we noted that some kittens that had received topical therapy had a worsening of lesions and it is possible that the mechanical rubbing of shampooing and dipping may actually worsen the clinical infection.

Although topical therapy alone has proven ineffective in altering the course of the infection, it has some value in killing spores on infected hairs that will not be killed by systemic agents or removed by grooming. Many of the commonly used antifungal agents are fungicidal *in vitro* studies. A recent study showed that lime sulphur (30 ml/gal water) and enilconazole (20 ml/gal water) were superior to chlorhexidine solution (25 or 50 cc/gal water), captan, povidine–iodine, ketoconazole shampoo and bleach in killing *M.canis* on infected hairs.

The major value of topical antifungal therapy is to limit environmental contagion by killing spores on the hair coat that may otherwise be shed into the environment. The decision to use topical adjuvant therapy is based upon the owner's ability and willingness to bath or dip their pet and the severity of the lesions. If it is felt that adjuvant topical therapy is

indicated to limit contagion, the author recommends lime sulphur (22g/l [4 oz/gal]) sponge-on dips or chlorhexidine shampoos. To date, enilconazole dip is not available in the US. If a dip is used, it is important to put an Elizabethan collar on the animal until the lime sulphur dries to prevent them from ingesting the dip. Irritant reactions, vomiting, and mild depression have all been reported when cats have ingested lime sulphur dip.

Another major consideration is the value of topical antifungal creams as adjuvant treatments. Topical therapy with creams is always difficult in animals because of the hair coat, which is poorly penetrated by ointments and creams. These agents are also vigorously groomed off by cats and are messy in both dogs and cats. Some agents can also be very irritating to the skin of cats and dogs. On the other hand, puppies and kittens less than 12 weeks of age are very difficult to treat with systemic agents (see below) because of the lack of information on safety, and the use of an ointment or antifungal cream may be a useful adjunct to lime sulphur dip or an alternative to no therapy at all in these young patients.

Systemic Therapy

Based upon our studies, systemic therapy is the treatment of choice for dermatophytosis. In our studies, cats with generalised *M. canis* infections receiving either griseofulvin (50 mg/kg *per os* once daily) or itraconazole (10 mg/kg *per os* once daily) as the sole therapy did dramatically better than the control group. Negative fungal cultures were seen as early as 7–8 weeks after the start of therapy in cats receiving itraconazole or griseofulvin. The cats receiving itraconazole were cured (three negative fungal cultures) after 12 weeks of therapy and the cats receiving griseofulvin were cured after 14 weeks of therapy.

Although these cats were clipped and we did see a worsening of lesions post-clipping, it was much milder than in the cats that had received only topical therapy. The infection sites healed much more rapidly and these two groups reached clinical cure (no visible lesions) and mycological cure (three negative fungal cultures) much faster than the control group.

Griseofulvin is the authors' drug of choice primarily because it is cheaper and easier to dose than itraconazole. Itraconazole is very expensive and is supplied in 100 mg capsules, requiring it to be suspended and reformulated for appropriate dosing. Animals should be treated until two to three negative fungal cultures are obtained.

Griseofulvin is a fungistatic drug that has enhanced absorption when administered in divided daily doses and with fatty meals. The most common side-effects are vomiting, diarrhoea and anorexia. These can be managed by dividing or slightly lowering the dose. Bone marrow depression (neutropenia, anaemia or pancytopenia) may occur in some patients but is idiosyncratic. This side-effect is most common in cats. Because severe neutropenic reactions have been associated with feline immunodeficiency virus (FIV), griseofulvin should not be used in cats with this infection. Ideally, all cats should be tested for FIV before griseofulvin is administered. Weekly or biweekly blood counts are recommended for these patients. **The use of griseofulvin is contraindicated for pregnant animals.**

Itraconazole is a newer antifungal that is related to ketoconazole. It appears to be better tolerated by cats than ketoconazole. We observed no side-effects in the kittens treated with this drug. This drug would be indicated in animals that cannot tolerate griseofulvin or have failed griseofulvin therapy. The authors consider that griseofulvin therapy has failed when the animal is still lesional and culture-positive after 100 days. If the animal is lesion free but still culture-positive, therapy should be continued with griseofulvin. **The use of itraconazole is contraindicated in pregnant animals.**

Fungal Vaccines

In eastern Europe, Russia and several Scandinavian countries, live fungal vaccines have been used successfully in cattle for the prevention of dermatophytosis caused by *Trichophyton* spp. The use of these vaccines has almost eradicated **clinical** dermatophytosis in cattle. The search for a fungal vaccine for the prevention of *M. canis* infections is currently underway in a variety of research laboratories.

An experimental fungal vaccine was tested in 12 kittens free of dermatophytosis in our laboratory (DeBoer and Moriello, 1993). In this study, six of the kittens were vaccinated with the experimental vaccine and six were vaccinated with a placebo. After 10 weeks, all kittens were challenged with live *M. canis* spores.

Although all of the kittens became infected, the vaccinated group had smaller, less inflammatory lesions. The infection did not resolve any faster in the vaccinated kittens. Immune function studies, which were performed on all of the kittens, showed that the vaccine stimulated antigen-specific immunity against *M. canis*. Although the failure of the vaccine to protect the cats against challenge was disappointing, we were not discouraged as we had used a very large number of spores. We have recently completed another study designed to test the efficacy of a killed *M. canis* vaccine to prevent infection under field conditions. This vaccine is not commercially available and was developed in our laboratory. In this study, two groups of kittens were vaccinated: one group received the vaccine and the other received a placebo. After 10 weeks of vaccination, a symptomatically infected cat was introduced into both rooms. After 4–6 weeks of contact, cats in both rooms developed classic lesions of dermatophytosis. At this time we are not optimistic that a killed *M. canis* vaccine will be protective against infection but it remains a very interesting option as a treatment modality and this needs further study.

Environmental Decontamination

Environmental contamination of the house is an under-recognised problem in multiple animal homes, especially in catteries and it requires control by means of good hygiene:

- The home should be thoroughly vacuumed each day to remove contaminated hairs and spores from surfaces.
- All surfaces should be thoroughly washed each day with a 1:10 dilution of household bleach. One application of this solution is not 100% sporicidal. Most chemicals advertised as antifungal are not effective against the infectious form of dermatophytes (i.e. infected hairs and spores).
- All furnace filters and heating vents should be thoroughly cleaned on a weekly basis.
- All brushes, combs and blankets should be discarded.

33

Topical Symptomatic Management of Canine Primary Keratinisation Disorders (Seborrhoea)

IAN MASON

The disorders of keratinisation affecting dogs are discussed in *Chapter 7*. In general, such disorders are associated with primary conditions such as ectoparasitism, hypersensitivity, endocrinopathy, metabolic disorders and autoimmune disease. Less commonly, primary idiopathic keratinisation disorders are encountered.

The management of disorders of keratinisation varies depending on the cause of the problem, which should always be investigated before long-term symptomatic treatment is introduced. Specific systemic and topical therapies are detailed in *Chapter 7*. Clearly, scaling disorders as diverse as cheyletiellosis and epitheliotropic lymphoma need quite different therapies and have completely different prognoses. Reliance on symptomatic treatment without making a diagnosis is doomed to failure.

Symptomatic topical therapy is indicated in those disorders which are idiopathic or where the underlying defect cannot be treated. Another indication for such treatment is as supportive therapy in the early management of a case where specific therapy has been introduced or where results of investigations are awaited; the aim is to hasten recovery. Topical therapy in domestic companion animals usually relies on shampoos and moisturising rinses because the lesions are often generalised or extensive and the hair coat obscures the underlying skin, limiting the use of ointments, gels, creams and sprays. However, localised lesions may be managed with such products (see later).

Treatment should be tailored to the specific case and selection of a topical agent is usually based on the morphological appearance of the skin and hair. Most therapeutic recommendations are based on clinical experience, anecdotal knowledge and extrapolation from the human literature as there have been no controlled studies in small animals.

A large number of veterinary shampoos are now available and practitioners are often bemused by the range of products. The aim of this chapter is to explain the actions of the active principle and constituents of antiseborrhoeic shampoos and to discuss the clinical applications of these substances. Sound advice is to use and stock only a limited range of veterinary shampoos and to ensure that all clinicians in the practice understand their uses, indications, contraindications and side-effects.

The mechanisms of action and potency of antiseborrhoeic substances vary. Some of the more potent products may be irritant or may sensitise the skin so that re-exposure to the substance leads to hypersensitivity. It is therefore recommended that animals under treatment should be monitored closely for the development of side-effects and that mild products, such as cleansers and moisturisers (Fig. 33.2), should be used initially. More potent agents should be reserved for those cases that are refractory to the beneficial effects of milder products. Once a patient's condition has been stabilised using more potent substances, it may subsequently be possible to return to milder products for maintenance therapy.

An essential early stage in the topical therapy of this group of disorders is good client communication. The client must be left in no doubt as to how difficult, expensive and time-consuming therapy will be.

Prolonged shampoo therapy requires considerable commitment on the part of the animal's owner, and also some products are expensive and difficult to use. It is often not easy—or even possible—to bath a large dog in the middle of winter where there are no adequate bathing and drying facilities. In addition, some shampoos are malodorous and some clients may object or even refuse to use them.

The clinician should determine as far as possible that the client is both willing and able to comply with instructions. Clients must also be educated regarding the correct use of shampoos—written instructions are very useful but are no substitute for a careful and clear explanation or even demonstration of how to bath the dog.

How to Shampoo Dogs

Bathing methods depend to a large extent on which product is being used and so may vary between cases. Veterinary surgeons should be very careful of terminology here: we may use the term 'a bath', but really we mean 'a shower'. Total immersion of the animal in water is seldom required and will lead to overdilution of the active principles in the shampoos. The clinician should consider the points listed in Fig. 33.1 before prescribing a shampoo and then provide the client with clear and complete instructions.

Antiseborrhoeic Shampoos

Numerous substances have been formulated into shampoos designed to treat keratinisation disorders in animal skin. Even water is said to be of value in hydrating the stratum corneum and removing debris, scales, crusts, micro-organisms and old medicaments from the skin surface. However, in practice water is seldom used alone and it is usual for it to be used as the vehicle for an actual shampoo. Figure 33.2 lists some of the most common active constituents of antiseborrhoeic shampoos, along with their indications and properties.

Mechanism of Action

Scale and grease form on the skin surface as a result of metabolic defects in keratinisation. These may be primary, or secondary to another disease process. The role of shampoo therapy is to remove scale, grease and other debris, hydrate the stratum corneum and restore normal epidermopoiesis and keratogenesis.

SHAMPOO THERAPY: FACTORS TO CONSIDER WHEN INSTRUCTING CLIENTS	
Clipping	In general, clipping is advised. Clipping hair to around 15 – 20 mm in length will enable the owner to wet, lather, rinse and dry the skin and coat more readily. Clipping also leads to enhanced penetration of the active principles of the shampoo into the outer layers of the epidermis and reduces the amount of shampoo that is needed
Pre-washing	In some instances where severe scaling, crusting and grease formation are present on the skin and within the coat, the use of a detergent such as washing-up liquid or human baby shampoo before the antiseborrhoeic bath will remove such debris from the skin surface and so enhance the penetration and efficacy of the medicated shampoo. This will reduce usage of the medicated product, reducing the cost
Frequency of treatment	Severe scaling disorders are best managed by using shampoos two or even three times weekly. Milder dermatoses need less frequent treatment. Once improvement is seen, then the frequency of application can be gradually reduced for maintenance. This will vary between cases, from twice weekly to monthly. The author has learned that owners are often the best judges of how frequently maintenance therapy is required
Skin contact time	Most shampoos are labelled with the optimum skin contact time. This varies with the active ingredients of the shampoo but is usually around 5 – 15 minutes. Owners should literally time themselves while they gently massage the shampoo into the skin surface. Timing should start as soon as the animal has been lathered. Clearly, the only opportunity for the active constituents of the shampoo to work is while they are actually on the skin. **Shampoos should then be thoroughly rinsed from the skin** Skin contact times of over 20 minutes are not recommended as they lead to maceration of the skin surface, which will damage cutaneous defence against micro-organisms
Water temperature	Pruritus is influenced by temperature. Cool baths are recommended where pruritus is a feature of the dermatosis. However, cold water should be avoided as both dogs and owners may be reluctant to allow or perform bathing if the water is too cold!
Drying methods	The author recommends the use of a towel rather than a hair-drier. Heating of the skin surface with a drier may lead to pruritus and may damage the hair and stratum corneum
The use of moisturisers	After bathing, the moisture content of the skin can be increased by the use of humectants and emollients

FIG. 33.1 Shampoo therapy: Factors to consider when instructing clients.

CONSTITUENTS OF 'ANTISEBORRHOEIC' SHAMPOOS			
	Properties	**Indications**	**Comments**
Cleansing and moisturising agents (sometimes called hypoallergenic shampoos). Examples of active ingredients and constituents are glycerin, lactic acid or sodium lactate, urea, oils (coconut oil, lanolin, essential fatty acids)	Removal of debris; moisturising the stratum corneum	Dry scaling, e.g. idiopathic seborrhoea, sebaceous adenitis, ichthyosis, scaling associated with low environmental humidity, endocrinopathy and hypersensitivity	These mild shampoos seldom irritate the skin and are a valuable addition to specific therapy (where such therapy is indicated and possible for those diseases listed above)
Sulphur	Keratolytic; keratoplastic; antifungal; antibacterial; antiparasitic; antipruritic	Dry and waxy scaling disorders poorly responsive to cleansing and moisturising shampoos. Examples of other diseases include ear margin dermatosis; zinc-responsive dermatosis; pemphigus foliaceus	May be irritant and drying although this usually occurs at concentrations much higher than those used in shampoos Malodorous Synergistic keratolytic activity with salicylic acid and is usually found in combination with this substance Poor degreasing agent
Salicylic acid	Karatolytic; keratoplastic; mildly antipruritic; bacteriostatic	As for sulphur	Very occasionally irritant reactions occur Synergistic keratolytic activity with sulphur and is usually found in combination with this substance
Benzoyl peroxide	Karatolytic, excellent antimicrobial and degreasing action. Reduces sebaceous gland activity and is said to 'flush' hair follicles. (The exact meaning of this term and its origin are unknown but it probably refers to the removal of scale, glandular secretions and bacteria that form comedones which plug the hair follicle ostia)	Primary keratinisation disorders associated with much grease, scale and secondary pyoderma. Follicular disorders, particularly those associated with pyoderma or *Malassezia* infection. Examples: Primary seborrhoea (Spaniels, Basset Hounds); vitamin A-responsive dermatosis; epidermal dysplasia (West Highland White Terriers); canine acne; ear margin dermatosis; Schnauzer comedo syndrome; follicular dystrophy	Extremely drying. Prolonged use requires post-treatment application of moisturiser Irritant reactions are not uncommon. Contact allergy may occur in some individuals after chronic exposure. These problems may also affect owners who do not wear gloves while bathing dogs Bleaches fabrics Can be unstable in solution — only purchase benzoyl peroxide that contains products from a reputable pharmaceutical company
Tar	Keratoplastic; antipruritic; degreasing	Primary keratinisation disorders associated with much greasy scale. Examples: Epidermal dysplasia of West Highland White Terriers; primary seborrhoea of Spaniels, Terriers, Basset Hounds and German Shepherd Dogs	**Contraindicated in cats** Rather drying and should be reserved for dogs with severe greasy scaling disorders. Prolonged use may need post-treatment application of a moisturiser. Irritant, urticarial-like reactions may occur. Tar will stain pale coats. Some clients object to the odour. Such side-effects increase with increasing tar concentration in the shampoo It is generally thought that the higher the concentration of tar within a shampoo, the greater the clinical efficacy of the shampoo. Whilst this is true, increasing the concentration of tar will lead to greater adverse effects. Higher concentrations are best reserved for severely greasy keratinisation disorders The interpretation of the tar concentration given on a bottle of shampoo must be made with caution. There is no standardised labelling system. 'Tar solution' , 'tar extract' and 'refined tar' are not synonyms. For

Continued

CONSTITUENTS OF 'ANTISEBORRHOEIC' SHAMPOOS			
	Properties	**Indications**	**Comments**
			example, a tar solution may contain only 20% tar; hence, a shampoo containing, say 3% of this tar solution will contain only 0.6% actual tar. If in doubt, practitioners should seek the advice of a recognised dermatologist
Selenium sulphide	Keratolytic; keratoplastic; degreasing. Has slight antifungal activity (*Malassezia pachydermatis*) and antiparasitic effects	As for tar. In addition, it may be helpful in some cases of *Malassezia* dermatitis (usually in combination with another antifungal agent)	**Contraindicated in cats** Selenium sulphide may be drying and irritating to mucous membranes and scrotum. This agent has fallen from favour amongst dermatologists in recent years, but it still has a role in the management of keratinisation disorders
Pyrithione zinc	There is no veterinary product containing this substance. Occasionally pet owners may use a human shampoo ('Head & Shoulders') on their pets, or veterinary surgeons may recommend it as an economical alternative to a shampoo specifically formulated for animals. There are anecdotal reports of quite serious neurological and ocular side-effects associated with the use of pyrithione zinc. The author has never encountered any animal that has had such a reaction to this product, but, in view of the wide range of effective alternatives, **it is recommended that pyrithione zinc is not used on dogs and cats**		

FIG. 33.2 Constituents of 'antiseborrhoeic' shampoos.

Normal development of the stratum corneum is discussed in detail in *Chapter 1*. Essentially, basal epidermal cells, or keratinocytes divide by mitosis; daughter cells migrate through the layers of the epidermis to form the flattened, dead, keratin-filled cells of the stratum corneum. These cells are then shed gradually in an organised manner with little gross scale formation. Lipids are also produced in parallel with and as a result of the process of keratinisation so that the normal stratum corneum is a lipid-rich structure in which the cells of the stratum corneum are embedded. In seborrhoea, this process is defective, leading to accelerated and disorganised keratinisation and the production of varying amounts of scale and grease on the skin surface. This disrupted skin surface is prone to opportunist microbial infections, particularly with staphylococci and *Malassezia*).

Virtually any shampoo will remove grease, scale and debris from the skin surface and facilitate rehydration of the stratum corneum. However, substances such as sulphur, salicylic acid, benzoyl peroxide, tar and selenium sulphide also have antimicrobial, keratolytic and keratoplastic properties. **Keratolytic** agents damage keratinocytes, leading to swelling and subsequent shedding of the cell and thereby reducing scaling. **Keratoplastic** agents affect epidermal cell kinetics, slowing cell production and reducing scale formation. It has been suggested that keratoplastic substances have a direct cytostatic effect on the epidermal basal cells.

Moisturising Agents

Moisturising agents play an extremely important role in the topical therapy of scaling disorders. The most common indications are:

1. Disorders associated with dry scaling ('seborrhoea sicca').
2. Instances where prolonged use of drying antiseborrhoeic agents such as benzoyl peroxide, tar or selenium sulphide is required.
3. To moisten the skin where drying flea dips are used.

Moisturising agents usually contain humectants or emollients, or both. An **emollient** is an agent which softens the stratum corneum and soothes the skin. Emollients are usually based on oils and waxes — examples include vegetable oils (olive, corn or safflower oil), animal fats (lanolin) or mineral oils (liquid paraffin). **Humectants** are oil-free substances which rehydrate the skin. Examples include urea, lactic acid and carboxylic acid. These agents attract and hold water within the stratum corneum. The source of this water is not the environment: it comes from transepidermal diffusion.

Moisturisers are most effective if applied to an animal when it is still wet after shampooing and rinsing. They should be mixed as directed, applied to the skin and coat and then the animal be gently towel-dried **without further rinsing**.

Topical Therapy of Localised Scaling Disorders

Topical therapy in canine scaling dermatoses usually relies on shampoos and moisturising rinses as the lesions are often generalised or extensive and the hair coat obscures the underlying skin. This limits the local use of ointments, gels, creams and sprays to a small group of disorders.

Tretinoin

Topical retinoid cream containing 0.05% tretinoin decreases epidermal turnover rate and reduces keratinocyte:keratinocyte adhesion. Indications for tretinoin therapy are localised scaling disorders such as canine (and feline) acne and canine idiopathic nasal hyperkeratosis. Daily application is required.

Salicylic Acid

Salicylic acid (6%) has been combined with urea (5%) and sodium lactate (5%) to form a keratolytic humectant gel. This product is not available in some countries. Indications are idiopathic nasal hyperkeratosis, acne and ear margin dermatosis. This product should be used daily until a beneficial response is seen and then as necessary for maintenance.

Cerumolytic Agents

Some dogs with severe greasy dermatoses may respond poorly to even the most potent antiseborrhoeic shampoos due to the build-up of thick, tightly adherent wax on the skin surface. The ventral neck of seborrhoeic Spaniels, West Highland White Terriers and Basset Hounds is an example of such a problem site. Aural ceruminolytic agents applied 15–20 minutes before shampooing will emulsify this greasy material, facilitating its removal during subsequent bathing.

34

Management of Psychogenic Disorders

IAN MASON

Little information is available on the treatment of psychogenic dermatoses. There have been open studies of some of the drugs mentioned in this chapter, but there have been few or no convincing published reports. Much of the information that follows is anecdotal.

Self-induced skin lesions as a result of psychological disease occur occasionally in veterinary medicine. The two most well-known disorders are canine acral lick dermatitis and feline psychogenic alopecia. The clinical features of the latter disorder is covered in *Chapter 8*.

Three risk factors are said to be involved in the aetiology and pathogenesis of psychogenic skin disease:

1. *Breed.* So-called 'highly-strung' breeds such as Abyssinian and Siamese cats or Dobermann Pinschers, Great Danes, Irish Setters and German Shepherd Dogs are more likely to develop these disorders.
2. *Management.* Stress, anxiety or boredom may lead to psychogenic dermatoses, even in non-predisposed breeds. Confinement, isolation, domination by the owner or another pet are examples of factors which may trigger psychogenic skin disease.
3. *Individual variation.* Irrespective of breed or management, some nervous or anxious cats and dogs may develop psychogenic disease.

A diagnosis of psychogenic skin disease is difficult to establish. There are no definitive tests for this group of disorders and the diagnosis is usually made on elimination of other possible causes of the clinical signs. These causes include trauma, pruritus (e.g. hypersensitivity), local pain (e.g. arthritis or penetration of a foreign body such as a grass seed), internal or endocrine disease, ectoparasitism, bacterial and fungal infection. An absolute diagnosis of, say, acral lick dermatitis can only be made where atopy, other hypersensitivities, demodicosis, other ectoparasitic disorders, carpel arthritis and foreign body, at least, have been eliminated as possible causes.

Psychogenic dermatoses recognised in dogs and cats include acral lick dermatosis, feline psychogenic alopecia, tail-sucking and biting, flank-sucking, foot-licking, 'self-nursing', and anal licking. Of these, the first two are the most common and will be discussed in detail.

Acral Lick Dermatitis

Figure 34.1 details one approach to the management of this problem. The prognosis varies from good to guarded. Once dogs have developed this habit, the problem appears to become entrenched in the dog's 'mind' and is difficult to cure, even if the underlying causes are identified and treated.

If the measures detailed in Fig. 34.1 fail to improve the condition, then a biopsy should be taken for histopathology. This may enable identification of the nature of the pathological process present (i.e. allergic, infectious, cicatrial or other).

If the information obtained from histology is unhelpful, there are four remaining options:

1. Management 'by crisis'

Physical restraint and antibiotics are applied whenever the problem is severe.

2. Behavioural or aversion therapy

The animal is referred to a behavioural consultant.

3. Local treatment

Glucocorticoids. Topical glucocorticoid creams, intra-lesional glucocorticoids and topical dimethyl sulphoxide mixed with various glucocorticoids have

CLINICAL MANAGEMENT OF CANINE ACRAL LICK DERMATITIS	
Prevent further self-trauma	The use of an Elizabethan collar or bandages or both may prevent or reduce the degree of self-trauma and allow the lesion to heal undisturbed. Healing is part of the inflammatory process and so is associated with pruritus. In dogs with acral lick dermatitis, this pruritus initiates further self-trauma. In rare instances, allowing the lesion to heal by the use of physical restraint is curative. However, the stress of such restraint may lead some individuals to self-traumatise another body region!
Control pyoderma	Secondary bacterial infection of acral lick lesions may lead to pruritus due to the production of bacterial toxins and enzymes. The authors of this book recommend that all cases of canine acral lick dermatitis be treated with antibiotics early in the investigation and management of the case. Systemic antibacterial therapy (*Chapter 32*) as an adjunct to physical restraint is usually necessary
Management changes	Boredom is blamed, often unfairly, for most cases of acral lick dermatitis. The author has seen many affected dogs from loving homes where exercise and attention are lavished on the animal. Traditionally, dermatology texts have recommended that more attention should be paid to affected dogs and that they should have longer and more frequent walks. Such an approach is seldom successful. This may be because the habit has become ingrained. Alternatively, the problem may be exacerbated by this increased attention as the dog uses its self-mutilation as an attention-seeking device. Some dogs prefer any attention, even chastisement, to being ignored Introduction of a companion animal into the household has been recommended. However, while this may reduce the level of boredom, it may also increase stress and so exacerbate the disorder

FIG. 34.1 Clinical management of canine acral lick dermatitis.

been recommended by some texts. These techniques may be successful in early cases but glucocorticoids impair healing and resistance to pyoderma, it is unlikely that they will be of long-term benefit, especially in chronic extensive lesions.

Surgery. Sharp surgical excision, cryosurgery and radiation therapy have been advocated by some. **In general, the authors do not recommend such treatments.** Early cases may respond to surgical excision provided that the suture line is protected from self-inflicted damage and that skin tension across the suture line is not excessive. Other forms of therapy are destructive to tissue and the danger exists that a moderate epidermal defect is replaced, after therapy, by a much larger one!

Miscellaneous therapies. Anecdotally, acupuncture is reported to be of value. The author has no experience of this technique nor knowledge of its success rate. Intra-lesional injections of modified cobra venom are expensive, ineffective and no longer readily available.

4. Mood-modifying drugs

Numerous sedatives and tranquillisers have been used in the past, including phenobarbitone, diazepam and primidone. Some clients may complain that a permanently drowsy, lethargic dog is not an acceptable pet. Progestagens have a calming effect

on some dogs, especially males. Megoestrol acetate has been used at 1 mg/kg daily to effect and then tapered but its use is contraindicated in intact females, due to the risk of inducing pyometra.

In recent years, more sophisticated drugs have been evaluated:

- The endorphin blocker **naltrexone** was given orally (2 mg/kg daily) to ten dogs with acral lick dermatitis. Seven dogs responded well but four of these relapsed when therapy was discontinued. One dog became much worse. Side-effects were not reported and so long-term maintenance treatment might be possible in dogs which respond to this drug.
- **Fluoxetine** is a serotonin-uptake inhibitor. Serotonin is believed to play a role in psychogenic dermatoses in humans. There has been one study using this drug in three dogs with acral lick lesions. Hyper-excitability and polyuria/polydipsia were observed as side-effects. Long-term clinical efficacy is unclear at this stage.
- **Clomipramine** is a serotonin uptake inhibitor and tricyclic antidepressant which has been used in human obsessive compulsive disorders. Six of nine dogs treated with this agent at an initial oral dose of 1 mg/kg daily showed a response to this agent. In some instances the dose was increased up to a maximum of 3 mg/kg per day.

The author has no experience of the use of these new mood-modifying drugs in the management of this disorder but suggests that their use be reserved for the last resort until more data concerning efficacy and long-term toxicity are available.

Feline Psychogenic Alopecia

The relevant details concerning the clinical features and differential diagnosis of this disorder are given in *Chapter 14*. The diagnosis of feline psychogenic alopecia can only be made if pruritic disorders and other causes of alopecia are ruled out (*Chapters 13* and *14*). A number of medical treatments have been described. All of these probably exert their effect via mood modification. However, the clinician should attempt to identify potential underlying causes before contemplating medical therapy. In some instances it may be possible to identify and correct a psychological trigger factor such as the introduction of an aggressive tomcat into the environment.

If the root cause of the problem cannot be identified and removed, then medical treatment is an option. However, most of the medicaments recommended for this disorder have been associated with side-effects and there is a good case for not treating these cats at all. The dermatological manifestations of the problem are often merely cosmetic.

If medical treatment is needed, then a number of drugs have been recommended in the veterinary literature. These are shown in Fig. 34.2.

Other Psychological Dermatoses

Other than canine acral lick dermatitis and psychogenic feline alopecia, psychogenic dermatoses are uncommon in cats and dogs. These disorders include tail-sucking in Siamese Cats. In dogs, tail-chasing, flank-sucking (especially in Dobermann Pinschers), foot-licking and anal licking (especially in Miniature Poodles) have been reported. The approach to these disorders is similar to that described for the diseases given above. Some clinicians recommend that Miniature Poodles which lick and bite at the anus and perianal area should be overfed so that the dog becomes so obese that it can no longer reach these sites. Physical diseases such as hypersensitivity, ectoparasitism, internal disease and pain should be eliminated from the differential diagnosis. If possible the psychological trigger should be identified. If this is not possible, then the treatments discussed above should be considered although it may be preferable not to treat the animal as the side-effects of some of the drugs given above are unknown and potentially severe.

MEDICAMENTS USED IN THE MEDICAL TREATMENT OF FELINE PSYCHOGENIC ALOPECIA	
The following information is anecdotal. No controlled studies have been undertaken. In many instances, the medicines listed are not licensed for use in cats	
Glucocorticoids	Oral or parenteral anti-inflammatory doses of glucocorticoids such as prednisolone (0.5–1.0 mg/kg) or methylprednisolone (0.4–0.8 mg/kg) may be effective. Prolonged therapy (up to a month) may be needed. The problem may relapse once therapy discontinues. **If cats respond to such therapy, then it is probable that a mis-diagnosis has been made and that the problem is primarily pruritic. Causes include hypersensitivity and ectoparasitism. See Chapter 13**
Sedatives and tranquillisers	Oral diazepam (1–2 mg per cat twice daily but usually ineffective), phenobarbitone (8–15 mg per cat daily) or primidone (12.5–25 mg per cat once to three times daily) have been recommended. None of these drugs are licensed for use in cats
Progestagens	Megoestrol acetate (2.5–5.0 mg per cat on alternate days for induction, then weekly for maintenance) is often highly effective in controlling this disorder but the use of progestagens in cats should be reserved for the last resort as a wide range of adverse effects has been associated with its use. **Again, response to this drug probably indicates that a primary pruritic disorder has been missed. The authors strongly advise against the use of megoestrol acetate in cats**
Miscellaneous agents	
Naloxone	An endorphin antagonist, has been evaluated in a group of five cats. Four of these five showed a beneficial response following one injection of naloxone (1 mg/kg subcutaneously). This effect lasted from 1 week to 6 months. There was often a lag period of some days after the injection and the apparent recovery, which might indicate that some other factor may have led to this improvement. Naloxone is not readily available; there are no toxicity data in this species and the route of administration is by injection
	There are anecdotal reports that **clompiramine**, the serotonin-uptake inhibitor and tricyclic antidepressant, may be of value in feline psychogenic alopecia. However, there is no information regarding dosage and toxicity
Busporine	5 mg/kg *per os* daily may be effective

Fig. 34.2 Medicaments used in the medical treatment of feline psychogenic alopecia.

Appendix

The following pages of tables are reproduced from Veterinary Clinics of North America: Clinical Management of the Cancer Patient Vol 20:14 with permission from W. B. Saunders Company.

COMMON SKIN TUMOURS OF DOGS AND CATS — EPITHELIAL TUMOURS

Tumour name	Breed predilections	Pertinent clinical and diagnostic findings	Behaviour	Treatment recommendation	Prognosis
Papilloma	Older dogs, especially males; Cocker Spaniels, Kerry Blue Terriers. Rare in cats	Single or multiple; predilection for head, face and feet; pedunculated or cauliflower-like, well circumscribed, usually smaller than 0.5 cm. Biopsy/surgical excision is most diagnostic	Usually benign	Surgical excision, cryosurgery, electrosurgery, or observation without treatment	Good to excellent
Viral papillomatosis	Young dogs, not reported in cats	Caused by a DNA virus; contagious; incubation period 30 days; almost always occurs as multiple lesions; papillomas vary from white flat plaques to pedunculated cauliflower-like masses; will affect the buccal mucosa, tongue, palate, pharynx, lips, skin, eyelids, cornea, conjunctiva. Patient profile, physical examination and biopsy are most diagnostic	Usually benign; however, severely affected dogs may have difficulty in eating. Some tumours may transform into squamous cell carcinomas	None—will usually resolve without treatment within 3 months. In severe cases, surgical excision electrocautery or cryotherapy may be necessary. Levamisole, thiabendazole and wart vaccines are ineffective. The use of autogenous vaccines should be avoided because malignant skin tumours may develop later at the site of inoculation	Good to excellent
Intracutaneous cornifying epithelioma	Dogs less than 5 years of age may be predisposed. May be hereditary. Norwegian Elkhounds and Keeshonds may be predisposed to generalised disease. Old English Sheepdogs, German Shepherd Dogs and Collies may also be at risk	Two patterns: single type more common in purebred dogs and located on the head, neck, thorax; generalised type most common in Norwegian Elkhounds. Clinically, lesions appear as a firm to fluctuant, well circumscribed mass with a pore that opens onto the skin. Keratin plugs that resemble cutaneous horns may be present. Some tumours do not communicate with skin surface. Biopsy is diagnostic	Usually benign tumours that do not recur at the site of removal. However, Keeshonds and Norwegian Elkhounds tend to develop new growths at different sites	Surgical excision, oral retinoids or intralesional 5-fluorouracil	Good

TABLE 1

Continued

COMMON SKIN TUMOURS OF DOGS AND CATS — EPITHELIAL TUMOURS					
Tumour name	Breed predilections	Pertinent clinical and diagnostic findings	Behaviour	Treatment recommendation	Prognosis
Squamous cell carcinoma	Common in dogs and cats. 'Sunbathing' individuals appear to be predisposed. White-haired-cats, Scottish Terriers, Pekingese, Boxers and Poodles are commonly affected	Solitary or multiple. In dogs, most common on the limbs and oral cavity. In cats, most common on the pinnae, lips, nose and eyelid. Lesions may be proliferative or ulcerative; cutaneous horns also may be present. Biopsy is diagnostic	Usually locally invasive but slow to metastasize. Tumours on the digits are locally invasive, but are cured by surgical excision. Black-skinned dogs are predisposed to subungual squamous cell carcinomas. Bull Terriers, Whippets and Dalmatians may develop multiple lesions on the chest and abdomen	Surgical excision, cryosurgery or radiotherapy. Radiotherapy is most useful for superficial lesions in dogs and cats. Chemotherapy has been ineffective	Guarded. Recurrence in white-faced cats is common
Basal cell tumour	Dogs and cats, may be more common in dark-skinned animals. Siamese Cats, Cocker Spaniels and Poodles may be predisposed	Usually single but may be multiple. Tumours are firm, elevated, round masses that may be ulcerated. Some tumours lie in the dermis and are freely movable. Tumours may or may not be cystic. Biopsy is diagnostic	Benign; local recurrence is very rare. In some cases tumours may be malignant	Cryotherapy, electrosurgery, surgical excision	Fair to good
Nodular sebaceous hyperplasia; sebaceous adenoma; sebaceous epithelioma	Common in dogs, especially Cocker Spaniels, Kerry Blue Terriers, Boston Terriers, Poodles, Beagles, Dachshunds, Norwegian Elkhounds and Basset Hounds. Rare in cats	Clinically, all tumours of sebaceous gland origin appear similar and are differentiated upon histological examination of tissue. Nodular sebaceous hyperplasia is most common and presents as a firm elevated, cauliflower-like lesion. Sebaceous adenomas are similar, but larger in size (>2cm). Sebaceous epitheliomas may appear similar to basal cell tumours. Diagnosis and differentiation are based upon biopsy	All benign	Surgical excision. May respond to oral retinoids	Excellent
Sebaceous adenocarcinomas	Primarily a tumour of dogs. Cocker Spaniels may be predisposed	Rapid rate of growth and early ulceration. Variable in size but often larger than 2 cm in diameter; poorly circumscribed. Biopsy is diagnostic	Malignant, locally invasive, but rarely metastasize. Inadequate surgical excision may result in local recurrence	Wide surgical excision	Good

TABLE 1

Continued

	COMMON SKIN TUMOURS OF DOGS AND CATS — EPITHELIAL TUMOURS				
Tumour name	**Breed predilections**	**Pertinent clinical and diagnostic findings**	**Behaviour**	**Treatment recommendation**	**Prognosis**
Apocrine cysts; eccrine cysts	Apocrine cysts are more common than eccrine cysts, especially in dogs	Apocrine cysts occur most commonly on head; may be single or multiple. Commonly recur. Eccrine cysts are uncommon. Biopsy is diagnostic	Benign	Surgical excision	Excellent
Apocrine adenomas; eccrine adenomas	Uncommon in dogs and cats	Apocrine adenomas are firm, elevated, well circumscribed masses 1 – 4 cm in diameter. Eccrine adenomas can appear similar, but are often less well circumscribed and are more often ulcerated. Eccrine tumours occur on the footpads. Biopsy is diagnostic	Benign	Surgical excision	Excellent
Apocrine adenocarcinomas; eccrine adenocarcinomas	Uncommon in dogs and cats	Apocrine adenocarcinomas may be indistinguishable from apocrine adenomas. They may be poorly circumscribed, ulcerated and infiltrative. They are commonly confused with areas of pyoderma or pyotraumatic dermatitis. Eccrine adenocarcinomas arise most commonly from the eccrine glands on the footpads. They are solitary, firm, poorly circumscribed tumours	Apocrine adenocarcinomas are malignant and may be highly invasive and metastasize. Eccrine adenocarcinomas may behave similarly	Wide surgical excision, cryosurgery, electrosurgery, radiotherapy	Guarded
Trichoepithelioma	Dogs and cats, no breed predilection	Tumours are usually solitary, may be multiple. Most common on the head. Firm, elevated, well circumscribed mass ranging in size from 0.5 – 10 cm. May be ulcerated. Biopsy is diagnostic	Benign, rarely invasive or metastatic	Surgical excision, cryotherapy, electrosurgery	Excellent

TABLE 1 Common skin tumours of dogs and cats — epithelial tumours.

COMMON SKIN TUMOURS OF DOGS AND CATS — MESENCHYMAL TUMOURS					
Tumour name	**Breed predilections**	**Pertinent clinical and diagnostic findings**	**Behaviour**	**Treatment recommendation**	**Prognosis**
Fibroma	Uncommon in dogs and cats. Boxers, Boston Terriers, Fox Terriers. Females may be predisposed	Solitary lesions on the extremities, flanks, and groin; usually well circumscribed, firm to soft masses; may be dome-shaped or pedunculated. Many tumours appear 'pinfeathered'. Biopsy is diagnostic	Benign, noninvasive and nonmetastatic	Surgical excision	Variable
Fibrosarcoma	Common tumours in dogs and cats. Fibrosarcomas in young cats are not common and may be caused by the feline sarcoma virus	Fibrosarcomas in older animals are solitary lesions with a predilection for the limbs. Lesions are poorly circumscribed, irregular in size and sometimes ulcerated. Tumours are slow or rapidly growing and infiltrative. Fibrosarcomas in young cats may be multiple. Fine needle aspirate or biopsy is diagnostic	Malignant, usually invasive: 25% of tumours will metastasize Vaccine-induced fibrosarcomas in cats are locally invasive and slow to metastasize	Wide surgical excision and/or amputation; recurrence may occur in 30% of canine cases. Radiotherapy plus hyperthermia post wide surgical excision Vaccine-induced fibrosarcomas are difficult to treat	Guarded Poor. Cats with sarcomas caused by feline sarcoma virus should not be treated due to potential human health hazard
Lipoma	Common in dogs, Cocker Spaniels, Dachshunds, Weimaraners, Labrador Retrievers, small Terriers. Obese females are predisposed. Uncommon in cats	Single or multiple tumours most commonly occurring over the thorax, ventrum, abdomen and proximal limbs. Lesions are dome-shaped or pedunculated, well circumscribed, soft to flabby, subcutaneous in location, and usually freely movable. Can present as an infiltrative benign mass that develops around muscle bellies and tendons. Fine-needle aspirate or biopsy is diagnostic	Benign	Surgical excision. Intralesional 10% calcium chloride is best avoided, owing to complications of infection and necrosis. Obese animals should be placed on a calorie-restricted diet Infiltrative form is impossible to excise	Excellent
Liposarcoma	Rare in dogs; Dachshunds and Brittany Spaniels, especially males, may be predisposed. Rare in cats	Usually solitary lesions; usually occurring on the ventral abdomen; poorly circumscribed, and subcutaneous in location. Biopsy is diagnostic	Malignant: 25 – 50% metastasize	Wide surgical excision	Guarded; likely to recur
Haemangioma	Uncommon in dogs, but Boxers may be predisposed. Rare in cats	Usually solitary lesions; most common on the head, neck, and limbs; well circumscribed;	Benign	Surgical excision, cryosurgery, electrosurgery or observation	Excellent

TABLE 2

Continued

COMMON SKIN TUMOURS OF DOGS AND CATS — MESENCHYMAL TUMOURS

Tumour name	Breed predilections	Pertinent clinical and diagnostic findings	Behaviour	Treatment recommendation	Prognosis
Haemangiosarcoma	Uncommon in dogs; German Shepherd Dogs, Golden Retrievers and Bernese Mountain Dogs may be predisposed. Rare in cats	firm to fluctuant; bluish to black in colour. Biopsy is diagnostic. There are two forms: 1) dermal form, which is locally invasive; 2) subcutaneous form, which is very invasive and may be part of the multifocal form of this disease. Tumours are usually firm and well circumscribed masses	1) First form is locally invasive but surgery is curative 2) Second form his highly metastatic	without treatment. Radical surgical excision. Possible combination chemotherapy with vincristine, doxorubicin and cyclophosphamide may be useful. Skin form may not respond to treatment	Good prognosis for the first form. Very poor prognosis for the second
Haemangiopericytoma	Common in dogs. Rare in cats	Solitary tumours, often on the limbs. Firm, multi-nodular, well circumscribed masses in the subcutaneous tissue. Can also be diffuse and poorly circumscribed	Locally invasive; rarely metastasize (5–15%)	Wide surgical excision or amputation; radiotherapy; radiotherapy and hyperthermia	Fair; 30 – 60% will recur
Lymphangioma; angioma	Rare in dogs and cats	Large, red, fluctuant solitary lesions in the axillary and inguinal regions. Biopsy is diagnostic	Benign	Wide surgical excision	Good
Amputation neuroma	Dogs that have had their tails docked	Historically, dogs have self-mutilated their tails since puppyhood. At the tail base there is a chronic, painful excoriated lesion on the tip of the tail. History and physical examination are most diagnostic	Benign	Surgical excision	Fair

TABLE 2 Common skin tumours of dogs and cats — mesenchymal tumours.

COMMON SKIN TUMOURS OF DOGS AND CATS — ROUND CELL TUMOURS

Tumour name	Breed predilections	Pertinent clinical and diagnostic findings	Behaviour	Treatment recommendation	Prognosis
Perianal gland adenomas/hyperplasia	Benign adenomas are primarily a tumour of intact male dogs. Cocker Spaniels, English Bulldogs, Samoyeds, Afghans, Dachshunds and Beagles are predisposed	Tumours may be single or multiple. Mostly occur near the anus but they may occur on the tail, perineum, prepuce, thigh, and along the dorsal or ventral midline. As they enlarge, tumours ulcerate and become lobulated. Biopsy is diagnostic	Benign	Castration is treatment of choice in male dogs, coupled with surgical excision of tumours. If tumour is very small it may regress without surgical excision. Surgical excision is treatment of choice for lesions in female dogs. Oestrogen therapy is *not* recommended. All female animals and males with recurrences should be evaluated for hyperadrenocorticism and elevated serum testosterone concentrations	Good to excellent, 95% of cases respond to castration and surgical removal
Perianal adenocarcinomas	May be more common in male than female dogs	May initially resemble perineal gland adenomas/hyperplasia, but grow much more rapidly and ulcerate more extensively	Malignant. Late onset of metastasis to local lymph nodes (20% spread)	Wide surgical excision, possible adjuvant chemotherapy or radiotherapy	Guarded. Tumours less than 5 cm may have a better prognosis
Anal sac adenocarcinomas	Most common in older female dogs	Affected dogs may present with obstipation, perianal irritation and tenesmus. Tumours vary in size to as large as 10 cm. One or both anal sacs may be affected and the skin may be ulcerated over the lesion. Commonly associated with pseudohyperpara-thyroidism. Anorexia, weight-loss, lethargy, polyuria and polydipsia associated with a rectal mass should arouse suspicion. Fine needle aspirate and/or biopsy is diagnostic. Serum bio-chemistry panel is recommended	Malignant and usually metastasize	Surgical excision, possible adjuvant chemotherapy or radiotherapy	Poor, 90% of dogs have metastasis to regional lymph nodes and 40% have distant metastasis
Melanoma	Common in dogs: Scottish Terriers, Boston Terriers, Airedales, Cocker Spaniels, Springer Spaniels, Boxers, Irish Setters, Irish Terriers, Chow Chows,	Tumours are usually solitary. In dogs they are most common on the face, trunk, feet and scrotum. The head, eyelids and pinnae are the most common sites	Benign or malignant	Wide surgical excision. Chemotherapy has been unrewarding; responses to immunotherapy have been inconsistent	Good to poor

TABLE 3

Continued

COMMON SKIN TUMOURS OF DOGS AND CATS — ROUND CELL TUMOURS

Tumour name	Breed predilections	Pertinent clinical and diagnostic findings	Behaviour	Treatment recommendation	Prognosis
	Chihuahuas, Dobermann Pinschers. Males appear to be predisposed. Uncommon in cats	in cats. Benign melanomas may be brown to black and vary in shape and size. Malignant melanomas grow rapidly, are larger than 2 cm and frequently ulcerate. Oral melanomas in dogs are usually malignant. Cutaneous melanomas in dogs are rarely malignant, except when found on the digits or in the mouth. Biopsy is diagnostic			
Canine mast cell tumours	Common in dogs. Boxers, Boston Terriers, English Bulldogs, Bull Terriers, Fox Terriers, Staffordshire Terriers, Labrador Retrievers, Dachshunds and Weimaraners are predisposed	Clinical appearance is extremely variable; therefore, any skin tumour should be suspect. Tumours are usually solitary but may be multiple. Tumours are most common on the trunk, perineum and limbs; frequently 'pinfeathered', oedematous and ulcerated. Non-cutaneous clinical signs may include gastric and duodenal ulcers, haemorrhagic diathesis. Fine needle aspirate is diagnostic	All tumours should be considered malignant, especially those arising on the perineum, digits or prepuce	Wide surgical excision, chemotherapy, radiotherapy. Treatment depends upon stage and grade	Guarded
Feline mast cell tumours	Common in cats, especially males (2:1 M:F ratio)	Two distinct subtypes. Type one is more common and usually occurs on the head, neck and limbs. Tumours are solitary, discrete dermal nodules and are benign; however, in some cases tumours may recur and spread. Type two is less common and occurs predominantly in Siamese Cats. These cats tend to be < 4 years of age and have multiple skin tumours. These lesions have been reported to regress spontaneously. In both	Feline mast cell tumours in non-Siamese Cats should be considered potentially malignant	Surgical excision or cryosurgery	Guarded in non-Siamese Cats

TABLE 3

Continued

COMMON SKIN TUMOURS OF DOGS AND CATS — ROUND CELL TUMOURS					
Tumour name	Breed predilections	Pertinent clinical and diagnostic findings	Behaviour	Treatment recommendation	Prognosis
		types, lesions may be firm or soft to the touch and may or may not be pruritic to the patient. Fine needle aspirate may be diagnostic; however, skin biopsy is recommended. Toluidine blue stain may be necessary to identify mast cell granules in some cats			
Cutaneous lymphosarcoma	Uncommon in dogs. Boxers, St Bernards, Basset Hounds, Cocker Spaniels, Beagles, German Shepherd Dogs, Golden Retrievers, Scottish Terriers. Rare in cats	Generalised or multifocal nodules, plaques, ulcers, erythroderma or exfoliative dermatitis. Pruritus is variable. Solitary tumours are rare. Cutaneous lymphosarcoma may be associated with a monoclonal or biclonal gammopathy, serum hyperviscosity and hypercalcaemia. Biopsy is diagnostic	Malignant	Not responsive to conventional combination chemotherapy. PEG-L-asparaginase may be beneficial for some. Topical nitrogen mustard may be effective, but this chemical is dangerous. Prednisolone 2 mg/kg may be effective. Surgery for solitary lesions	This disease may have a very long clinical course and temporary remission may be induced in dogs with prednisolone
Epitheliotropic lymphoma	Rare in dogs and cats	There are four common clinical presentations: generalised pruritic erythema and scaling; mucocutaneous ulceration and depigmentation (commonly misdiagnosed as pemphigus vulgaris, bullous pemphigoid, lupus erythematous); solitary or multiple cutaneous plaques or nodules; infiltrative and ulcerative oral mucosal disease. Animals may or may not have systemic illness. Multiple biopsies are required for definitive diagnosis	Malignant	Generally non-responsive to conventional chemotherapeutic agents. High doses of prednisolone 2 mg/kg in addition to 3–4 mg isotretinoin *per os* daily may alleviate some of the animal's discomfort	Grave
Histiocytoma	Common in young dogs, Boxers, Dachshunds, Cocker Spaniels, Great Danes, Shetland Sheepdogs	Solitary tumours on the head, pinnae and limbs. They are usually small, well circumscribed, dome-shaped, red alopecic lesion tumours with a rapid rate of	Benign; most will regress within 3 months	Surgical excision for diagnostic purposes	Excellent

Continued

TABLE 3

	COMMON SKIN TUMOURS OF DOGS AND CATS — ROUND CELL TUMOURS				
Tumour name	Breed predilections	Pertinent clinical & diagnostic findings	Behaviour	Treatment recommendation	Prognosis
Cutaneous histiocytosis	Dogs	growth. Fine needle aspirate is diagnostic. Benign proliferative disorder of dogs. Clinically presents as multiple, erythematous dermal or subcutaneous plaques or nodules on the body. Lesions may wax and wane. Systemic involvement or lymphadenopathy is not present	Benign	Systemic glucocorticoids and cytotoxic drugs may be useful	Good
Malignant histiocytosis	Rare in dogs, may be hereditary. Bernese Mountain Dogs, Golden Retrievers, especially males	Cutaneous lesions are rare and consist of multiple, firm, dermal to subcutaneous nodules on the body. Ulceration and alopecia of lesions may be present. Systemic signs of disease include weight-loss, lymphadenopathy, hepatosplenomegaly, pancytopenia	Malignant, rapidly fatal course	None proven; doxorubicin, cyclophosphamide and vincristine may be useful	Grave
Systemic histiocytosis	Rare disorder of dogs, may be hereditary. Bernese Mountain Dogs, especially males 2 – 8 years of age	Cutaneous signs include papules, plaques, nodules that ulcerate over the entire body, but especially on the face. Non-cutaneous signs include respiratory stertor, weight-loss and anorexia. Clinical signs may be prolonged and fluctuating with periods of remission or rapidly progressive and fatal. On necropsy, histiocytic infiltrates of the lungs, spleen, lymph nodes and bond marrow are common	Malignant	No effective treatment; chemotherapy and glucocorticoid therapy have been ineffective	Grave
Fibrous histiocytoma	Uncommon in dogs; rare in cats. Collies	Usually multiple and occur most commonly on the face. Lesions are usually firm and well circum- scribed. Overlying skin may be haired or alopecic. Lesions can occur on the cornea	Benign	Surgical excision or intralesional glucocorticoids	Good

Continued

TABLE 3

COMMON SKIN TUMOURS OF DOGS AND CATS — ROUND CELL TUMOURS					
Tumour name	**Breed predilections**	**Pertinent clinical and diagnostic findings**	**Behaviour**	**Treatment recommendation**	**Prognosis**
Malignant fibrous histiocytoma	Rare neoplasms of dogs and cats	Solitary, firm, poorly circumscribed, variably sized masses in the skin and subcutaneous tissues. Most common on the limbs and neck. May be locally invasive, but slow to metastasize. Biopsy is diagnostic	Malignant with local invasion to underlying muscle and bone. May metastasize in rare cases	Radical surgery or amputation. The role of adjuvant chemotherapy is unclear	Guarded

TABLE 3 Common skin tumours of dogs and cats — round cell tumours.

	COMMON SKIN TUMOURS OF DOGS AND CATS — NON-NEOPLASTIC TUMOURS			
Tumour name	Breed predilections	Pertinent clinical and diagnostic findings	Behaviour	Treatment recommendation	Prognosis
Epidermoid cysts	Common in dogs, rare in cats	Cysts may be single or multiple; usually smooth, round, well circumscribed, elevated masses, firm to fluctuant. Cysts may open and discharge material onto the surface. Occur most commonly on the extremities	Benign	Surgical excision	Excellent
Dermoid cysts	Congenital; most common in Rhodesian Ridgebacks, Kerry Blue Terriers, Boxers	Single or multiple. Dermoid cysts of Rhodesian Ridgebacks occur as single or multiple sinuses along the dorsum. Hair, keratinous material and adnexa may be visible grossly. Biopsy is diagnostic. Dermoid cysts in Rhodesian Ridgebacks should be evaluated radiographically to be sure that they do not communicate with the subarachnoid space	Benign	Surgical excision	Excellent
Follicular cysts	Common in dogs, may be congenital or acquired	Small, 2–5 mm in size, white to yellow in colour, may resemble calcinosis cutis or pustules	Benign	Surgical excision	Excellent
Calcinosis cutis	Dogs	Clinically appears as firm papules to plaques in the skin. Most commonly observed on the dorsal neck region and inguinal region; may be generalised. Lesions are usually non-pruritic; may be ulcerated or infected. Can occur as a result of a variety of diseases; however, overzealous administration of glucocorticoids or naturally occurring hyperadrenocorticism are the most common underlying causes. Can be caused by the percutaneous absorption of calcium chloride. Biopsy is diagnostic. Evaluate the dog for	Benign	Lesions will resolve over a period of months once the underlying disease is controlled	Good

TABLE 4

Continued

COMMON SKIN TUMOURS OF DOGS AND CATS — NON-NEOPLASTIC TUMOURS				
Tumour name	Breed predilections	Pertinent clinical and diagnostic findings	Behaviour	Treatment recommendation	Prognosis
Cutaneous mucinosis	Dogs and cats. Shar Pei	Generalised cutaneous mucinosis may occur in dogs with hypothyroidism, lupus dermatomyositis, mycosis fungoides, lupus erythematosus; considered normal in the Shar Pei. Cutaneous mucinosis has been seen in cats with alopecia mucinosis and mycosis fungoides. Focal cutaneous mucinosis can occur in dogs. Lesions are solitary asymptomatic, rubbery soft nodules. Biopsy is diagnostic; however, Alcian blue or colloidal-iron positive stains are required for definitive diagnosis underlying diseases	Benign	Treat underlying disease, if present	Good
Naevi	Dogs and cats. Collagenous naevi in German Shepherd Dogs	Naevi are congenital defects of the skin. There are many types of naevi including collagenous, organoid, vascular, sebaceous, epidermoid, melanocytic. German Shepherd Dogs with multiple collagenous naevi on the extremities frequently develop nodular dermatofibrosis and bilateral multifocal renal cystadenocarcinomas. This disease is hereditary. Dogs initially present with collagenous naevi, but develop renal disease over months to years	Benign except for nodular dermatofibrosis and renal cystadenocarcinomas of German Shepherd Dogs	Surgical excision. No known successful treatment for the disease of German Shepherd Dogs	Good

TABLE 4 Common skin tumours of dogs and cats — non-neoplastic tumours.

Selected Bibliography

General References

Becker, A., Janik, T. A., Smith, E. *et al.* (1989) *Propinio-bacterium acnes* immunotherapy in chronic recurrent canine pyoderma. An adjunct to antibiotic therapy. *J. Vet. Intern. Med.* **3**, 26–30.

Cowell, R. L. and Tyler, R. D. (1989) *Diagnostic Cytology of the Dog and Cat.* American Veterinary Publications, Goleta, CA.

DeBoer, D. J. (1990) Strategies for the management of recurrent pyoderma in dogs. In: *Veterinary Clinics of North America — Small Animal Practice* (Editor DeBoer, D. J.), **20**, pp. 1509–1524.

DeBoer, D. J. and Moriello, K. A. Experimental feline dermatophytosis — Effect of a fungal cell wall vaccine. *J. Med. Vet. Mycol.* (submitted for publication).

DeBoer, D. J., Moriello, K. A., Thomas, C. B. *et al.* (1990) Evaluation of a commercial staphylococcal bacterium for management of idiopathic recurrent superficial pyoderma in dogs. *Am. J. Vet. Res.* **51**, 636–639.

Dunstan, R. W. (1990) A user's guide to veterinary surgical pathology laboratories. Advances in veterinary dermatology. In: *Veterinary Clinics of North America — Small Animal Practice* (Editor DeBoer, D. J.), **20**, pp. 1397–1417.

Ferguson, E. A. (1993) Glucocorticoids, use and abuse. In: *Manual of Small Animal Dermatology* (Editors Locke, P. H., Harvey, R. G. and Mason, I. S.), pp. 233–243. BSAVA, Cheltenham, Glos.

Georgi, J. R. and Georgi, M. E. (1992) *Canine Clinical Parasitology.* Lea and Febiger, London.

Griffin, C. E., Kwochka, K. W. and MacDonald, J. M. (1993) *Current Veterinary Dermatology: The Science and Art of Therapy.* Mosby Year Book, St. Louis, MO.

Gross, T. L., Ihrke, P. J. and Walder, E. J. (1992) *Veterinary Dermatopathology: A Macroscopic and Microscopic Evaluation of Canine and Feline Skin Disease.* Mosby Year Book, St. Louis, MO.

Halliwell, R. E. W. and Gorman, N. T. (Editors) (1989) *Veterinary Clinical Immunology.* W. B. Saunders Co., Philadelphia, PA.

Horobin, D. F. (1982) *Clinical Uses of Essential Fatty Acids.* Eden Press, Montreal.

Kirk, R. W. (1989) *Current Veterinary Therapy*, **X.** W. B. Saunders Co., Philadelphia, PA.

Kirk, R. W. and Bonagura, J. D. (1992) *Current Veterinary Therapy*, **XI**. W. B. Saunders Co., Philadelphia, PA.

Koch, H. J. and Vercelli, A. (1993) Shampoos and other topical therapies (Workshop Report). In: *Advances in Veterinary Dermatology*, Vol. **2**, pp. 409–411. Pergamon Press, Oxford.

Lloyd, D. H. (1989) Essential fatty acids and skin disease. *Journal of Small Animal Practice*, **30**, pp. 207–212.

Morgan, R. V. (1992) *Handbook of Small Animal Practice* (2nd edn). Churchill Livingstone, New York.

Muller, G. H., Kirk, R. W. and Scott, D. W. (1989) *Small Animal Dermatology* (4th edn). W. B. Saunders Co., Philadelphia, PA.

Olivry, T., Prelaud, P., Heripet, D. and Atlee, B. (1990) Allergic contact dermatitis in the dog: Principles and diagnosis, advances in clinical dermatology. In: *Veterinary Clinics of North America — Small Animal Practice* (Editor DeBoer, D. J.).

Shelton, G. H., Grant, C. K., Linenberger, M. L. and Abkowitz, J. L. (1990) Severe neutropenia associated with griseofulvin therapy in cats with feline immunodeficiency virus. *J. Vet. Int. Med.* **4**, 317–319.

Sousa, C. A. and Noeton, A. L. (1990) Advance in methodology for diagnosing allergic skin diseases. Advances in clinical dermatology. In: *Veterinary Clinics of North America — Small Animal Practice* (Editor DeBoer, D. J.), **20**.

White-Weithers, N. (1993) Evaluation of topical therapies for the treatment of dermatophytosis in cats and dogs. In: *9th Proceedings of the Annual AAVD/ACVD Meeting*, p. 29. San Diego, CA.

Willard, M. D., Tvedten, H. and Turnwald, G. H. (1989) *Small Animal Clinical Diagnosis by Laboratory Methods*, pp. 207–212. W. B. Saunders Co., Philadelphia, PA.

References for Section IV: Problem-Oriented Approach to Skin Disease of Non-Domestic Pets

The authors would like to acknowledge gratefully the following authors and sources, from which much of the information in this section has been summarised:

Brue, R. N. (1994) Nutrition. In: *Avian Medicine: Principles and Applications* (Editors Ritchie, B. W., Harrison, G. J. and Harrison, L. R.), pp. 63–95. Wingers Publishing, Inc., Florida.

Burke, T. J. (1992) Skin diseases of rodents, rabbits, and ferrets. In: *Current Veterinary Therapy* (Editors Kirk, R. W. and Bonagoura, J. D.), **XI**, pp. 1170–1175. W. B. Saunders Co., Philadelphia, PA.

Campbell, T. W. (1994) Cytology. In: *Avian Medicine: Principles and Applications* (Editors Ritchie, B. W., Harrison, G. J. and Harrison, L. R.), pp. 199–222. Wingers Publishing, Inc., Florida.

Collins, B. R. (1993) The common dermatological diseases of small mammals. *Proceedings of the 1993 University of Wisconsin WEZAM Conference.*

Collins, B. R. (1986) Dermatologic disorders of common small nondomestic animals. In: *Contemporary Issues in Small Animal Practice: Dermatology* (Editor Nesbitt, G.), pp. 235–294. Churchill Livingstone, New York.

Cooper, J. E. and Harrison, G. J. (1994) Dermatology. In: *Avian Medicine: Principles and Applications* (Editors Ritchie, B. W., Harrison, G. J. and Harrison, L. R.), pp. 607–639. Wingers Publishing, Inc., Florida.

Crawshaw, G. J. (1992) Amphibian medicine. In: *Current Veterinary Therapy* (Editors Kirk, R. W. and Bonagoura, J. D.), **XI**, pp. 1219–1230. W. B. Saunders Co., Philadelphia, PA.

Crawshaw, G. J. (1993) Amphibian medicine. In: *Zoo and Wild Animal Medicine, Current Therapy* (Editor Fowler, M. E.) **2**. W. B. Saunders Co., Philadelphia, PA.

Gerlach, H. (1994) Viruses. In: *Avian Medicine: Principles and Applications* (Editors Ritchie, B. W., Harrison, G. J. and Harrison, L. R.), pp. 862–948. Wingers Publishing, Inc., Florida.

Graham, D. L. (1985) The Avian Integument: Its Structure and Selected Diseases. *Proceedings of the 1985 Annual Meeting of the Association of Avian Veterinarians*, pp. 33–52.

Harkness, J. E. (Editor) (1987) Exotic pet medicine. In: *Veterinary Clinics of North America — Small Animal Practice*, Vol. **17**. W. B. Saunders Co., Philadelphia, PA.

Harrison, G. J. (Editor) (1984) Caged bird medicine. In: *Veterinary Clinics of North America — Small Animal Practice*, Vol. **14**. W. B. Saunders Co., Philadelphia, PA.

Harkness, J. E. and Wagner, J. E. (1982) *The Biology and Medicine of Rabbits and Rodents* (3rd edn). Lea and Febiger, Philadelphia, PA.

Harrison, G. J. (1986) Disorders of the integument. In: *Clinical Avian Medicine and Surgery* (Editors Harrison, G. L. and Harrison, L. R.), pp. 509–524. W. B. Saunders Co., Philadelphia, PA.

Hillyer, E. V. (1992) Ferret endocrinology. In: *Current Veterinary Therapy* (Editors Kirk, R. W. and Bonagoura, J. D.), **XI**, pp. 1185–1189. W. B. Saunders Co., Philadelphia, PA.

Hillyer, E. V., Quesenberry, K. E. and Baer, K. (1989) Basic avian dermatology. *Proceedings of the Association of Avian Veterinarians*, pp. 101–121.

Hoff, G. L., Frye, F. L. and Jacobson, E. R. (Editors) (1984) *Diseases of Amphibians and Reptiles*. Plenum Press, New York.

Jacobson, E. R. (1993) Viral diseases of reptiles. In: *Zoo and Wild Animal Medicine, Current Therapy* (Editor Fowler, M. E.), **3**, pp. 131–139. W. B. Saunders Co., Philadelphia, PA.

Jenkins, J. R. and Brown, S. A. (1993) *A Practitioner's Guide to Rabbits and Ferrets*, Animal Hospital Associates.

Lennox, A. M. and Van Der Heyden, N. (1993) Haloperidol for use in treatment of psittacine self-mutilation and feather plucking. *Proceedings of the 1993 Annual Conference of the Association of Avian Veterinarians*, pp. 119–120.

Macwhirter, P. (1994) Malnutrition. In: *Avian Medicine: Principles and Applications* (Editors Ritchie, B. W., Harrison, G. J. and Harrison, L. R.), pp. 842–861. Wingers Publishing, Inc., Florida.

Marcus, L. C. (1981) *Veterinary Biology and Medicine of Captive Amphibians and Reptiles*. Lea and Febiger, Philadelphia, PA.

Perry, R. A., Gill, J. and Cross, G. M. (1991) Pet avian medicine. In: *Veterinary Clinics of North America — Small Animal Practice* (Editors Rosskopf, W. J. and Woerpel, R. W.), pp. 1307–1328. W. B. Saunders Co., Phildaelphia, PA.

Petrak, M. L. (Editor) (1982) *Diseases of Cage and Aviary Birds* (2nd edn). Lea and Feabiger, Philadelphia.

Post, G. (1987) *Textbook of Fish Health*. T. F. H. Publications, Neptune City, NJ.

Raphael, B. L. (1993) Amphibians. In: *Veterinary Clinics of North America — Small Animal Practice* (Editors Quesenberry, K. E. and Hillyer, E. V.), pp. 1271–1286. W. B. Saunders Co., Philadelphia, PA.

Quesenberry, K. E. and Hillyer, E. V. (Editors) (1993) Exotic pet medicine I. In: *The Veterinary Clinics of North America — Small Animal Practice*, Vol. **23**. W. B. Saunders Co., Philadelphia, PA.

Quesenberry, K. E. and Hillyer, E. V. (Editors) (1994) *The Veterinary Clinics of North America — Small Animal Practice: Exotic Pet Medicine II*. Vol. **24**, W. B. Saunders Co., Philadelphia, PA.

Reeves, D. E. (1993) *Care and Management of Miniature Pet Pigs*, Veterinary Practice Publishing Co., Santa Barbara, CA.

Rosskopf, J. R. and Woerpel, R. W. (Editors) (1991) Pet avian medicine. In: *The Veterinary Clinics of North America — Small Animal Practice*, Vol. **21**. W. B. Saunders Co., Philadelphia, PA.

Schmidt, R. E. (1993) The use of biopsies in the differential diagnosis of feather picking and avian skin disease. *Proceedings of the 1993 Annual Conference of the Association of Avian Veterinarians*, pp. 113–115.

Stoskopf, M. K. (Editor) (1988) Tropical fish medicine. In: *Veterinary Clinics of North America—Small Animal Practice*, Vol. **18**. W. B. Saunders Co., Philadelphia, PA.

Stoskopf, M. K. (Editor) (1992) *Fish Medicine*. W. B. Saunders Co., Philadelphia, PA.

Turner, R. (1993) Trexan use in feather picking in avian species. *Proceedings of the 1993 Annual Conference of the Association of Avian Veterinarians*, pp. 116–118.

Index

ORDER FORM

☐ Please enter my subscription to Volume 5 of *Veterinary Dermatology* (00946) (00946) at the special rate of **£42.00 (US$63.00)**

☐ Please send me information of veterinary medicine titles published by Elsevier

Name _____

Position _____

Organization _____

Department _____

Address _____

_____ Post/Zip Code _____

Country _____

E-Mail/Internet No. _____

Order value sub-total £/US$ _____

EU residents must either: state VAT number here

_____

or: VAT, or equivalent tax, @ ___%   £/US$ _____
(see table for appropriate tax rate)

Total Payment £/US$: _____

Payment details
☐ Please send a proforma invoice

☐ Cheque/money order/UNESCO coupon made payable to Elsevier Science enclosed.

Payment by credit card
☐ I wish to pay by credit card
Visa/MasterCard/American Express/Diners Club
(delete as appropriate).

Issuing Bank _____
(MasterCard only)

Card No. _____ Expiry Date _____

Signed _____ Date _____

EU (European Union) Countries, VAT equivalents and tax rates:

Belgium:	BTW 6%
Denmark:	MOMS 25%
Eire:	VAT 21%
France:	TVA 5.5%
Germany:	MWST 7%
Greece:	FPA 4%
Italy:	VA 4%
Luxembourg:	TAV 0%
Netherlands:	BTW 6%
Portugal:	IVA 5%
Spain:	IVA 3%
UK:	VAT 0%

Tax rates quoted are correct at time of going to press, but may be subject to change at any time by individual governments.
Elsevier Science UK VAT number: GB 490 6384 25 000.

Prices include postage and insurance.
Sterling price quoted applies worldwide, except in The Americas. US dollar price quoted applies in The Americas only.

Where to send your order and requests:

Elsevier Science Ltd
The Boulevard
Langford Lane
Kidlington
Oxford OX5 1GB, UK
Telephone:
+44 (0) 1865 843479/843781
Fax: +44 (0) 1865 843952

Elsevier Science Inc.
660 White Plains Road
Tarrytown
NY 10591-5153, USA
Telephone: +1914 524 9200
Fax: +1 914 333 2444

VE419 12/94